Immunology
In
Medical Practice

Edited by

GEOFFREY TAYLOR, MD

Reader in Immunology, University of Manchester;
Consultant in Immunology, United Manchester Hospitals,
Manchester.

Marie G. Graber

Immunology In Medical Practice

1975

W. B. Saunders Company Ltd London · Philadelphia · Toronto

W. B. Saunders Company Ltd: 12 Dyott Street
London WC1A 1DB

West Washington Square
Philadelphia, Pa. 19105

833 Oxford Street
Toronto, Ontario M8Z 5T9

Library of Congress Cataloging in Publication Data

Taylor, Geoffrey, 1929–
Immunology in medical practice.

1. Immunopathology. I. Title. [DNLM: 1. Immunity. QW504 T24li]
RC585.T35 616.07'9 74-4592
ISBN 0–7216–8767–9

Printed by The Whitefriars Press Ltd, London and Tonbridge

Print Number: 9 8 7 6 5 4 3 2 1

Contributors

J. F. ACKROYD, DSc, FRCP, Honorary Physician, St. Mary's Hospital; Senior Lecturer in Medicine, St. Mary's Hospital Medical School, London.

C. G. BEARDWELL, BSc, MB, MRCP, Honorary Lecturer in Medicine, University of Manchester; Consultant Physician, Withington and Christie Hospitals, Manchester.

RODNEY H. BLUESTONE, MB, MRCP, Associate Professor of Medicine, University of California, Los Angeles; Chief, Rheumatology Section, Wadsworth VA Hospital, Wilshire and Sawtelle Boulevards, Los Angeles, California, U.S.A.

JONATHAN BROSTOFF, MA, BM, MRCP, Senior Lecturer in Immunology, Middlesex Hospital Medical School, London.

JERRY DOLOVICH, MD, Associate Professor, Department of Pediatrics, McMaster University, Hamilton; Active Staff, Pediatrics, McMaster University Medical Center and St. Joseph's Hospital, Hamilton, Ontario, Canada.

MALCOLM W. GREAVES, MD, PhD, FRCP, Professor of Dermatology, Institute of Dermatology, Lisle Street, London and St. John's Hospital for Diseases of the Skin, London.

FREDERICK E. HARGREAVE, MD, MRCP, Assistant Professor, Department of Medicine, McMaster University, Hamilton; Active Staff, St. Joseph's Hospital, Hamilton, Ontario, Canada.

ANTHONY R. HAYWARD, MB, PhD, Lecturer, Department of Immunology, Institute of Child Health, London.

N. P. MALLICK, BSc, MB, ChB, MRCP, Senior Lecturer in Medicine, University of Manchester; Physician in Renal Disease, Manchester Royal Infirmary, Manchester.

HYLTON McFARLANE, PhD, MRCPath, Senior Lecturer in Biochemistry, Medical School, University of Manchester; Senior Lecturer in Chemical Pathology, United Manchester Hospitals, Manchester.

W. McN. ORR, ChM, FRCSE, FRCS, Senior Lecturer in Surgery, University of Manchester; Consultant Surgeon, Manchester Royal Infirmary; Director, Renal Transplantation Unit, Manchester Royal Infirmary, Manchester.

GEOFFREY TAYLOR, MD, Reader in Immunology, University of Manchester; Consultant in Immunology, United Manchester Hospitals, Manchester.

GEOFFREY WALKER, MD, FRCP, Consultant Gastroenterologist, St. Mary's Hospital, London.

Preface

The immunological literature has been expanding at a considerable rate for the past few years. This not only includes an increase in both frequency and number of journals, but also monographs and textbooks. It has become difficult, if not impossible, for even a specialist immunologist to keep fully abreast of this vast output; much less so an individual whose interest is only peripheral. Yet the importance of immunology in clinical medicine has also increased and there is clearly a need for all clinicians to have at least a nodding acquaintance with this science. There are several excellent textbooks available, but either they become unduly large in an effort to be all-embracing or deal at great length with the scientific aspects of immunology to the relative neglect of the clinical applications. This book attempts to provide only a summary of the fundamentals of immunology and to concentrate on the value of immunology in the diagnosis and treatment of patients. To this end the contributors are all directly involved in clinical work.

No attempt has been made to provide a complete coverage of the subject and the topics considered have been deliberately restricted. Subjects such as immunity to infectious diseases and the uses of immunological methods in their diagnosis are not included, as such information is readily available elsewhere. Likewise, the immunology of haemolytic anaemia is not considered in detail as this subject is well provided for in textbooks of haematology and of general medicine. Investigations which are still largely experimental, e.g., the immunology of malignant disease, and diseases in which the evidence for the involvement of immunological processes is still debatable, are also not presented.

After an initial chapter, the aim of which is to present a concise account of immunological principles, each chapter considers a major clinically-applied subject. Where appropriate to the topic additional basic immunology is included to supplement that presented in Chapter 1. The aim is to help clinicians to select and to interpret immunological investigations which are of value in the diagnosis, prognosis and treatment of patients. Chapters on immunodeficiency, paraproteinaemia, and connective tissue disorders are followed by systematic chapters on the endocrine glands, the gastro-intestinal tract including the liver, the kidneys, the upper and lower respiratory tracts, the skin, and finally chapters on drug hypersensitivity and tissue transplantation.

I would like to thank the contributors and the publishers for their forbearance at the inevitable delays involved in producing a multi-author book, and finally my colleagues in Manchester for many helpful discussions.

Geoffrey Taylor

Contents

1. Introduction: Basic Immunology

GEOFFREY TAYLOR

At the outset, it is probably necessary to attempt a definition of immunology. This is particularly so because an individual's views of the science may be very much coloured by which aspects he has studied. To one person it represents a study of the chemistry of immunoglobulins, to another it is very closely linked with microbiology and concerns itself with protection from and responses to infectious agents. Others see it as a basic science involving the study of the reactivity of lymphocytes (usually of mouse origin) with antigens (preferably chemically defined), and yet another group are concerned with the response of humans to environmental allergens. All are indeed involved in aspects of immunology. The science has advanced greatly in the recent past both with respect to the basic understanding of immunological phenomena, and with respect to the application of this knowledge and technique to medicine as a whole. There must scarcely be any medical speciality into which immunologists have not delved to some extent.

In essence immunology concerns itself with functions involved in the differentiation of self from non-self thus detecting that which is foreign; with the specificity of this recognition mechanism and with the laying down of immunological memory of the past experience of foreignness. These basic functions result in a specifically altered state of reactivity which may become manifest in a variety of ways—from protection to destruction. It is the expression of specific changes in reactivity rather than the fundamental mechanisms involved in inducing them which most concerns immunology in its relation to clinical medicine. In addition, as with most if not all biological functions, both congenital and acquired defects may occur in the immunological apparatus. Thus the capacity of an individual to recognise foreignness may be impaired—he is to some extent immunodeficient. An individual may fail to recognise self as self and thus respond as he would against foreign material. This is the situation in autoimmunity. From a therapeutic viewpoint manipulation of a normal or abnormal immune response, as in the immunotherapy of allergic disease or the immunosuppression used to prevent rejection of a allograft, must be considered. Finally, and somewhat peripheral to the main theme, immunological technique, because of its great sensitivity and specificity, is of great value in medical practice in the specific assay of very small quantities of antigenic molecules such as peptide hormones in tissue fluids.

Manifestation of the immune response

For historical reasons, the phenomena which arise from the immunological recognition of foreignness are usually collectively known as the immune response. It has been recognised that in many ways this is a bad term because an immune, i.e. protected, state need not necessarily derive from a particular response. The response may result in a state which, far from conferring protection against re-exposure to foreign material, is positively damaging. Anaphylaxis is probably the most obvious example. The immunological apparatus, though recognising and responding against foreignness very efficiently, fails to differentiate between potentially harmful foreignness and 'neutral' foreignness. In the context of the beneficial response against potentially harmful foreignness, as for instance infectious agents, part of the immunological sequelae may well be damaging to the host, but will be partially hidden by the infectious process and will be considered usually to be an integral part of the infectious disease. When the foreign material is normally non-harmful per se—a pollen grain for instance—we see the whole response as being damaging. Similar mechanisms do operate in both types of situation and hence a division into harmful and potentially beneficial is scientifically illogical. For this reason it has been suggested that the term *allergic* response should replace *immune* response: allergic having its original meaning of altered reactivity. This logical suggestion has not unfortunately reached common usage and I therefore propose to continue to use the term immune response. It will mean the specific changes in responsiveness which result from experience of foreignness irrespective of whether the change is beneficial or detrimental to the animal concerned.

The various manifestations of the immune response appear to be very diverse when observed at the level of the patient. It is thus difficult to see any relationship between the acquisition of immunity to an infectious agent following a natural infection or the administration of a vaccine, the rejection of a kidney allograft and the development of serum sickness following a dose of horse anti-toxin. In order to appreciate that each is a direct result of an immune response it is necessary to examine the changes which take place when an animal responds to a material foreign to itself.

THE IMMUNE RESPONSE

A highly complex sequence of events takes place during an immune response, and at many points in the sequence one reaction may interfere with another. The following simple account divides the sequence into the 'input'—which initiates the response; the 'output'—the specific products of the immune response; the 'central' mechanisms which connect the two, and finally how the specific products of the immune response modify the reactivity of an animal—the immunological effector systems. It should be noted that this rather artificial compartmented view of the immune response is used as an aid to understanding. The reactions in each 'compartment' will often influence reactions in another. Thus the change in responsiveness brought about by the immunological effector system will alter the way in which the 'input' is handled by 'central processing' and hence may alter subsequent 'output'.

The material against which an animal mounts an immune response is usually referred to as an *antigen.* This term requires greater qualification and is defined as a molecule which is capable of inducing an immune response in an animal and which is further able to react specifically with the products of the response. The terms *immunogen* and *immunogenicity* are used sometimes to refer to the immune response-inducing properties of a molecule and *antigen* and *antigenicity* to the reactivity of the molecule with the products of the immune response. Usually the same molecule will exhibit both immunogenicity and antigenicity. It should be noted that a molecule which is immunogenic for one species need not be so for another. In addition, varying degrees of immunogenicity will be exhibited by a single immunogen in different animal species.

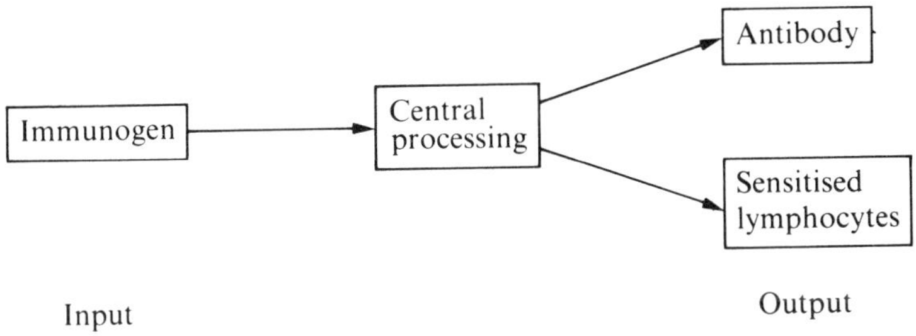

Figure 1.1. Simple model of immune response.

The products of an immune response with which an antigen will specifically react are of two types. These are sometimes referred to as the *humoral* and *cellular* aspects of the response. The former are *antibodies*, a non-uniform group of globulins present in serum and in some secretions and the latter are lymphocytes which have specific receptors on their surfaces—*specifically sensitised lymphocytes.*

In its simplest form an immune response may be illustrated as in Figure 1.1.

In order that the immune response shall be expressed as an altered state of reactivity, the products of the immune response must react specifically with antigen. Thus the specificity of the immune response involves two points of 'contact'.

1. In the *afferent arc* of the response during which *cognition* of the foreignness of the immunogen takes place.
2. In the *efferent arc* where the *recognition* of the same foreignness takes place by its reaction with the products of the response.

The specific reaction between antigen and antibody or antigen and sensitised lymphocyte in itself behaves only as a specific trigger. The reactions trigger complex sequences of events involving both soluble molecules and other cells which collectively can be considered as immunological effectors. It is the effectors—both cellular and humoral—which largely produce the effects which we observe at the level of the whole animal. We can add this effector stage to the model of the immune response, as in Figure 1.2.

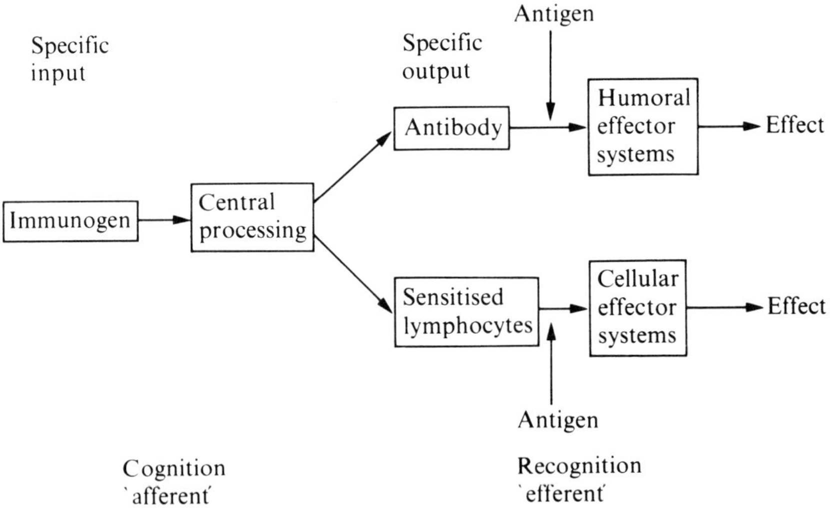

Figure 1.2. Model immune response with effector systems.

The Input

Immunogenic substances are usually of high molecular weight; usually the larger the molecule the greater is the degree of immunogenicity. It is difficult to define a lower limit, but molecules as small as angiotensin (mol.wt 1031) and glucagon (mol.wt 3800) behave as immunogens, nonetheless of a low order. Immunogens are usually natural macromolecules and as such are protein, polysaccharide or are complex such as lipoprotein, lipopolysaccharide etc. They are normally required to be foreign to the animal producing the response and in general the greater the degree of phylogenetic difference between the source of the immunogen and the responding animal, the greater is the apparent immunogenicity.

The work of Landsteiner in investigating the immunogenicity of molecules to which small known chemical groupings had been attached has indicated that the immune response is not directed against the whole molecule but against small specific portions of its structure. Such portions of the molecule are known as *determinants*. Experiments using artificially added determinants have indicated that it is the overall three-dimensional shape and to some extent the distribution of ionised groups on the determinant against which an immune response is raised. In naturally occurring molecules the size of a determinant is of the order of up to six monosaccharide units or up to four or five amino acid units. They may, however, be smaller than this maximum size on some immunogens. A natural immunogenic molecule will contain multiple determinants, some of which may be repeated several times on the same molecule. The immune response to a single molecular species will be therefore made up of responses to several or many different specific determinants. An antiserum raised against a single molecular species will not contain antibodies of a single specificity when considered at the level of reactivity with determinants. Often one determinant may be more immunogenic than others on the same molecule and therefore a large portion of any immune response will be directed against this *immunodominant* determinant.

Whilst an antibody may be capable of reacting with an isolated small molecular weight determinant, the administration of such a determinant unattached to its *carrier* molecule will not normally induce an immune response. Thus we have a small molecule which is non-immunogenic but in its ability to react with antibody raised against determinant and carrier is antigenic. Such a molecule is known as a *hapten*. The chemically defined artificial substituents used by Landsteiner can be considered as haptens. Chemically reactive haptens may combine with a carrier molecule in vivo after administration and so become capable of eliciting an immune response. Therapeutic agents used in medicine may behave in this way.

Because determinants are relatively small and are made up of a limited range of sugars and amino acids, it is not surprising that very similar or identical determinants may occur on unrelated macromolecules. In this circumstance with respect to the 'shared' determinants an animal or an antiserum will react with both in a similar manner. This is the basis of *cross-reactivity*. Although cross-reactivity appears to imply a lack of immunological specificity when considered at the molecular level, no such lack exists at the level of reactivity with determinants. Cross-reactivity is relatively common. Macromolecules which subserve a similar function in different species will often cross-react. Human blood group determinants are present on some bacteria, and some determinants, notably those of the Forssman antigen, are very widely distributed in nature. It is very important to take into account the possibility of cross-reactivity when interpreting the results of any immunological system.

A number of terms are used to describe the properties of various groups of antigens. Antigens of the type which possess cross-reacting determinants with molecules derived from a wide range of species are described as exhibiting *heterogenetic specificity*. Determinants which are present on different molecular types derived from the same species are exhibiting *species specificity*. Thus an antiserum may react with a range of human proteins by virtue of their 'human' determinants. *Allospecificity* implies determinants which are present on a specific molecular type, but only in a proportion of members of a particular species. The human ABO blood group system provides an example of allospecificity, as does the HLA antigen system used in tissue-typing. The allospecificity is directed against *allotypic* determinants, which are inherited characters. *Organ specificity* refers to determinants shared by antigens derived from the same tissue of a number of species. Thyroglobulin derived from a number of species has determinants in common, as does central nervous tissue.

The Output

As already mentioned the specific output of the immune response consists of antibody molecules and specifically sensitised lymphocytes. Both have the ability to react with the antigen which invoked their formation. The dose and the type of antigen and the route of administration will influence whether the antibody or sensitised lymphocyte output predominates. In many circumstances both types of output will occur.

First experience of an antigen gives rise to a *primary response* which is different in several ways from the response to subsequent exposure to the same antigen—a *secondary response.* Although such differences do occur in the output of sensitised lymphocytes, they are best exhibited by the antibody response.

1. The delay between antigen administration and first demonstration of antibody is much greater in a primary response than in a secondary.
2. The total amount of antibody output is less in a primary response.
3. The duration of antibody synthesis is less in a primary response.
4. The type of antibody produced differs in the two responses; the ratio of IgM:IgG is greater in a primary than in a secondary response.

The fundamental reason for these differences is that specific *immunological memory* has been established following the primary dose of antigen (p. 16).

Antibodies

Antibody activity is found in a group of γ globulins present in plasma, in the extravascular compartment, and in some secretions. The molecules exhibiting antibody activity are not homogenous but vary in molecular weight, in isoelectric point, in amount of carbohydrate present in the molecule, and in many of their biological properties. With a clearer understanding of the basic structure of the molecules showing antibody activity it has become possible to classify them into five classes. Collectively these proteins are known as immunoglobulins (Ig).

By breaking disulphide bonds at reduced pH, immunoglobulins can be split into their component polypeptide chains. The chains derived from all immunoglobulins fall into two major size ranges and are known as heavy

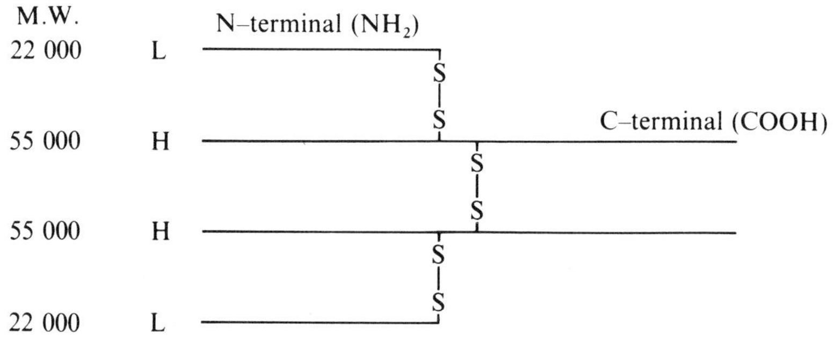

Figure 1.3. The basic chain structure of the Ig molecule. H = heavy chain; L = light chain.

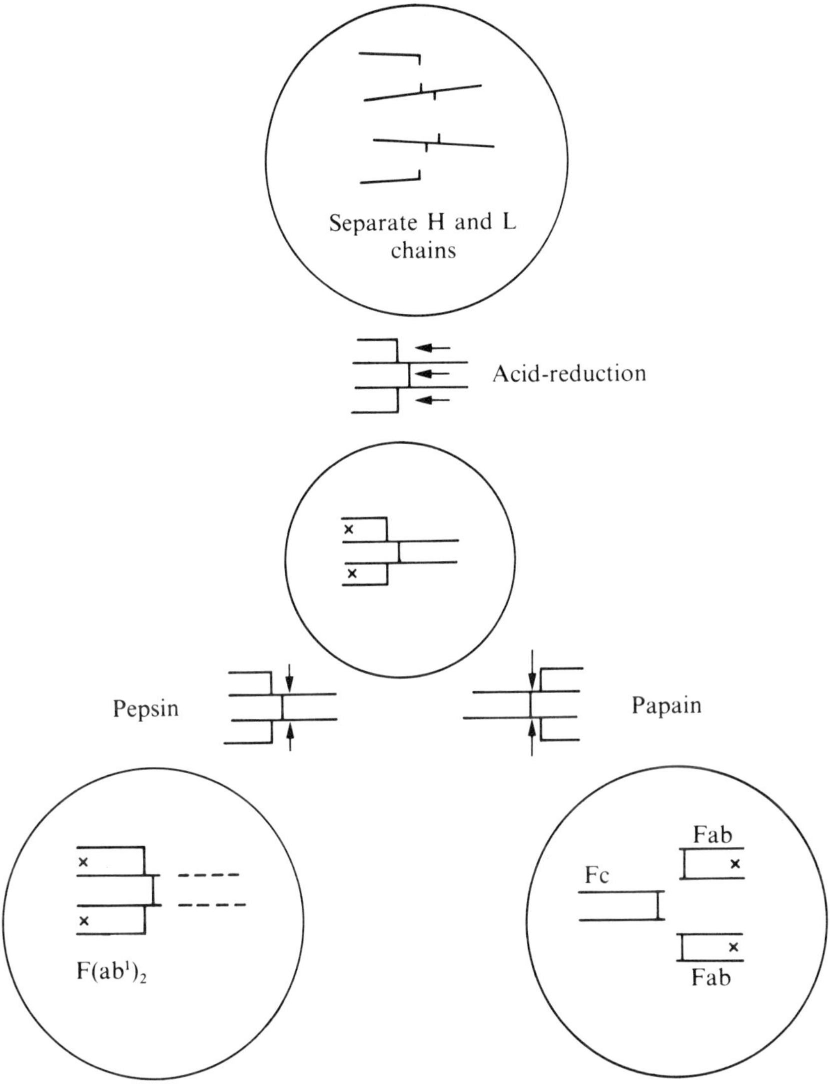

Figure 1.4. The effects of acid-reduction and of proteolytic enzymes on the Ig molecule to show the fragments produced. X = antigen binding site.

chains and light chains. If the products of cleavage of all classes of immunoglobulin are studied by immunochemical means there are two different types of light chains, designated kappa (κ) and lambda (λ) and five different heavy chains designated alpha (α), gamma (γ), delta (δ), epsilon (ϵ) and mu (μ). The heavy chains largely influence the biological characteristics of antibodies and it is according to the type of heavy chain that the immunoglobulins are divided into classes. Thus α chains are found in immunoglobulin A (IgA), δ chains in IgD, γ chains in IgG, ϵ chains in IgE, and μ chains in IgM. All immunoglobulin molecules have either κ or λ chains; never both on the same molecule.

The structure of Ig has also been investigated by splitting the molecules using the enzymes papain and pepsin. The chains are linked by disulphide bonds and in the IgG molecule two heavy and two light chains are linked as shown in Figure 1.3. This model of the structure which was derived from study of the products of breakdown of the molecule in experiments illustrated in Figure 1.4 has been confirmed by electron-optical examination of Ig molecules in combination with divalent haptens. These studies have shown that on combination with a determinant the antibody molecule is capable of undergoing a conformational change. It is flexible about a '*hinge region*' situated between the points of chain breakage produced by the two enzymes pepsin and papain. The part of the molecule which is capable of binding with

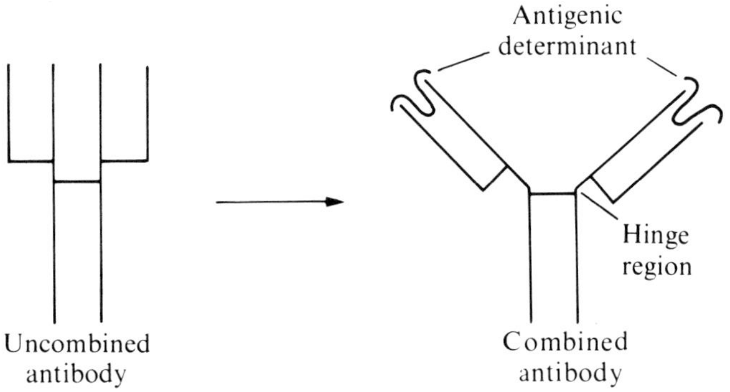

Figure 1.5. Diagram to show steric change in Ig molecule by bending about the hinge region on combination with antigenic determinants.

an antigenic determinant—the *antigen-binding site*—is situated towards the N-terminal ends of the heavy and light chains, both of which probably contribute to the binding. Thus the IgG molecule has two binding sites. During combination with a determinant the antibody molecule changes its shape. This conformational change may confer new properties on the molecule, e.g. ability to fix complement.

Further information on the structures of Ig molecules has derived from an investigation of the properties of myeloma proteins. These Ig, derived from malignant plasma cells, are homogeneous and allow amino acid sequences to be determined. In addition isolated homogeneous light chains are usually found in the urine of these patients as Bence-Jones protein. Comparing the sequences from different myeloma and Bence-Jones proteins some parts of the chains are found to have a constant sequence whilst others have considerable variation from protein to protein. These *variable* and *constant* regions are arranged as in Figure 1.6. As well as the *inter*-chain disulphide bonds there are also *intra*-chain bonds which produce 'loops'. These are arranged and designated as in Figure 1.7. Thus both heavy and light chains have one

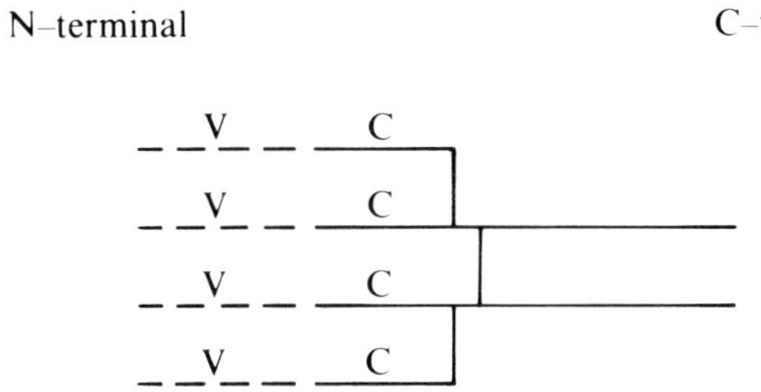

Figure 1.6. Diagram to show the positions of the variable (V) and constant (C) parts of the heavy and light chains.

variable 'loop'—the VL and VH loops. The specificity of the antigen binding site is probably determined by the variable loops on both the heavy and light chains acting together.

The loops in the constant portion of the molecule may also have important properties, but so far, although various biological activities of Ig such as passage across the placenta and fixation to mast cells and macrophages have been localised to the Fc portion of the heavy chains, their precise position on the chains is not known.

Other sites on the Ig molecule within the 'constant' regions have been shown to vary from individual to individual. These are allotypic determinant sites, are inherited characters, and involve very minor changes in amino acid

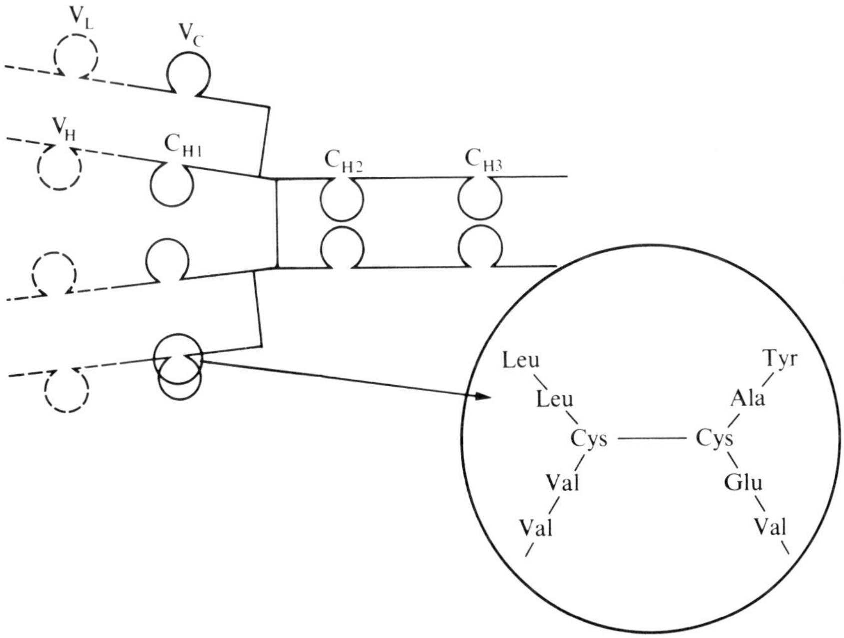

Figure 1.7. Diagram to show the arrangement of intra-chain disulphide (Cys–Cys) bonds to produce loops. The amino acid sequence is of the human κ chain.

sequence. In man the two main systems are known as the Gm and Inv and are situated on the heavy and light chains of IgG respectively. It is possible for an individual to produce an immune response against allotypic determinants following the administration of Ig of a different allotype to his own.

Further heterogeneity of heavy chain structure gives rise to intra-class variation. IgG heavy chains are found to fall into four *subclasses*, IgG 1, IgG 2, etc. Whilst these four subclasses have very much in common, minor variation in amino acid sequence, and in particular differences in the arrangement of inter-chain disulphide bonds, give rise to differences in biological properties. IgA and IgM also exhibit intra-class variation and each has two subclasses. Subclasses of Ig are considered further in Chapter 3.

Studies of the IgG molecule have helped considerably in understanding the structure and properties of Ig in general, but other classes do present important differences. The following brief notes present some of the more important of these differences.

IgA is produced mainly in lymphoid tissue in close relationship to mucosal surfaces. It is present in many secretions where it provides the major immunoglobulin. IgA possesses an additional *J chain* which is believed to be important in dimerisation. In serum, IgA is present mainly but not exclusively as a monomer with two α chains and two light chains per molecule, whereas in secretions the dimer form is predominant. In secretions an additional protein is also associated with the molecule—the *secretory piece* or component. This component is produced in the cells of the epithelial surface and presumably attaches to dimeric IgA on its passage through the mucosal surface. Secretory IgA (SIgA) is important in mucosal defence against microorganisms, and may act as an antigen-specific barrier. Thus individuals deficient in SIgA have been shown to produce circulating IgG antibody in large amounts to ingested antigens implying greater systemic antigenic stimulation. IgA does not fix complement in the conventional manner by activating the first component of complement (C1) but may activate complement through the C3 bypass (p. 25). It may also 'collaborate' with lysozyme and complement in killing Gram-negative organisms.

IgD is present in only low concentrations in serum. Its structure is essentially similar to that of IgG. Although some antibody activity has now been demonstrated to be present in the IgD class no special biological function has yet been discovered.

IgE is, like IgA, produced in lymphoid tissue in close association with mucous surfaces. The basic structure is similar to that of IgG. The special biological property of IgE is its ability to bind to mast cells which thereby become specifically sensitised. Thus IgE is able to mediate mast cell degranulation and is the main Ig class responsible for the initiation of local and systemic anaphylactic reactions.

IgM has a much higher molecular weight than the other Ig. It is essentially a pentameric form of the basic 4-chain structure. Like IgA, IgM possesses the J chain and also may appear in secretions. IgM is however found mainly in serum where it represents the major Ig class of the primary response. Possibly because of its multivalancy it is a very 'efficient' antibody especially where complement activation is involved. IgM does not cross the placenta, and IgM class antibodies in cord blood have been used as an index of fetal infection in utero.

The specific cellular output

It has long been recognised that some types of immunologically specific reaction, both protective and damaging, do not depend on the production of circulating immunoglobulin. These include immunity to infection caused by microorganisms which are found in intracellular sites, cutaneous delayed hypersensitivity to bacterial and fungal antigens, contact sensitivity and the rejection of allografts. Passive transfer of such types of sensitivity from one animal to a non-sensitised recipient cannot be carried out by means of serum but only by means of lymphoid cell populations. The immune output responsible for determining the specificities of such types of reaction resides in the lymphocyte. Because the antigen-specific trigger is cellular rather than an isolated macromolecule, this type of immune reactivity is often known as *cell-mediated immunity* (CMI). As with antibody mediated responsiveness both protective and destructive effects may be mediated by CMI.

Animal experiments and studies of human immunodeficiency states have shown that the responsibility for CMI resides in part of the lymphocyte population—*thymus dependent* or *T lymphocytes*. There is some evidence that the antigen binding site on the surface of a sensitised T lymphocyte is immunoglobulin-like, but that it is firmly bound and is not secreted by the cell.

The organisation of the immune system

Although there is some evidence of acquired changes in responsiveness in invertebrates, an immune response resembling the mammalian type is found, at its most primitive, in the cyclostomes. The lamprey is able to produce high molecular weight antibody but only to a limited range of antigens. Long-term immunological memory is probably not present, but efficient CMI demonstrable by graft rejection is well developed.

Through the higher fishes, amphibians and reptiles immune responses remain temperature-dependent but become more mammalian in character showing both high and low molecular weight immunoglobulins and the development of memory. The avian immune response is very similar to that of the mammal. The immunoglobulins produced by a wide variety of vertebrates show considerable similarity of structure. Thus, from a phylogenetic viewpoint, CMI and IgM production are the most primitive with a diversification of Ig classes produced appearing as a later evolutionary development.

The increase in complexity in the immune response from the simplest cyclostome response to the complex avian and mammalian responses is related to the appearance and development of the thymus, the spleen and other lymphoid tissue. In the bird a further lymphoid organ, the *bursa of Fabricius*, is present. This is a lympho-epithelial organ situated near to the cloaca. Like the thymus, the bursa of Fabricius develops early during embryogenesis; the 'peripheral' lymphoid tissue, lymph nodes and spleen, becoming cellular at a much later stage. The 'central' lymphoid tissue has a profound effect on the development of immune responsiveness.

Removal of the thymus in the neonatal mouse results in a loss of the ability to mount a CMI response, whilst the ability to produce antibody is impaired to some extent in response to some antigens but not to others. In the bird the bursa of Fabricius is responsible for the development of ability to produce antibody. Removal or destruction of the bursa before or shortly after hatching results in a bird able to mount a CMI response, but failing to produce antibody on antigenic stimulation. As in the mouse the thymus is necessary for the development of CMI.

There is no clear-cut bursa-equivalent organ in mammals, but it is likely that the lymphoid tissue of the appendix, the sacculus rotundus and the Peyer's patches—*gut associated lymphoid tissue*—performs a similar function. Considering the experimental data along with a study of human immunodeficiency states (Chapter 2) there can be little doubt that the development of the ability to mount the antibody and cell-mediated responses are separately controlled in man.

The cell type central to the production of both the cell-mediated and the antibody responses has been shown by a variety of experimental procedures to be the lymphocyte. The evidence derived from thymectomy and bursectomy experiments and supported by work on human immunodeficiency states would therefore indicate two populations of lymphocytes, one responsible for CMI, and the other for antibody production. These are usually known as *T lymphocytes*—thymus dependent and involved with the induction of CMI responses, and *B lymphocytes*—bursa or bursa-equivalent dependent and involved with antibody production.

Lymphocytes are found in the developing fetus first in the embryonic haemopoietic tissues where they arise from stem cells. Later they are to be seen in the central lymphoid organs, in man the thymus, and later still in the spleen, lymph nodes and in the circulation. In the adult, lymphocytes are produced mainly in the bone marrow and in the thymus. The majority of those produced in the latter organ are relatively short-lived and remain within the thymus. Their function is not clear. Those produced in the bone marrow ultimately give rise to T and B lymphocytes. There is evidence that the bone marrow lymphocytes require 'processing' by the thymus and the bursa-equivalent tissue to become functional T and B cells respectively. Lymphocytes continuously recirculate, passing from the lymphoid tissue to the circulation via the lymphatics. They re-enter lymphoid tissue by passing through the endothelium of the post-capillary venules. By studying the effect on lymphoid tissue of selective depletion of either T or B cells and also the responses of lymph nodes in which either a predominantly T-cell or B-cell response is taking place it has been shown that these cells tend to be spatially separate within the node. B cells are found in the cortical germinal follicles and in the medullary cords whilst T cells are present in the deeper cortex—the paracortical thymus-dependent area. Thus in a lymph node draining an allograft or an area of skin subjected to a contact sensitiser, both procedures which result in CMI, the thymus-dependent paracortical region will be the site of cell proliferation. This contrasts with the response of a node to stimulation by a polysaccharide antigen. Antibody is formed but no detectable CMI and the predominant area of proliferation is of the germinal centres in the superficial cortex. With many antigens which induce both antibody formation and CMI this distinction is not seen. A similar spatial separation of lymphocyte populations is to be found in the spleen.

Considerable effort has been directed towards developing methods to differentiate between T and B cells. In the mouse a surface antigen (θ) has been demonstrated on the surface of T cells which is absent from B cells. This has been very valuable in experimental work, but so far the analogous human antigen has not been so well defined. A number of differences have been demonstrated which are applicable to human lymphocyte populations. Thus, B cells have Ig on their surfaces which is easily demonstrable by immunofluorescent techniques; T cells may possibly have Ig on the surface, but this is debatable and certainly not easily demonstrable. B cells, unlike T cells, also have receptors on their surfaces to which the Fc portion of IgG will bind, also receptors for complement (p. 23). T cells will, under appropriate conditions, bind sheep erythrocytes onto their surface to form rosettes. The mechanism of this presumably immunologically non-specific binding is not clear, but it has been used to quantitate the number of T cells in a mixed population (see p. 58). The response of living lymphocytes to non-specific mitogens has also been used in attempts to quantitate the two lymphocyte compartments. Phytohaemaglutinin (PHA) and conconavalin A (con-A) appear to be T-cell mitogens whilst in man pokeweed mitogen (PWM) stimulates both B and T cells to mitotic activity.

Central interactions in the immune response

As already mentioned histological examination of lymphoid tissue subjected to antigenic stimulation shows increased cellularity implying a proliferative response. There is a considerable increase in the proportion of more 'primitive looking' lymphoid cells—*lymphoblasts* and also usually an increase in *plasma cells*. Both cell types can be stained with the dye, pyronin, suggesting a high synthetic activity and the former are accordingly sometimes known as large pyroninophil cells. Localisation of antibody by fluorescent and other tracer techniques has demonstrated that the major source of immunoglobulin is the plasma cell. Ferritin studies indicate that antibody is synthesised in the abundant endoplasmic reticulum of the plasma cell. Other studies in which the antibody production by single isolated lymphoid cells has been examined shows that a proportion of large lymphocytes also produce antibody. These also possess 'rough' endoplasmic reticulum, but not in the profusion found in the plasma cell.

Fluorescent antibody techniques have also demonstrated that a single plasma cell will usually contain only one light chain type (κ or λ) and only one heavy chain type. Rarely, cells with more than one heavy chain type have been observed. The question of whether an antibody producing cell can switch from the production of one class to another has not been fully resolved. As far as the specificity of the antibody produced by a cell is concerned some evidence suggests that one cell—one specificity—is the usual situation with only occasional cells producing antibody of two specificities. The evidence of some workers is in direct conflict with this view and suggests that more than one specificity of antibody may be produced by a single cell quite commonly. As many different methods and different antigens have been used to investigate this question, it is impossible to reach a satisfactory conclusion.

Depletion of an animals' recirculating pool of small lymphocytes greatly impairs its ability to produce antibody and CMI whilst replacement of these cells will restore this ability implying that both antibody forming cells and those involved in CMI are derived directly or indirectly from the small lymphocyte. Passive transfer studies have indicated that small lymphocytes carry immunological memory. With respect to both a primary and a secondary antibody response, the key cell is therefore clearly the lymphocyte. If small lymphocytes from a presensitised animal or human are incubated with antigen, a proportion of the cells will increase in size and change in cytology to become lymphoblasts. Such cells also undertake active synthetic activity and will divide. This in vitro phenomenon is known as transformation and the cells produced resemble those seen in an antigen-stimulated lymph node. Similar changes are induced in lymphocyte populations by the action of the non-specific mitogens such as PHA, but very many more cells are activated than by specific antigen. Although antigen-induced lymphocyte transformation results in the development of cells, some of which have endoplasmic reticulum, the actual production of antibody by these cells has not been unequivocally demonstrated. The presence of some of the effector substances of CMI (p. 26) in cultures of small lymphocytes stimulated with an antigen of which the cell-donor has had previous experience, clearly relates in vitro lymphocyte transformation to CMI. Under the conditions in which antigen-induced lymphocyte transformation is carried out it is likely that the T rather than the B lymphocyte is the major responder.

So far the immune response has been presented as though a complete separation existed between the humoral and cellular responses; the bursa-equivalent processed lymphocytes proliferating in response to antigen, transforming into larger lymphocytes, lymphoblasts and plasma cells and producing antibody whilst the thymus-processed lymphocytes are also proliferating to produce lymphoblasts with CMI function. There is, however, considerable evidence to show that whilst T lymphocytes do not produce antibody themselves they are necessary for an efficient antibody response to many so-called thymus-dependent antigens. This *cellular cooperation* has been demonstrated both in vivo and in vitro by studying the antibody forming capabilities of T cells and B cells separately and together either in cell culture or when used to 'reconstitute' an animal rendered immunologically incompetent. Cooperation seems to be important in the production of antibody when small doses of antigen are given. Other studies have suggested that the T cells may act to concentrate antigen and to 'present' it in a suitable manner for B-cell activation. Alternatively there is also some evidence to suggest that primed T cells may produce a soluble factor on contact with specific antigen which either directly or indirectly activates primed B cells to produce antibody. A major problem in interpreting the work on cell–cell cooperation is the difficulty in clearly defining the populations of cells used. Thus, whilst it is often possible to show that a population contains, say, T cells but few or no B cells, it is often impossible to determine what other cells are present in addition. This is particularly relevant if macrophages are present as these cells are also involved in the immune response.

The distribution and fate of antigens, following administration, have been investigated in considerable detail. The distribution clearly depends on the route of administration but essentially antigens are taken up by the reticulo-endothelial system, mainly by liver and spleen if given by intravenous injection, and by draining lymph nodes if given locally and in small doses. In a draining lymph node antigen is found in the phagolysosomes of macrophages of the medullary cords and in the perifollicular zones on first experience of an antigen, but the distribution of an antigen in a primed animal is strikingly different. Here the localisation is in the lymphoid follicles where it is present between rather than inside cells and is associated with the processes of 'dendritic' cells. The precise nature of these cells is uncertain, but as their function does not seem to be one of phagocytosis they are probably not macrophages. In the cell-membrane-bound state the antigen is associated with Ig, and is probably in the form of antigen–antibody complexes. A similar difference in distribution of antigen between 'virgin' and primed animals is found in the spleen.

A large portion of antigen taken up by macrophages is degraded, but some macrophage-associated antigen remains immunogenic as demonstrated by transfer to other animals, for long periods after administration.

The role of the macrophage and macrophage-associated antigen in the induction of the immune response has been investigated in many ways. Whilst there is no doubt that macrophages alone do not produce antibody there is good evidence, derived from in vivo and in vitro experiments, that they are involved. Thus reticulo-endothelial blockade using colloidal particles impairs macrophage function and also depresses antibody formation. There is good correlation between the efficiency of macrophage uptake of an antigen and its immunogenicity and in vitro model systems have demonstrated the need for both macrophages and lymphocytes in order to induce a primary response to an antigen. In such mixed cultures clusters of macrophages and lymphocytes develop which appear to be necessary for antibody production in that breaking up the clusters early in the incubation period diminishes antibody formation. Precisely what is involved in this cell–cell relationship is still not clear. Antigen fragments associated with RNA have been extracted from macrophages and are found to be more immunogenic than native antigen. It has been claimed that such RNA-antigen complexes will stimulate immunologically 'virgin' lymphocytes to produce specific antibody in vitro. This has led to the suggestion that the macrophage RNA may be instructional with respect to antibody specificity—'a long distance' messenger RNA; the interaction taking place in the cell clusters would be interpreted on this hypothesis as the transfer of such informational RNA. The RNA found in association with processed antigen is not newly synthesised following phagocytosis. If the RNA were to be informational it would therefore need to be an integral part of the macrophage's stock of coded information and imply either the possession of the capability to produce a vast range of different mRNA molecules; one per antigen determinant, or the production of a specific mRNA only in response to one or a limited number of antigens. There is no evidence that macrophages are so discriminating in their phagocytosis and neither possibility seems likely.

More likely roles for the macrophage are the presentation of concentrated antigenic determinants in a suitable form for interaction with T and B lymphocytes and also the partial breakdown of antigen molecules to reveal 'hidden' inaccessible determinants which would otherwise not be able to contact lymphocytes. A third possible role is to reduce antigen concentration. A state of specific unresponsiveness known as tolerance (see below) may be induced by high concentrations of antigen. This may result from direct action of the antigen on lymphocytes; the macrophage population serving to prevent antigen concentration reaching sufficiently high levels to induce tolerance except under unusual circumstances.

Thus three cell types, the macrophage, the T and the B lymphocyte, all interact with antigen resulting in a proliferation of B lymphocytes to produce plasma cells and antibody and T lymphocytes to produce a population of sensitised effector cells. A further result of this interaction is the development of immunological memory. This will result in a change in character (from the primary to the secondary type) of immune response on subsequent exposure to the antigen. Memory is relatively long lived and almost certainly resides in the small lymphocyte. It is assumed that such memory-carrying lymphocytes arise during the proliferative response to antigen. Memory is probably carried as antigen-specific receptors on the lymphocyte surface. There is evidence that both B and T lymphocytes can carry immunological memory.

Once an immune response is established more complex interactions become possible. The antibody and sensitised T cells generated can alter the distribution of antigen giving rise to positive and negative feedback systems which will modulate the response. Passively transferred antibody can 'switch off' antibody production by competing for antigen with lymphocyte receptors. This mechanism may also operate with actively produced antibody as a negative feedback system. Antibody will also affect the distribution of antigen by forming complexes which will usually be rapidly phagocytosed and also by inducing binding to the surfaces of the dendritic cells of the germinal follicles. Small quantities of antibody may augment the subsequent antibody response by this mechanism. The population of sensitised T cells generated will also influence future responses. Under some circumstances they serve to potentiate the response and may be involved in the switch from IgM to IgG production. Other experimental evidence shows that under some conditions sensitised T cells may inhibit antibody production. The possible interactions involved in the central control of the immune response are many and undoubtedly very complex. A clearer understanding could be very valuable in that it might allow a more rational approach to modifying responses for therapeutic reasons.

Under some circumstances the administration of an antigen will not result in an immune response but will render the animal specifically unresponsive to that antigen on future presentation. This is *immunological tolerance.* Not only does an immune response not occur but a 'negative' memory is established, that is, the capability of developing 'positive' memory is removed. Antigens to which an animal is tolerant are treated as 'self' antigens. The phenomenon was initially investigated by administering antigens in the form of living cells from a donor strain to a different recipient strain before or very shortly after birth. On subsequent challenge by grafting cells from the donor strain rejection did not occur. General depression of immune responsiveness was not present as the tolerant animals could reject grafts from animals other than the original donor strain. This phenomenon has been considered important in self-recognition; a tolerant state to self antigenic determinants being established during embryological development.

Immunological tolerance can be induced to non-living and hence non-self-replicating antigens, but not quite so easily, and also may be produced in adult animals. In adults two dose levels will produce tolerance. These are very large doses and relatively small doses. The states produced are usually known as *high zone* and *low zone* tolerance. The term immunological paralysis, used in the past to denote the former state, is now rarely used. Doses of antigen between those required to produce low and high zone tolerance are immunogenic.

It has been observed that if an antigen is fractionated by ultracentrifugation into native, unaltered molecules and partially altered 'aggregated' material, then the former is highly tolerogenic and the latter is immunogenic. Aggregated antigens are very rapidly cleared from the circulation by phagocytosis as compared with unaltered molecules which recirculate for long periods unless antibody is present. This suggests that antigen presented to the immunological apparatus via the macrophage is immunogenic, but if macrophage phagocytosis does not occur and antigen is presented directly to other cells, presumably lymphocytes, then tolerance may result. Tolerance does not persist indefinitely but gradually wanes. The state may be maintained permanently if the antigen is given repeatedly or if the antigen is self-replicating. This does not necessarily mean that persistence of antigen is required to maintain tolerance as the state may persist for some time after antigen has been reduced below the level of detectability.

The cellular changes involved in the induction of tolerance have been examined by passive transfer studies into x-irradiated recipients and by in vitro methods. Macrophage function appears not to be affected and changes in both T and B lymphocyte populations have been demonstrated. T-cell tolerance is much easier to induce and persists for long periods whereas B-cell tolerance is only achieved with difficulty and is shortlived. B-cell tolerance can be produced more easily in a partially immunosuppressed animal which may explain the difference in the ease of tolerance induction in the neonate as compared with the adult. Low zone tolerance is believed to operate through T lymphocytes and high zone to involve both lymphocyte populations. Both types result in failure of antibody production because of the lack of T–B cell cooperation in the T-cell tolerant animal. Precisely what happens to 'tolerised' lymphocytes has not been determined.

As already mentioned tolerance may be the mechanism preventing responses against self-antigenic determinants and hence, failure of tolerance could be implicated in those situations where responses against self-antigens do occur. This view is discussed in relationship to autoimmune diseases in Chapter 5.

Factors influencing the quantity and quality of the output

There is considerable variation between normal individuals with respect both to quantity and quality in the immune response obtained following a given dose of antigen. This applies to apparently normal individuals and excludes those with congenital and acquired abnormalities of immunological function considered in Chapter 2. This biological variation is to be expected in any population, but must be taken into consideration when determining the optimal number and size of doses of a vaccine for prophylactic purposes. The dosage schedule must cater for those who produce the poorer responses. Other factors relating to the individual will also influence his immune response. Age is important, for although a neonate is capable of mounting a response this is usually far poorer than that of an adult. There is also probably some decrease in capability in old age. The health of the individual will also influence his responsiveness. Starvation impairs antibody production, and may also interfere with the cellular response to a lesser extent. Following some virus infections, e.g., measles, responsiveness may be depressed for a period, and some serious diseases; carcinomatosis, leukaemia, myelomatosis and uraemia are associated with acquired immunodeficiency.

The route of administration, dose and formulation, will also greatly influence the output produced by a given immunogen. Within limits, the concentration of antigen which reaches lymphoid tissue is important rather than the total dose given. Thus a dose of some immunogens given by intravenous injection will produce a poor response because part may be catabolised, part taken up by macrophages in the liver, an organ with little or no capacity to respond, and in the case of small molecules, part may be excreted. When a dose of immunogen is given by intradermal injection a large proportion will reach the regional lymph nodes via the dermal lymphatics and a proportionately greater response may be expected. Subcutaneous injection usually falls midway. In experimental animals, injection directly into a lymph node is probably the most efficient method if only very small amounts of antigen are available.

The dose of antigen greatly influences both the quantity and the quality of an immune response. The size of the primary dose has a greater effect in the response than any subsequent doses given. In general, small doses produce a response of 'good quality' high association constant antibody (see below) whilst larger doses, though producing more total antibody, have the effect of decreasing its average association constant.

The formulation of the antigen will also influence the response; particulate materials will tend to be better immunogens than soluble molecules. Immunogens are often formulated with adjuvants. These are agents which augment and usually also modify qualitatively the immune response. The use of alum and aluminium hydroxide precipitated immunogens, e.g. bacterial toxoids, in the immunoprophylaxis of infectious disease is a common example. Oil in water emulsions with or without the addition of killed *Mycobacteria* to the oil phase are known respectively as complete and incomplete Freund adjuvants. The immunogen is present in the water phase and will not only behave as a slow release preparation but will also induce a greater local inflammatory response with greater cellular uptake of immunogen. Freund's adjuvants are very commonly used in inducing immune responses in experimental animals. In addition to augmenting the response, the *Mycobacteria* in complete Freund adjuvant also tend to produce a much greater cell-mediated response. *Bordetella pertussis* used as an experimental adjuvant tends to induce a much greater anaphylactic antibody response than is produced by an immunogen in its absence. Similar augmentation of the anaphylactic antibody response occurs in the presence of infection by nematodes and also if the immunogen is coupled chemically to a nematode extract. The mechanism of this effect is not known.

The interaction of antibody with antigen

The reaction between a specific antibody and the antigen which induced its formation can be considered at essentially three levels:

1. at a molecular level by which the binding between the antigenic determinant and the antibody combining site is studied;
2. by observation in vitro of the secondary effects of the combination of antigen and antibody as in precipitation, agglutination, neutralisation and the activation of serum factors such as the complement cascade;
3. by observing the effects of antigen–antibody interaction either in the whole animal or in isolated tissues. This approach is very much more complicated and indirect in that both humoral and cellular events are involved and will be discussed in the section on immunological effector systems.

Reaction at molecular level. The binding between an antigenic determinant and antibody has been investigated mainly by the use of haptens which in this context behave as isolated determinants. The binding does not involve permanent chemical change in either reactant. The physical forces holding the determinant to the antigen binding site depend on 'closeness of fit,' i.e. very short intermolecular distances, and include the attraction of opposite charges on ionised groups, hydrogen bonding, hydrophobic interaction and van der Waal's forces. The reaction has been shown to be reversible as

$$H + A \rightleftharpoons HA$$

where H represents the hapten and A the antibody. At equilibrium an association constant K can be determined if the molar concentrations of antibody and bound [HA] and unbound [H] hapten are known. This is analogous to the dissociation constant familiar in the law of mass action.

$$K = \frac{[HA]}{[H]\,[A]}$$

Although several methods of investigating the association constant K of antibodies have been used, most data are available for the equilibrium dialysis method in which dialysable hapten and non-dialysable antibody reach equilibrium across a dialysis membrane. Bound hapten is restricted to one side of the membrane by the non-dialysable antibody to which it is bound. Unbound hapten will reach equal concentration on both sides of the membrane. The important points which arise from this and other related work are that:

1. The valency of the IgG molecule is confirmed as 2.
2. The population of antibody molecules in an antiserum directed against a hapten is not uniform with respect to association constants. An average association constant K_0 can be measured which is the reciprocal of the molar concentration of free hapten which maintains half the antibody binding sites in combination with hapten. This is measured in litres/mole.
3. The K_0 of an antiserum is influenced by the immunisation schedule used.
4. There is biological variation in the K_0 of antisera produced by different strains of animal given similar immunisation courses. Biological variation almost certainly occurs in man and may be important in determining the 'quality' of an antibody response and also the likelihood of developing a situation in which circulating soluble complexes may occur (p. 30). Methods for determining the K_0 of human antibody directed against a whole antigen molecule are unreliable because of multiple and potentially interfering determinants. A relative association constant K_{rel} has been measured in animal antisera directed against whole antigen molecules and such studies with human sera could be very useful.
5. The concept of cross-reactivity between related though non-identical determinants can be quantified as differences in K_0 obtained with inducer and cross-reacting determinants.

Secondary effects of antigen–antibody combination in vitro. A very wide range of techniques has been developed either to demonstrate the presence of, or to quantitate with, various degrees of sensitivity, either antigen or antibody. The systems either involve only the two reactants or also involve secondary reactants such as complement; or a secondary system to demonstrate changes in properties of the antigen, e.g. the neutralisation of a biological property of the antigen. A detailed account of such methods is not within the scope of this chapter, and only those aspects which demonstrate important principles will be considered.

The two simplest methods of visualising an antigen–antibody reaction are precipitation if the antigen is soluble or agglutination if the antigen is particulate. The same principle applies in both cases providing the soluble antigen has multiple antigenic determinants. Antibody molecules link like determinants on either molecules or antigenic particles to produce insoluble complexes or clumps of particles. The reaction is reversible and at equilibrium will depend on the relative concentration of the reactants. An excess of antigen, relative to the antibody concentration, in a precipitation reaction will result in the generation of smaller complexes. In this situation the smallest complexes formed will be made up of one molecule of divalent antibody and two of antigen ($AbAg_2$). Such complexes are usually soluble. It follows that unless the ratio of antigen to antibody is within certain limits precipitation may not be seen but *soluble complexes* will be formed. The most rapid and efficient precipitation takes place at optimal proportions. Just as precipitation is inhibited by the addition of excess antigen so agglutination may be inhibited by adding the appropriate non-particulate antigen or isolated haptenic group. Such inhibition reactions provide useful measuring systems. There is a limit to the amount of precipitate that may be seen, and many methods are available to increase the sensitivity and to make possible the demonstration of soluble complexes. The use of radiolabelled antigen or antibody to increase sensitivity is further considered in Chapter 5 as radioimmunoassay. The precipitin reaction may be visualised in the detection of antigen or antibody in tissues by the use of fluorescent labelling or, at the electron-optical level, by the use of electron-dense or enzyme labels.

Systems in which antigen and antibody are diffused towards each other in a gel matrix also provide an increase in sensitivity by allowing a somewhat greater latitude of relative concentrations and by concentrating the precipitate in one site. Using such double-diffusion systems directly (Ouchterlony) or combined with electrophoresis (immuno-electrophoresis), information concerning the number and relative importance of the reacting systems can be obtained. Increased sensitivity may be achieved by radioactive labelling either reactant followed by autoradiography. Precipitation reactions are in general less sensitive and less flexible than agglutination. The reaction between an antibody and a soluble antigen can be converted to a passive agglutination system by coating the antigen onto a non-reacting particle such as an erythrocyte or a latex particle. Soluble antigens may also be rendered insoluble by binding onto cellulose or a cross-linked dextran (sephadex). The uptake of antibody can then be measured. Insolubilised antibody may be used in a similar manner to measure antigen.

Two main groups of techniques depend on effects secondary to the combination of antigen and antibody. These are neutralisation and complement fixation. If an antigen possesses biological properties such as toxic, infective or enzymic activity, the combination of antibody with the antigen will often remove this property. A toxin will lose its toxic properties as demonstrable by injection into an animal; a virus will not infect a suitable tissue culture system and an enzyme may be unable to bind to its appropriate substrate. Because of the need for a secondary detection system which may often be complex, such techniques are used only where simpler methods are not possible.

Complement is a complex system of serum globulins which operate in cascade fashion; activation of the initial component resulting in sequential activation of the other components. There are nine components designated as C1–C9. Activation of the cascade is brought about by steric changes in an antibody molecule, usually consequent upon binding with antigen.

If the antigen is at the surface of a cell, the complement system results in activated complement components binding to the cell and ultimately producing a membrane lesion which results in cell lysis. From the view point of complement fixation the complexities of the reaction are best ignored. A more detailed account of the complement system is given under effectors (p. 23).

The first stage of a complement fixation test allows for the possibility of the interaction of antigen and antibody in the presence of C. If such a reaction occurs C will be fixed and the concentration of C activity in the reaction mixture will fall. The second stage of the test utilises erythrocytes onto which specific antibody is bound to act as a complement detection system. In the presence of complement they will lyse. Either the amount of complement initially present in the system may be limited and the reaction declared positive if this quantity is removed by the antigen–antibody reaction, or the decrease in complement activity may be measured. Very many methods have been developed, differing in detail and resulting in greater or lesser sensitivity.

Immunological Effector Systems

Immune effector systems comprise part of the efferent arm of the immune response. The specific output either as antibody or sensitised lymphocyte on combination with antigen initiates a biological amplification system which results in an inflammatory response. The inflammatory response evoked may be of a variety of types and may confer advantages in the form of resistance to infective organisms, or may be entirely detrimental if the antigen per se was incapable of producing harm. Precisely the same mechanisms apply in either case. Effector systems involve the participation of cellular 'intermediates' including polymorphs, mast cells, platelets and macrophages and non-cellular factors such as complement. 'Final' mediators include a wide range of molecules. These either have activity within participating cells, e.g. enzymes, or after release, on tissues, e.g. histamine. The effectors involved in antibody-mediated responsiveness are different from those in cell-mediated immune reactivity although in many clinical situations both types may be involved together. Tables 1.1 and 1.3 list the intermediates and final mediators of the antibody and sensitised lymphocyte systems.

The data available on immunological effector systems have been derived by attempting to dissect the processes, often by using in vitro methods. A bewildering number of systems have been revealed, usually having complex inter-relationships. It has become obvious that there exist considerable differences from species to species. It should be appreciated that whilst it may be possible to demonstrate the existence of a particular system under special conditions in the laboratory, its relevance to the phenomenon observed in the whole animal is often debatable. It is even more difficult to relate laboratory data on effector systems in the case of naturally occurring human disease. This applies even if the experiments are carried out using human material. What is needed is information to rank the inter-relating systems in some order of importance in human diseases. This would require the capacity to block a system specifically without influencing others and without untoward effects. At the moment this is not possible.

Antibody-mediated Effector Systems

One very obvious difference between an animal with circulating antibody and one without is in the handling of administered antigen. The presence of the antibody results in accelerated clearance of the antigen. Antigen–antibody complexes are much more rapidly removed by the cells of the reticulo-endothelial system (RES) than are free antigen molecules. After capture by the RES the antigen is usually catabolised. Small soluble complexes are less efficiently cleared and may remain in the circulation with the potentiality of producing tissue damage (vide infra). Accelerated clearance is very similar to opsonisation in which particulate antigen (usually on the surface of a bacterium) is more readily phagocytosed in the presence of antibody and particularly if complement is also present. Opsonisation occurs with both polymorphs and macrophages and depends on cell surface receptors which can bind the Fc portion of an antibody molecule hence capturing and/or holding antigen in close contact with the cell surface by means of the antibody combining sites in the Fab portion of the molecule. Receptors which can bind the third complement component (C3) will also cause complexes or particles which have activated the complement cascade to bind to the surface. Following surface binding of a particle phagocytosis is greatly facilitated.

Both accelerated antigen clearance and opsonisation involve the collaboration of specific antibody and a phagocytic cell, and will tend to destroy bacteria and neutralise and remove toxic materials. In this sense they can be seen to confer advantages. Similar mechanisms will however cause accelerated removal of autologous erythrocytes coated with antibody as in haemolytic

Table 1.1. The 'intermediates' and mediators of antibody mediated effector systems

Intermediates		Mediators
Cellular	Non-cellular	
Mast cells Neutrophils Platelets Macrophages Eosinophils ? a subpopulation of lymphocytes	complement kinin-forming system blood clotting factors	histamine slow-reacting substance (SRS-A) eosinophil chemotactic factor (ECF-A) serotonin prostaglandins kinins lysosomal enzymes neutrophil polypeptides anaphylatoxins $C3_a$, $C5_a$

disease of the newborn and autoimmune anaemia. A similar situation, with increased destruction of cells by the RES, is found in some patients with thrombocytopenia and leucopenia.

Combination of IgM and some subclasses of IgG antibody (IgG 1, IgG 2 and IgG 3) with antigen will activate the complement cascade. The first complement component C1 is a tri-molecular complex of C1q, C1r and C1s whose integrity depends on the presence of calcium ions. C1q reacts with a site on the Fc part of the Ig molecule which is either revealed or altered following combination of antigen with the Fab portion. This particular reaction has been exploited to demonstrate the presence of soluble complexes which will precipitate with C1q. Following reaction with Ig the C1 becomes activated and is designated $C\bar{1}$. The activity resides in the C1s portion which can be demonstrated to have esterase activity. $C\bar{1}$ acts sequentially on C4 and C2 in each case cleaving the molecules into two. One C4 fragment will bind either to a cell surface or to Ig and in the presence of magnesium ions one fragment of C2 will also bind to form an active complex $C\overline{42}$. Once this has occurred it is no longer necessary for $C\bar{1}$ to remain bound. $C\overline{42}$ has activity directed against C3 and is known as C3 convertase. C3 is split into two fragments C3a and C3b, one of which (C3a) is released and has important biological characteristics, while the C3b joins C42 to form the complex C423.

The active C423 cleaves C5 into two fragments C5a and C5b; the former having similar though not identical properties to C3a. The next two components, C6 and C7, react with C4235; each step being subject to decay. The tri-molecular complex C567 again has biological properties; it is chemotactic to polymorphs and can bind to the surface of cells which have neither antibody nor earlier complement components on their surfaces. The final two components C8 and C9 may react with the tri-molecular complex to become activated. At the surface of a cell they are taken up by the cell membrane and produce a lesion. Permeability changes across the membrane lesion result in cell lysis.

It is not only the end result of this classical complement cascade, i.e., cell lysis, which is important. At each stage of the reaction new properties are conferred on the complex whether it is free or at the surface of a cell. In addition, the cleaved fragments, particularly C3a and C5a, have the properties of releasing histamine from mast cells and are highly chemotactic for polymorphs. The combination of 'early' complement components enables attachment of the complex to leucocytes which facilitates opsonisation. Also by a phenomenon known as immune adherence they may attach to erythrocytes and to platelets. This again may produce a more readily phagocytosable particle.

Two serum factors known as conglutinin (K) and immuno-conglutinin (IK) will also link together particles having early complement components on their surfaces. These two factors behave like antibodies to activated complement components although K is not an immunoglobulin. The former appears to be naturally occurring only in *Bovidae* whilst the latter is probably induced when considerable in vivo complement activation is taking place, i.e. is an auto-antibody to altered complement.

Thus the activation of complement may result in cell lysis, increased phagocytosis, leucotaxis and local increase in vascular permeability. In addition activated C may act on platelets and initiate the blood clotting system and also through this system induce the generation of kinins from plasma precursors. In the context of an infection the activation of complement will thus rapidly induce an acute inflammatory reaction which will be advantageous. On the other hand a similar inflammatory reaction will ensue if complement is activated by antibody combination with an 'innocent' antigen. Such a situation exists in the Arthus reaction and in damage to blood vessels produced by complement activation by circulating soluble complexes. The polymorphs attracted to the area of complement activation will tend to phagocytose antigen–antibody–complement complexes and will liberate lysosomal enzymes. These will have the capacity to produce tissue damage in their own right subject to the anti-enzyme activity of naturally occurring serum globulins. In addition polymorph polypeptides have inflammation-inducing activity and also will cause fever.

More recently attention has been devoted to alternative mechanisms of C3 activation other than by $C\overline{42}$ in the classical cascade. These are known as alternative pathways of C activation or the C3 shunt. Activation at the C3 level will be capable of inducing many of the effects of classical activation. It may be brought about via the properdin system which may therefore operate as a non-specific defence mechanism. This system is complex and involves properdin activation by some polysaccharides. This reacts via serum factors C3 proactivator (C3PA) and C3PA convertase to cleave C3 to C3a and C3b. The alternate pathway may also be activated by bacterial lipopolysaccharides (endotoxins) and this mechanism may be important in the Schwartzman reaction. Immunoglobulins may also activate complement at the C3 level. Of particular importance in this respect is the ability of IgA so to do, in that it will not activate via the classical pathway. The activation site for the alternate pathway appears to be in a different situation on the Ig molecule than the classical activation site.

A further mechanism whereby IgG antibody molecules may produce effects is by collaborating with a subpopulation of lymphocytes. These do not appear to be T cells, are probably not B cells, and have been named as K for 'killer' cells. In vitro such cells have the ability to kill target cells having antibody on their surface. Complement is not necessary. It has been suggested that this system may be involved in defence against malignant tumours, and it could have a role in the tissue damage in some autoimmune diseases. The status of the system in human diseases is still to be determined.

Antibody of the IgE class has the special property of binding to tissue mast cells and blood basophils. The binding is via the Fc part of the molecule and the association constant between antibody and cell is very high. The IgE-mast cell system provides the initiating mechanism for anaphylactic type reactivity. IgE antibody is almost exclusively produced in lymphoid tissue in close association with the mucous membrane of the respiratory and gastro-intestinal tracts; both of which are rich in mast cells. Circulating IgE may bind to mast cells elsewhere in the body, but because of the high association constant for mast cells IgE will tend to bind first to cells in the region of its production. Steric change, probably in two adjacent IgE molecules, induced by combination with antigen, activates a sequence of events which results in the release of mast cell granules. The intracellular sequence is probably complex, can be modulated by the intracellular concentrations of the two cyclic nucleotides c-AMP and c-GMP and may involve actomyosin contraction.

The mast cell granules contain histamine which is released during degranulation. Other pharmacologically active agents can also be demonstrated following antigen challenge of sensitised tissues in vitro. These may either be derived from the mast cell or be generated consequent upon the degranulation. Other mediators demonstrable include slow-reacting substance of anaphylaxis (SRS-A), prostaglandins, 5-hydroxytryptamine, and eosinophil chemotactic factor of anaphylaxis (ECF-A). In different animal systems investigated differing proportions of the mediators are found. Thus in the rat 5-HT is predominant, whilst in the guinea pig histamine and SRS-A appear to be more important. The effects produced by the mediators results in eosinophil infiltration (ECF-A) and spasm of smooth muscle and increased capillary permeability (the others). The reaction takes place very rapidly (SRS-A is only given the designation 'slow' relative to histamine) and will tend to be transient.

In many animal species two different Ig classes can mediate reactivity of this type. These are either IgE-like as described above or due to IgG anaphylactic antibody. Unlike IgE, IgG anaphylactic antibodies are heat stable, do not bind so firmly to mast cells but will sensitise mast cells much more rapidly. Like IgE, the IgG anaphylactic antibody will exhibit specificity as to the species of mast cells to which it will bind. Anaphylactic antibodies of both classes have therefore been termed homocytotropic antibodies. Human IgG homocytotropic antibody has been demonstrated, but its role in allergic reactions still needs clarification. Table 1.2 indicates the differences in the two types of antibody.

Table 1.2. Properties of homocytotropic antibodies

Property	IgE	IgG
Heat stability (56°C)	labile	stable
Time for tissue sensitisation	long (days)	short (hours)
Duration of sensitisation	long (weeks)	short (days)
Placental transmission	no	yes

Anaphylactic reactivity is often interpreted as a purely destructive phenomenon. Such reactivity is however represented in many species and therefore may have some survival value. It is possible that reactivity of this type taking place at a mucosal surface may aid in the shedding of parasites such as nematodes. It is noticeable that very many parasitic infestations induce particularly good anaphylactic antibody responses, and although the antibody is unlikely to have any direct effect on the parasite, the acute inflammatory reaction induced by mast cell release of granules may allow other Ig classes and possibly sensitised lymphocytes to gain easier access to the parasite. As a mechanism of tissue damage the anaphylactic antibody–mast cell system is involved in generalised anaphylaxis, and the allergic disease of the respiratory tract, gut and skin.

Cell-mediated Effector Systems

The specificity of cell-mediated effector systems depends on T lymphocyte surface receptors. Although proof has been difficult to obtain these are probably Ig-like yet are not secreted. Combination of antigen with the specific receptor results in a stimulus to synthesise DNA, RNA and new proteins and to multiply. This is seen in vitro as lymphocyte transformation and is often used as a laboratory parameter of cell-mediated immunity. The transformed lymphocytes resemble lymphoblasts. During the reaction between antigen and sensitised lymphocyte proteins with biological activity are released which have been called lymphokines and are named after the activity they possess. They are proteins of molecular weights from 20 000 to 80 000, i.e. are smaller than immunoglobulins, and can be released from stimulated lymphocytes well before cell division takes place.

The lymphokine most studied is macrophage migration inhibition factor (MIF) which slows or stops the normal movement of macrophages across glass or plastic surfaces in tissue culture. It is usual to measure MIF by packing macrophages in a small capillary tube and placing this within a tissue culture chamber. Normally a fan-shaped area of migration away from the end of the capillary tube is observed. In the presence of MIF this is either absent or reduced in size. The demonstration of MIF activity following incubation of human lymphocytes with antigen has been used as another laboratory parameter of cell-mediated reactivity. MIF does not have species specificity and guinea pig peritoneal macrophages are usually used as indicator cells. A related system, the inhibition of migration of whole peripheral blood leucocytes

Table 1.3. The 'intermediates' and mediators of sensitised lymphocyte mediated effector systems

Intermediates		Mediators
Cellular	Non-cellular	
'Recruited' lymphocytes	skin reactive factor	? lymphotoxin
Macrophages	lymphocyte mitogenic factor	direct effect of lymphocyte-target cell contact
	macrophage chemotactic factor	
? polymorphs	macrophage migration inhibition factor	macrophage enzymes
	macrophage agglutination factor	
	macrophage activating factor	

in a one-stage test, has also been used. The lymphocytes in the system provide the specific trigger and the effect is measured on the migrating leucocytes. Whilst under some circumstances this test appears to reflect lymphocyte mediated reactivity the results should be viewed with some caution as antigen–antibody complexes can also inhibit migration in this system. Macrophage agglutinating activity has also been observed in stimulated lymphocyte supernatants and this may represent another activity of MIF.

Other lymphokines with activity directed against macrophages are a chemotactic factor (MCF) and possibly an activation factor. Activated or 'angry' macrophages have a considerably augmented ability to kill micro-organisms and probably also greater phagocytic ability. They have a greater content of hydrolases and alterations in respiration. Although the activating sequence operates through the T lymphocyte and hence has immunological specificity the augmented macrophage activity is non-specific.

A lymphokine with the capability to induce cell multiplication in 'uncommitted' lymphocytes—mitogenic factor (MF)—has been demonstrated. This may serve to recruit uncommitted lymphocytes and so increase the output of lymphokines. A lymphotoxin (LT), capable of killing some cells in tissue culture has also been demonstrated. The role of this factor in disease states is unclear. Other activities demonstrable in lymphocyte culture supernatants include a skin reactive factor (SRF) producing redness and thickening of the skin several hours after injection and interferon which can interfere with virus replication.

As well as the capacity to produce effects by the release of lymphokines, T lymphocytes appear to be able to operate directly. This is most readily demonstrable in the killing of target cells in tissue culture. Most of the work has been carried out in the context of tumour immunity. T lymphocytes from both experimental animals and from patients with malignant tumours may kill the appropriate tumour cell in tissue culture. The reaction requires contact between lymphocyte and tumour cell but this need not be prolonged. There is no evidence that lymphotoxin release is involved as non-tumour cells in the immediate vicinity of a tumour-cell-lymphocyte pair are not damaged. The mechanism is not known.

Thus combination of a sensitised T lymphocyte with antigen will cause accumulation of macrophages (MCF), which will remain in the area (MIF), may become activated by activation factor so that they will readily take up and destroy a microbial invader. In addition lymphocyte proliferation both of committed and uncommitted lymphocytes (MF) will take place. If the reaction occurs in the skin, as in a delayed hypersensitivity reaction, redness and induration will be observed (SRF). The picture described is as in a granulomatous form of inflammation and as in a positive delayed skin response to tuberculin. From the viewpoint of defence against microorganisms, particularly intra-cellular parasites, e.g. tuberculosis, brucellosis, these mechanisms are very important. It is also likely that the liberation of interferon and the capacity to kill cells with virus determinants on their surfaces is important in immunity to virus infections, particularly during the recovery phase which often takes place before circulating antibody is detectable. T-lymphocyte mediated reactivity is also involved in the rejection of allografts, in skin contact sensitivity, and has been thought to account for the inflammatory reaction in organ specific autoimmune diseases. T lymphocytes are postulated to have an immuno-surveillance role by which abnormal cells including neoplastic cells are destroyed. The degree of efficiency of tumour cell killing by T lymphocyte and by other mechanisms may determine the pace of tumour development and hence have an influence on prognosis in human malignant disease.

Transfer factors

The passive transfer of cell-mediated reactivity in experimental animals has been achieved by transfer of large numbers of lymphoid cells obtained from peripheral blood, lymph nodes, spleen or peritoneal exudates. In man it is possible to transfer cell-mediated reactivity between individuals by the passive transfer of relatively small numbers of peripheral blood white cells. By this means delayed hypersensitivity to tuberculin PPD, coccidioidin, streptococcal M protein and diphtheria toxoid has been observed in the previously negative recipient of cells from a positive donor. Positivity is not permanent but may sometimes last for more than one year. Similar transfer may be achieved by using lysed peripheral blood leucocytes and by a small molecular weight material present in the lysate. This material will pass through a dialysis membrane and is therefore known as dialysable transfer factor. The nature of this material is unclear, indeed there may well be more than one type of transfer factor. Transfer factor probably operates through uncommitted lymphocytes. This is supported by the observation that the capacity of lymphocytes to respond to specific antigen by transformation can be induced by transfer factor in vitro. Repeated doses of transfer factor have been used in attempts to restore cell-mediated responsiveness in human immunodeficient states, particularly in mucocutaneous candidiasis.

Classification of Tissue-damaging Reactions

Although cell or tissue damage of some degree is the inevitable cost of activating immunological effector systems in the defence against infection, this is considered to be a 'good bargain'. If the same effector systems are activated via an immune response to an 'innocent' or to a 'self' antigen tissue damage will also result, but this will confer no concomitant advantage. The individual will suffer from either a hypersensitivity or autoimmune disease. In some situations the relationship between immunity and hypersensitivity may become blurred when the response to an infective organism is considered. One individual may produce a response which results in immunity with little tissue damage whilst another, in responding against the same antigens, may exhibit both immunity and a hypersensitivity disease. Differences in the total output of Ig, its association constant, its distribution between the Ig classes and in the output of sensitised lymphocytes probably account for this variation. It should be stressed that the same immunological effector systems are involved irrespective of whether immunity or hypersensitivity results.

Tissue damage associated with hypersensitivity is best classified by the immuno-pathogenetic mechanisms operating and the classification of Gell and Coombs into four types is most commonly used. On occasion a hypersensitivity reaction may involve more than one type of mechanism. A brief account of this classification is given below and reference should be made both to the section on immunological effector systems and to later chapters for additional detail.

Type 1—Anaphylactic

This type of reaction depends on the sensitisation of mast cells by homocytotropic antibody which becomes bound to the surface. Combination of antigen with this antibody causes secretion of mast cell granules and the entry into the tissues of vasoactive and smooth muscle contracting agents. The homocytotropic antibody is usually of IgE class; IgG homocytotropic antibody has been demonstrated but its importance is undecided. Type 1 reactions may be divided into systemic and local depending on dose and route of entry of antigen and sometimes on differential sensitivity of target tissues. Type 1 reactions are involved in allergic asthma, rhinitis, urticaria, food allergy, as well as systemic anaphylaxis.

Type 2—Cytotoxic or cytolytic

The mechanism depends on the effects produced by the binding of antibody to a determinant on a target cell surface. The antibody may be directed against a structural antigen of the cell surface or against an antigen from some other source attached to the surface, e.g. drug, microbial antigen. The cell may be phagocytosed after adhesion to a phagocyte, may be lysed by activation of the whole complement cascade or maybe destroyed by a non-T lymphocyte (K cell, p. 25). Type 2 mechanisms are involved in autoimmune haemolytic anaemia, some cases of leucopenia and thrombocytopenia, haemolytic disease of the newborn, immunological reactions to some drugs and possibly in some autoimmune conditions.

Type 3—Arthus type or antigen–antibody complex mediated

This type depends on the activation of the complement cascade by antigen–antibody complex. The result is an acute inflammatory response initiated by C3a, C5a and C567. Activation of blood clotting mechanisms, kinin liberation and the effects on tissues of released polymorph enzymes may be involved in the ensuing tissue damage. A type 3 reaction may take place locally or systemically. This will depend on the route of entry of the antigen and also on the relative proportions of antigen and antibody. In antibody excess the insoluble complexes produced will tend to be localised. This applies in a skin Arthus reaction and probably also in allergic alveolitis. In antigen excess, small soluble complexes will be produced which can be disseminated in the circulation. This is more likely to occur if antibody of low association constant is involved. Complexes may become arrested in vessels and may be filtered by the renal glomerulus. Activation of C at these sites will result in vasculitis and glomerulonephritis respectively. The antigens involved may be administered therapeutically, e.g., horse antitoxin, may be microbial, or may be autoantigens as in systemic lupus erythematosus.

Ag + Thymocyte

Type 4—Cell-mediated or delayed hypersensitivity

Unlike the preceding three types of tissue damaging reactions which are antibody dependent, type 4 involves combination of an antigen with a sensitised T lymphocyte. The effects are produced either by means of released lymphokines or by direct T-lymphocyte mediated cell destruction. Type 4 reactivity is involved in delayed skin reactivity, best exemplified in the tuberculin skin test, but present in other bacterial, fungal, viral and protozoal diseases. Type 4 reactivity is also involved in skin contact sensitisation in which the sensitiser acts as a hapten attached to a 'self' carrier, in rejection of allografts and possibly in organ-specific autoimmune diseases.

Selected Reviews, Monographs and Reference Works

Immunoglobulins

Bennich, H. & Johansson, S. G. O. (1971) Structure and function of human immunoglobulin E. *Advances in Immunology*, **13,** 1.

Cohen, S. & Milstein, C. (1967) Structure and biological properties of immunoglobulins. *Advances in Immunology*, **7,** 1.

Green, N. M. (1969) Electron microscopy of the immunoglobulins. *Advances in Immunology*, **11**, 1.
Metzger, H. (1970) Structure and function of γM macroglobulins. *Advances in Immunology*, **12**, 57.
Nezlin, R. S. (1970) *Biochemistry of Antibodies*. New York: Plenum.
Tomasi, T. B. & Bienenstock, J. (1968) Secretory immunoglobulins. *Advances in Immunology*, **9**, 1.

Antigens and antigen–antibody reactions

Kabat, E. A. (1968) *Structural Concepts in Immunology*. New York: Holt, Rinehart and Winston.
Kabat, E. A. & Mayer, M. M. (1961) *Experimental Immunochemistry*. 2nd edition. Springfield, Illinois, U.S.A.: Thomas.
Karush, F. (1962) Immunologic specificity and molecular structure. *Advances in Immunology*, **2**, 1.
Sela, M. (1966) Immunological studies with synthetic polypeptides. *Advances in Immunology*, **5**, 30.
Weir, D. M. (Ed.) (1973) *Handbook of Experimental Immunology*. Vol. I. 2nd edition. Oxford: Blackwell.
Williams, C. A. & Chase, M. W. (Eds.) (1971) *Methods in Immunology and Immunochemistry*. Vol. III. New York: Academic Press.

Cellular basis of the immune response

Cunningham, A. J. (1973) In *Progress in Allergy* (Eds.) Kallos, P., Waksman, B. H. & de Weck, A. Basel: Karger.
Landy, M. & Braun, W. (Eds.) (1969) *Immunological Tolerance*. New York: Academic Press.
Miller, J. F. A. P., Basten, A., Sprent, J. & Cheers, C. (1971) *Cell Immunology*, **2**, 469.
Nossal, G. J. V. & Ada, G. L. (1971) *Antigens, Lymphoid Cells and the Immune Response*. New York: Academic Press.
Playfair, J. H. L. (1971) Cell cooperation in the immune response. *Clinical and Experimental Immunology*, **8**, 839.
Playfair, J. H. L. (1974) The role of antibody in T cell responses. *Clinical and Experimental Immunology*, **17**, 1.
Siskind, G. W. & Benacerraf, B. (1969) Cell selection by antigen in the immune response. *Advances in Immunology*, **10**, 1.
Weigle, W. D. (1973) Immunological unresponsiveness. *Advances in Immunology*, **16**, 61.

Immunological effector systems

Austen, K. F. & Becker, E. L. (Eds.) (1971) *Biochemistry of the Acute Allergic Reactions; Second International Symposium*. Oxford: Blackwell.
Becker, E. L. & Henson, P. M. (1973) In vitro studies of immunologically induced secretion of mediators from cells and related phenomena. *Advances in Immunology*, **17**, 93.
Bloom, B. R. (1971) In vitro approaches to the mechanism of cell-mediated immune reactions. *Advances in Immunology*, **13**, 102.
Lawrence, H. S. & Landy, M. (Eds.) (1969) *Mediators of Cellular Immunity*. New York: Academic Press.
Lepow, L. H. & Ward, P. A. (Eds.) (1972) *Inflammation, Mechanisms and Control*. New York: Academic Press.
Muller-Eberhard, H. J. (1968) Chemistry and reaction mechanisms of complement. *Advances in Immunology*, **8**, 1.
Osler, A. G. & Sandberg, A. L. (1973) Alternate complement pathways. *Progress in Allergy*, **17**, 51.
Perlmann, P. & Holm, G. (1969) Cytotoxic effects of lymphoid cells in vitro. *Advances in Immunology*, **11**, 117.
Pick, E. & Turk, J. L. (1972) The biological activities of soluble lymphocyte products—a review. *Clinical and Experimental Immunology*, **10**, 1.

2. Immunodeficiency

ANTHONY HAYWARD

Immunodeficiency describes a clinical state of increased susceptibility to infection. This is a common situation but in practice those patients labelled as having 'immunodeficiency' are recognised because they form part of a polar group usually characterised by a specific and clearly demonstrable defect. There is no reason to suppose, however, that there is a sharply demarcated boundary which separates them from other less severely affected individuals who suffer from frequent colds or sore throats.

The physiological means which the body has available for defence against infection can broadly be divided into specific and non-specific, each with humoral and cellular components.

Non-specific immunity mechanisms

The vast majority of an individual's contacts with microorganisms are dealt with by non-specific mechanisms. In most cases this protection depends initially on a mechanical barrier to prevent invasion together with a decontamination mechanism to remove organisms which are excluded. The upper respiratory tract, for example, has an epithelial surface as a barrier which is kept decontaminated by a constant stream of mucus. The barrier afforded by the skin is similarly decontaminated by the antibacterial action of fatty acids in sebaceous secretions. Deficiency of decontamination or disruption of the mechanical barrier usually leads to repeated episodes of infection at that site, thereby differing from the generalised immunodeficiency syndromes in which multiple sites are usual.

The outcome of an encounter with an organism which, by virtue of its invasiveness or failure of the mechanical barrier, does gain access to the body depends both on pathogenicity and the individual resistance. The humoral components of non-specific resistance are present in the intravascular and extravascular fluids. The capacity of fresh serum for direct bactericidal action depends on many factors such as antibody, complement and lysozyme. The extent to which natural antibodies can be regarded as non-specific is debatable as many bacteria have antigenic determinants in common. Antibody cross-reacts weakly between these and in experimental conditions Gram-negative bacteria are the most affected.

Lysozyme, which is widely distributed in the body, is another protein with a non-specific action. It functions as a mucolytic enzyme which can kill bacteria by interacting with the muramic acid of cell walls. It is present in many secretions including tears where it contributes to decontamination mechanisms.

Complement activation by the alternative pathway is also a non-specific mechanism which may bypass the need for specific antibody. One serum protein which can mediate this activation is properdin and a number of Gram-positive and Gram-negative bacteria as well as some viruses are susceptible to it. Non-specific factors in resistance to viruses include interferon which can be released by many types of cell. It limits the spread of virus to surrounding cells but disappointingly has been of little therapeutic value.

Cellular mechanisms play a major role in non-specific immunity by the phagocytosis and intracellular digestion of particles. Polymorphs and macrophages are recruited to areas of inflammation by soluble mediators and interaction with specific mechanisms is important here. Some bacteria can be phagocytosed directly in the absence of antibody but others, particularly those with polysaccharide capsules, are resistant unless opsonised. In some instances, suitable surfaces such as fibrin can substitute for specific antibody opsonins. The ability of phagocytes to ingest and destroy organisms in the absence of specific factors is sometimes responsible for innate or species immunity. The importance of this non-specific resistance is illustrated by innoculation of mice with herpes simplex virus. Although not naturally susceptible to this infection, mechanical bypass of macrophages by intracerebral injection is followed by fatal encephalitis.

Specific immunity mechanisms

Specific immunity depends on adaptive mechanisms by which the individual modifies his response to a pathogen as a result of experience: it is mediated by antibodies and by cells.

Antibody must be directed against appropriate antigenic determinants on the surface of the pathogen if it is to be effective. This is not an invariable finding, for example the anti-salmonella O antibody readily demonstrable after salmonella infection is not associated with enhanced resistance. Antibodies are not able to penetrate living cells so that intracellular pathogens such as *Brucella* and *Listeria* are able to proliferate inside macrophages despite a high titre of circulating antibody. The localisation of antibody production is particularly important. IgM, because of its large molecular size, is virtually confined to the intravascular space while IgG can in addition diffuse into tissue spaces. Antibody is most effective against extracellular viruses and can effectively quench a viraemia. Some viruses, such as rubella, can be directly neutralised by antibody in the plasma, but for herpes simplex virus early complement components are involved as well. The antibacterial actions of antibody are also often mediated by complement acting either as an opsonin or by effecting lysis directly.

In recent years the importance of local immunity has been increasingly recognised. The protection of mucosal surfaces is closely associated with the secretion of a dimeric form of IgA which is composed of two linked IgA molecules and a secretory piece, the addition of this piece protecting the molecule from digestion by proteolytic enzymes. IgA-containing plasma cells are found under many mucous membranes and the site of secretory IgA synthesis is closely linked to the route of antigen administration. This can be exploited clinically: strains of rubella vaccine which can be administered nasally result in more effective protection than other vaccines which are given intramuscularly. Similar secretory IgA-mediated local immunity mechanisms are probably important in the protection of the gut from organisms such as *Salmonella* or *Vibrio cholerae*.

The effector mechanisms of specific cellular immunity are complex. Thymus-derived lymphocytes interacting with an antigen to which they are sensitive can become directly cytotoxic leading to lysis of specific target cells. They can liberate pharmacologically active substances which recruit other lymphocytes and also act on macrophages, giving rise in vivo to the cellular infiltration typical of a type 4 allergic reaction.

The immune response to an infection usually has both cell-mediated and humoral components but they may not be equally important. Toxins can be neutralised by antibody and so, in the case of *Clostridium tetani*, prevent clinical disease. Eradication of the bacteria, however, depends on phagocytosis so that for active immunity an intact blood supply, opsonising antibody and phagocytes are all necessary. Resistance to intracellular pathogens such as measles virus depends in the first place on circulating antibody which can prevent the virus from entering susceptible cells. However, once the virus is inside cells, other—especially cellular—mechanisms are of major importance.

Experimentally, resistance to tuberculosis and *Listeria* infection can be transferred by lymphocytes but not by serum. In both cases opsonising antibodies have no protective function because the organisms are able to multiply inside the phagocyte. The macrophage response to intracellular pathogens can be modified by specifically sensitive lymphocytes so that multiplication is stopped and the organisms are killed instead. Such 'macrophage arming' is immunologically non-specific in its efferent limb and unrelated intracellular organisms are also killed.

Elimination of viruses can probably be achieved by two lymphocyte effector mechanisms. Specifically sensitive T cells can be metabolically stimulated by virus antigens and in this process become cytotoxic to cells with the virus antigens on their surface. If the virus surface antigens are coated with IgG antibody other lymphocytes can also be stimulated to become cytotoxic, in which case the specificity of target cell killing is dictated by the antibody and not by the lymphocytes.

With increasing clinical experience both single and multiple defects of defence mechanisms are being recognised. Many of these are secondary to other pre-existing conditions or arise as a consequence of drug therapy. The primary immunodeficiencies will, however, be discussed first as they illustrate some of the consequences of relatively clearly defined defects. Some of the primary immunodeficiency syndromes are congenital, and many of those which arise in childhood and adult life appear to be genetically determined. A clear classification in terms of aetiology is not yet possible although a start

Table 2.1. Classification of primary immunodeficiency disorders (Fudenberg et al, 1971)

	Suggested cellular defect		
	B cells	T cells	Stem cells
Infantile X-linked agammaglobulinaemia	+		
Selective immunoglobulin deficiency (IgA)	+ (some)		
Transient hypogammaglobulinaemia of infancy	+		
X-linked immunodeficiency with hyper-IgM	+	?	
Thymic hypoplasia (pharyngeal pouch syndrome, DiGeorge's syndrome)		+	
Episodic lymphopenia with lymphocytotoxin		+	
Immunodeficiency with normal or without hyperimmunoglobulinaemia		+ (sometimes)	
Immunodeficiency with ataxia telangiectasia	+	+	
Immunodeficiency with thrombocytopenia and eczema (Wiskott–Aldrich syndrome)	+	+	
Immunodeficiency with thymoma	+	+	
Immunodeficiency with short-limbed dwarfism	+	+	
Immunodeficiency with generalised haematopoietic hypoplasia	+	+	+
Severe combined immunodeficiency			
(a) autosomal recessive	+	+	+
(b) X-linked	+	+	+
(c) sporadic	+	+	+
Variable immunodeficiency (common, largely unclassified)	+	+ (sometimes)	

has been made by a WHO group (Table 2.1). It is based on the T and B cell classification of immunological response (Fudenberg et al, 1971).

Most of the conditions listed in the table are extremely rare and have been recognised on account of their severity. A large number of patients fall into the group 'variable immunodeficiency' and a better understanding of immunity mechanisms will be required to classify them.

Deficiencies of Specific Humoral Immunity

Complete failure of immunoglobulin production rarely, if ever, occurs. Even in X-linked hypogammaglobulinaemia, in which serum levels may be less than 10 per cent of normal, some immunoglobulin can be detected by sensitive assay methods. It is likely that genetically determined hypogammaglobulinaemias are due to failures of normal cell development rather than a deficiency of genes coding for immunoglobulin molecules. The defect may be in cells of the B lymphocyte series or it may affect their inductive environment. On clinical grounds four major types of immunoglobulin deficiency due to decreased synthesis can be recognised.

X-linked hypogammaglobulinaemia

This condition affects boys and has an incidence of about 1 in 100 000 live male births. The first description by Bruton in 1952 was of a boy aged eight years who had a four-year history of recurrent pneumonia and pneumococcal septicaemia (Bruton, 1952). Serum electrophoresis showed an almost complete lack of gamma globulins and no antibody synthesis could be detected following immunisation with diphtheria toxoid or typhoid organisms. Most importantly the child improved clinically following injections of gamma globulin. Subsequent descriptions were predominantly of boys and an X-linked recessive inheritance was suggested. In practice this inheritance can only be demonstrated in an individual case where appropriate maternal relatives have been available. In affected individuals the lack of immunoglobulin is associated with a lack of plasma cells. The reticular structure of lymph nodes is normal but they do not contain germinal centres and the medullary cords are devoid of plasma cells. The blood lymphocyte count is usually normal but there is a deficiency of lymphocytes with cell surface associated immunoglobulins and the capacity to bind antigens: both of these are characteristics of B cells.

Although the failure of immunoglobulin synthesis is congenital, clinical symptoms do not develop until the IgG passively acquired from the mother at the end of pregnancy is exhausted. Presentation is generally between four and eight months of age but may be sooner or later. The infections typical of hypogammaglobulinaemia are caused by pyogenic organisms, most often pneumococci, *Haemophilus influenzae* and streptococci. The respiratory tract is usually involved with recurrent episodes of pneumonia. Although these respond readily to appropriate antibiotic treatment, further episodes may lead to irreversible lung damage, especially bronchiectasis. Other common problems are recurrent ear and skin infections, such as boils and cellulitis. The lack of a normal inflammatory response facilitates the spread of the microorganisms giving rise to septicaemia or metastatic abscesses.

In contrast to their susceptibility to bacterial infections these patients respond normally to many virus infections. Recovery from measles, mumps and varicella takes place spontaneously but, since virus-neutralising antibodies do not develop, repeated attacks may occur.

Apart from the consequences of infection the other major complication is arthritis. This affects predominantly large joints, typically the knees first, less commonly the ankles and hands (Lawrence, 1971). The Rose–Waaler and latex tests are negative and the systemic manifestations of Still's disease are lacking. The arthritis usually responds rapidly to adequate immunoglobulin replacement unless chronic joint damage has occurred.

Diagnosis is based on the demonstration of low levels of immunoglobulins in the serum. In infancy the first pointer is a persisting low level of IgM at a time when IgG would still be derived from the mother. Salivary IgA does not become detectable at the normal time—about six weeks of age. In fact, the actual serum immunoglobulin levels found in boys with this condition are variable. IgG deficiency is the rule but the IgM level is often normal and may rarely be raised. This observation has led some workers to propose a separate category of 'X-linked hypogammaglobulinaemia with normal IgM' for such patients. However, the existence of families with siblings having IgG deficiency in common but low or normal IgM in different individuals suggests that the division may be an artificial one. Immunoglobulin is virtually never undetectable in any individual with X-linked hypogammaglobulinaemia and there is no reason to suppose that the condition can be defined arbitrarily. Even when IgM levels are normal the patient's antibody function remains severely depressed and isohaemagglutinins are absent. Failure to demonstrate blood lymphocytes with surface immunoglobulin may be a useful confirmatory and prognostic test as this defect appears to be characteristic of boys with the sex-linked form of hypogammaglobulinaemia affecting all immunoglobulin classes.

Management. With early diagnosis and adequate management these children often have a reasonably satisfactory prognosis. The major hazard they face is the development of chronic lung disease secondary to tissue damage sustained during recurrent attacks of pneumonia. Consequently prompt and effective antibiotic management of any episode of infection is essential.

Immunoglobulin injections at a dose of 25 mg/kg/week have been shown to reduce the incidence of infection in some of these children (M.R.C. Report, 1971). Others have not benefitted unless they were given 50 mg/kg/week or more. Because these injections are painful and expensive the smallest dose which provides adequate prophylaxis should be used.

Reactions to intramuscular immunoglobulin injections are exceptionally rare in boys with X-linked hypogammaglobulinaemia.

Physiological hypogammaglobulinaemia of infancy

A physiological trough in the infant's immunoglobulin levels usually occurs between the fourth and sixth month of life. At this time the contribution of maternal immunoglobulin has decreased because of dilution and catabolism before the child has achieved adequate compensation. Symptoms arise if the trough is accentuated either because the initial supply of maternal immunoglobulin was deficient or when there is delay in the maturation of the infant's own plasma cells. The first situation is a common complication of premature birth as most of the passive transfer of maternal immunoglobulin takes place in the last month of pregnancy. Delay in immunoglobulin production is seen in the siblings of some cases of hypogammaglobulinaemia, suggesting that the degree of phenotypic expression in these conditions can be variable.

The clinical features of children with physiological hypogammaglobulinaemia resemble those of boys with the X-linked form; respiratory infections are predominant. The differential diagnosis can be made with serial immunoglobulin measurements, which show maturation of IgM and IgA levels and the presence of secretory IgA in the saliva. The distinction is an important one as infants with physiological hypogammaglobulinaemia will mature to normal immunoglobulin production and do not often require replacement injections.

Primary acquired hypogammaglobulinaemia

This forms part of the variable immunodeficiency group in the WHO classification. The condition is characterised by low levels of one or more immunoglobulin classes; onset is at any age and both sexes are affected. Many cases have relatives with collagen disorders suggesting a genetic basis but concordance in identical twins is not invariable. Unlike children with X-linked hypogammaglobulinaemia these patients do not always lack lymphocytes with surface immunoglobulin determinants and cells with the ultrastructural characteristics of B lymphocytes have been found in the blood. The cellular basis of this immunodeficiency appears to be a failure of immunoglobulin secretion by B cells although their proliferative response to antigen stimulation has remained intact. This proliferation could account for the nodular lymphoid hyperplasia which sometimes occurs and which may be mistaken for a leukaemic process. In one report, in vitro stimulation of blood lymphocytes with the non-specific stimulant pokeweed mitogen resulted in immunoglobulin synthesis and release, suggesting that the failure of B-cell maturation is not irreversible and providing possible prospects for treatment.

The clinical features are variable because not all the immunoglobulin classes are equally affected. Recurrent infections are usually of the respiratory tract and the skin. In addition, these patients are liable to diarrhoea leading to malabsorption and anaemia. This is probably due to chronic low-grade infection of the gastrointestinal tract; *Giardia lamblia* has been isolated from some cases.

Immune disturbances, particularly autoimmune haemolytic anaemia, systemic lupus erythematosus and amyloid disease have an increased incidence both in the patients and in their relatives.

In addition to the immunoglobulin abnormalities, in vitro tests of lymphocyte function often give abnormal results. Impaired phytohaemagglutinin (PHA) response as measured by thymidine uptake or cytotoxicity point to a degree of cellular immunodeficiency which may contribute to the clinical picture.

Management. Susceptibility to infection can to some extent be mitigated by immunoglobulin injections but adverse reactions to these occur, occasionally of such a severity that more reliance has to be placed on antibiotic treatment. These patients have a worse prognosis than those with other types of antibody deficiency.

IgA deficiency

This has been found as an isolated immunoglobulin deficiency in approximately 0·1 per cent of the population; many of these individuals are perfectly healthy (Tomasi, 1972). Symptoms, when they do occur, are related predominantly to the respiratory and gastrointestinal tracts with recurrent sinusitis and diarrhoea. Plasma cells secreting IgA are normally widely distributed in the lamina propria and it is possible that symptomless cases of IgA deficiency have been able to compensate for their defect by increased mucosal production of IgM as both these immunoglobulins are actively transported across mucous membranes. A combined lack of IgM and IgA is commonly associated with diarrhoea and malabsorption.

The cellular basis of isolated IgA deficiency is not understood but it appears to be a fault in cell differentiation. Affected individuals do not lack circulating lymphocytes with surface IgA determinants but these cells do not mature into plasma cells. Chromosomal abnormalities, particularly of the C18 group have been reported in some patients with isolated IgA deficiency.

In some patients the clinical picture is complicated by apparently autoimmune diseases. Up to one-third of children with IgA deficiency have been found to have antithyroid antibodies and in both children and adults overt thyroiditis is relatively more common than in normals. The pathogenesis of the malabsorption syndrome to which IgA-deficient individuals are prone is disputed. Sometimes it remits with withdrawal of gluten from the diet but in others it appears to be due to infection. One organism which has frequently been implicated is *Giardia* and a lack of mucosal protection by antibody would clearly leave the patient at risk from such opportunists.

As many as one-half of the patients with IgA deficiency have antibodies in their serum which would react with IgA. It is possible, however, that this is a cross-reaction, as precipitation with constituents of cow's milk has also been described. The presence of antibody to IgA in an individual who also had circulating lymphocytes with cell surface IgA would be surprising.

Management. The place of immunoglobulin injections in these patients is dubious. Immunoglobulin preparations at present available contain very little IgA and it is doubtful whether even purified IgA reaches the secretions when injected. Since the susceptibility to infection in these cases is presumably related to a lack of mucosal protection it is unlikely that immunoglobulin preparations composed mainly of IgG would be helpful. They may well, however, give rise to systemic reactions and are possibly implicated in provoking IgA antibodies. An alternative has been the infusion of large volumes of fresh plasma consistently obtained from one donor (Buckley and Durham, 1972).

Combined Immunodeficiency

The association of severe lymphopenia and extensive *Candida* infection with a downhill course and death before the age of one year was recognised in 1950. The first cases were described in Switzerland and the term 'Swiss type agammaglobulinaemia' was applied to them. Family studies of these suggested an autosomal recessive inheritance. Further series from America indicated that the disease could also be transmitted as an X-linked trait. Both types are now included in the term 'severe combined immunodeficiency' (SCID) and these infants differ from those with X-linked hypogammaglobulinaemia in a number of ways (Hitzig, Barandum and Cottier, 1968).

Recurrent infections had an earlier onset, often only in the first weeks of life. In addition to bacterial infections, there was liability to severe candidiasis, persistent diarrhoea and progressive lung disease, responding poorly to antibiotics. Skin rashes were usual, and there was failure to thrive. Investigation showed a low blood lymphocyte count and biopsy material was deficient in both lymphocytes and plasma cells. Death occurred in the first years, and at post-mortem the thymus was small, depleted of lymphocytes and without Hassall's corpuscles.

About half of affected infants lack erythrocyte adenosine deaminase (ADA). This enzyme is an aminohydrolase which converts adenosine to inosine, a pathway by which purines could be reutilised. It is uncertain whether ADA deficiency has any aetiological significance. Lower ADA levels have been found in the mothers of some children with SCID than in controls, so enzyme assay may become useful in genetic counselling.

It is now apparent that this syndrome can vary enormously in severity, particularly regarding the time of onset and duration till death. These differences are to some extent associated with different modes of inheritance but the distinctions are not absolute. Successively affected infants in a family often run the same course.

Onset in the most severe form is in the first month of life and, without successful treatment, most cases die within a year. The presenting symptoms are usually persistent diarrhoea and failure to thrive. A pleomorphic skin rash is common; it may be due to superficial *Candida* infection or sometimes possibly to a graft-versus-host reaction. Some children have presented with generalised vaccinia following a vaccination attempt. Opportunistic infections of the lungs are common, especially with the protozoan *Pneumocystis carinii.*

Investigation shows a lymphopenia, the serum levels of IgM and IgA are very low and there is no antibody response to immunisation. Skin tests are negative and foreign skin grafts are retained.

Death usually results from lung infection or persistent diarrhoea. Post-mortem findings are of total hypoplasia of lymphoid tissues.

Less severe forms of combined immunodeficiency often have a delayed onset and for the first six to nine months the infant may gain weight normally. Recovery from infections may also take place spontaneously during this period. The onset of the disease is usually with failure to gain weight and then diarrhoea; the downhill course can be more gradual than in the severe form.

The immunological findings at any stage are variable and the lymphocyte count is commonly normal. Immunoglobulins, especially IgM, may be normal initially but progressively decline. Death usually follows in the first few years.

The association of normal or near-normal serum immunoglobulin concentrations with the clinical picture of SCID was described by Nezelov et al (1964) in a family where four of eight siblings had died in infancy. The propositus, studied at the age of 14 months, suffered from diarrhoea and recurrent chest infections. Investigation showed that the child had normal gamma globulins detected by serum electrophoresis and had numerous plasma cells in the marrow. There was, however, a persistent lymphopenia in the blood. Antigenic challenge was not followed by antibody production and the serum immunoglobulins did not appear to have any useful information.

The post-mortem findings in children dying with severe combined immunodeficiency have included a generalised lack of lymphocytes in the blood, lymph nodes and spleen. The thymus is small, it is composed mostly of connective tissue and epithelial cells and the medulla does not contain Hassall's corpuscles. These findings were sufficiently typical for the retrospective diagnosis of 20 cases in a consecutive series of 1000 paediatric post-mortems; although most centres have found a lower incidence it is likely that the condition is often missed clinically. Most of these retrospective diagnoses were made in children who had been admitted with gastrointestinal complaints including diarrhoea and failure to thrive.

The abnormal thymus histology led early investigators to believe that this defect was causative in the aetiology. In the light of subsequent experimental work in animals, the combined deficiency of both thymus-derived and antibody-producing cells is better interpreted as failure of differentiation of precursor cells. The most severely affected infants lack blood lymphocytes with the surface characteristics of T or B cells. The cause of this deficiency (which might be inherent in the precursor cell or reflect an abnormal inductive environment) is obscure and probably varies in individual families. In less severely affected individuals, some of whom have had detectable serum immunoglobulins, blood T lymphocytes have been lacking but B cells were present in normal or high numbers. In this case the developmental defect must have been at a later stage than a common T and B stem cell. A functional deficiency of T cells might result in failure of lymphocyte cooperation dependent antibody production, though this is not borne out by the observation of normal immunoglobulin levels in DiGeorge's syndrome. The occasional presence of complement deficiencies or chromosome abnormality suggests that there may be multiple different pathological processes involved.

The successful treatment of some children with severe combined immunodeficiency by bone marrow grafts suggests that the thymus at least is capable of processing appropriate precursor cells normally. These results, which have been extensively reviewed (Van Bekkum, 1972), illustrate some of the problems of immunological reconstitution in man. The recipients themselves are immunologically incompetent and will retain foreign skin grafts. This is a hazardous situation because in addition to liability to infection they are unable to destroy foreign lymphocytes. Consequently a transfusion of foreign immunologically competent cells will usually result in a fatal graft-versus-host reaction. This outcome has been seen following blood transfusion and attempts at grafting marrow derived from non-HL-A identical donors. At present routinely successful marrow grafts are only possible when an HL-A identical sibling is available as a donor. Even then many of the recipients have experienced a transient graft-versus-host reaction, recovery from which may depend on the production of specific blocking factors.

Reticular dysgenesis

This rare condition was described by de Vaal and Seynhaeve (1959) and is characterised by agranulocytosis and lymphopenia with normal red cell and platelet production. It is presumed to be due to a failure of leucocyte stem cells and at post-mortem no lymphoid tissues were present. In a case described by Gitlin, Vawter and Craig (1964) leucocytes were infused but disappeared from the circulation after 15 minutes, apparently without clinical benefit. Affected infants have died rapidly of overwhelming infection.

Primary Deficiencies of Cell-mediated Immunity

DiGeorge syndrome

This is an exceptionally rare condition characterised by maldevelopment of the thymus and parathyroid associated with abnormalities of the aortic arch (DiGeorge et al, 1967). It is not thought to be hereditary as affected individuals have lacked a family history. The developmental defect occurs in intrauterine life and involves predominantly the third brachial arch. The cause is unknown. In addition, some cases have micrognathia, low-set, malformed ears and a cleft palate or nose. Because the epithelial component of the thymus is deficient, the circulating pool of thymus-derived lymphocytes fails to develop and affected children have a primary deficiency of cell-mediated immunity. Most of the blood lymphocytes have surface immunoglobulin, plasma cells develop normally and serum immunoglobulins are present in normal concentrations.

Affected infants present with neonatal tetany due to hypocalcaemia secondary to lack of parathormone. In early life their main problems are cardiovascular ones, because of heart or great vessel malformations. The susceptibility to infection may be a relatively minor problem; the commonest pathogen isolated is *Candida albicans* giving rise to widespread candidiasis.

Diagnosis has been made from the association of neonatal tetany with cardiovascular malformation. It must be confirmed by demonstration of lack of T cell function, failure of PHA-induced lymphocyte transformation for example, because hypocalcaemia can complicate some congenital cardiac lesions.

Management. Rapid restoration of the PHA response with subsequent clearing of the *Candida* rash has followed the grafting of human fetal thymus tissue (August et al, 1968). In two cases the recovery of PHA response occurred within days suggesting that a potentially immunocompetent pool of cells was already available. The children did not become chimaeric in their blood lymphocyte population so benefit from the fetal thymus tissue was probably conferred by a humoral factor, possibly a thymic hormone. Other cases of DiGeorge's syndrome treated with thymus grafts have had a much slower rate of recovery, which would be consistent with the delay observed in experimental animals while stem cells migrate to the thymus to be processed before emerging as immunocompetent cells. The spontaneous though gradual recovery of immunocompetence in children who at birth had no detectable thymus function has also been observed. It is likely that at least some of these children had a partial rather than total deficiency of thymus tissue so that their immunological maturation was only delayed.

Immunological reconstitution is only one part of the management of these children and cardiac surgery may sometimes be required. Blood transfusions, if given, should probably be depleted of immunocompetent lymphocytes (see page 64).

The DiGeorge syndrome is interesting because the defect in development appears to result in an isolated deficiency of thymus-derived cells. A high population of blood lymphocytes in this condition have surface immunoglobulin determinants and the ultrastructural features of B cells; the blood count is usually normal. The tonsils and Peyer's patches are macroscopically normal although their paracortical regions are depleted of lymphocytes. Because of the resemblance this condition has for the neonatally thymectomised mouse, affected children have been studied in detail to determine their antibody-forming capacity. Experimental work in laboratory animals (see Chapter 1) suggests that thymus-derived cells play an important role in co-operating with B cells in the production of antibody to most antigens. In the

DiGeorge syndrome normal antibody responses have been found following immunisation with diphtheria and tetanus toxoids, ϕX 174 and pneumococcal polysaccharide. There is, however, a failure to mount a normal secondary response following further challenge, implying a lack of immunological memory.

Familial thymic aplasia

One family in which two siblings lacked both thymus and parathyroids, in the absence of cardiovascular abnormalities, has been described. One infant, studied before death, had a grossly impaired PHA response and a partial similar defect was observed in the parents (Steele et al, 1972).

Tests at present available probably only detect severe degrees of cell-mediated immunity deficiency. Other evidence, such as liability to lepromatous leprosy, suggests that partial degrees of immunodeficiency are very much commoner but are mostly unrecognised.

Miscellaneous Deficiencies Involving Cell-mediated Immunity

Wiskott–Aldrich syndrome

This is a rare and incompletely understood syndrome characterised by thrombocytopenia, eczema and an increased susceptibility to infection (Cooper et al, 1968). The clinical features were originally described by Wiskott and the inheritance, which is X-linked recessive, was defined by Aldrich et al. The components of this syndrome are variably expressed and often do not arise simultaneously; their onset may be delayed into childhood. In the absence of eczema it is likely that some cases are diagnosed as idiopathic thrombocytopenic purpura.

Melaena and haemorrhage are the commonest presenting features, with an onset in infancy or early childhood. The eczema has the characteristics and distribution of atopic eczema and is sometimes very mild. With the associated thrombocytopenia, however, the skin lesions are very liable to bleed. The commonest infections are of the skin and again the eczematous areas are particularly vulnerable. Otitis media, pneumonia and meningitis occur with increased frequency. Resistance to virus infection has generally been normal though severe cytomegalovirus and herpes simplex infections are exceptions to this.

Most cases die in childhood, usually of infection or haemorrhage. An increased incidence of malignancy, predominantly reticuloendothelial in origin, has been observed.

Investigations. The platelet count is low and in many cases the platelets are abnormally small. The thrombocytopenia is probably due to reduced platelet formation as the survival of homologous platelets transfused back into patients has been normal. In the marrow megakaryocytes are reduced in number and may be morphologically abnormal.

Immunoglobulin levels. Most case reports have described normal levels of IgG with low to normal levels of IgM. IgA and IgD levels have been normal or raised. Consistently raised IgE levels have been reported, a finding in keeping with a possible atopic aetiology for the skin lesion.

Antibodies: Isohaemagglutinins are very low or absent, an observation which is helpful in diagnosis. The antibody response to a variety of protein antigens is normal but the response to carbohydrate antigens is depressed.

Cellular immunity. The blood lymphocyte count may be normal or low. A selective depletion of the thymus-dependent areas of lymph nodes has been observed so there may be quantitative abnormalities of the lymphocyte population. This probably involves the blood lymphocytes too, as few of these cells are capable of forming E rosettes. Functional tests are also often abnormal —in particular it may be difficult to demonstrate delayed hypersensitivity with skin tests. In vitro tests of blood lymphocytes have shown a subnormal response to PHA and grossly impaired response to antigens. An observation of apparent clinical usefulness is that a proportion of these patients lack monocytes with receptors for IgG.

Management. Until recently relatively little treatment had been available for these patients. The thrombocytopenia is resistant to steroids and to splenectomy, which is best avoided as it is usually followed by death from infection.

Some cases have now been described which have improved considerably following transfer factor treatment. It appears that this helps mainly those who lack monocytes with IgG receptors. Those who do respond have a diminished susceptibility to bruising as well as fewer infections.

The cause of the abnormalities in the Wiskott–Aldrich syndrome is obscure. The failure to make antibody to polysaccharide antigens would be compatible with a defect in antigen processing by macrophages, as would the lack of lymphocyte response to protein antigens in vitro. However, it has not been possible to demonstrate an abnormality of macrophage function in these patients and the abnormalities of their in vitro tests are not corrected by adding normal donor macrophages.

Recent studies on immunoglobulin turnover in Wiskott–Aldrich patients has shown markedly reduced half-life for many serum proteins, including IgG, IgA and albumin. Consequently, normal levels are only maintained as a result of increased synthesis and this compensation may be least effective for IgM.

Ataxia telangiectasia

This condition is characterised by a progressive ataxia which develops in early childhood; the telangiectasia of the bulbar conjunctivae with which it is associated may not develop until some years later (McFarlin, Strober and Waldmann, 1972). A family history of affected siblings is common and the disease is probably inherited as an autosomal recessive.

The immunological abnormalities in ataxia telangiectasia are only a part of a multi-system disorder with effects as varied as glucose intolerance and raised α fetoprotein levels. The susceptibility to infection may be slight and the infections are more easily managed than the progressive ataxia and weakness. They commonly result in chronic lung damage and death in the teens is usual. An increased incidence of lymphoma has been found.

Investigation has revealed low serum IgA and IgE levels in 50 per cent or more of cases. In most reports salivary IgA could not be detected in patients with low or absent serum IgA. These patients have also lacked IgA-containing plasma cells in the marrow or the lamina propria. However, lymphocytes with surface IgA are present in normal or raised proportion. Low molecular weight IgM has been detected in the serum of cases with low IgA levels. This form of IgM can diffuse faster than the 19S form and can give spuriously high values when measured by the Mancini technique. Other immunoglobulin classes, where measured, have been normal and isohaemagglutinins are present in normal concentrations.

A proportion of cases have impaired cell-mediated immunity, demonstrated by delayed rejection of foreign skin grafts and failure to become sensitised to dinitrochlorobenzene (DNCB). T cell function measured by PHA response may be grossly impaired when the proportion of blood T lymphocytes detected by the rosette technique is only slightly reduced. At necropsy the thymus and thymus-dependent areas of lymph nodes may be atrophic.

Immunological amnesia

Some children have been described who suffered from periodic episodes of severe lymphopenia. This has been traced to the presence of a complement-dependent antilymphocyte antibody which has been most active against thymus-derived cells. During periods of lymphopenia there is a loss of the PHA response and there is subsequently a defect of immunological memory so that secondary antibody responses are lost. In some cases the condition has terminated in lymphoma.

Mucocutaneous candidiasis

Candida albicans is a yeast which is widely distributed in the environment and which is carried on the skin of many healthy people. The commonest form that *Candida* infection takes is superficial and is transient. In individuals who have a defect in cell-mediated immunity mechanisms, as seen in DiGeorge syndrome or severe combined immunodeficiency, *Candida* can establish itself as an opportunistic pathogen. A liability to *Candida* infection is also seen where there is an endocrine disorder such as diabetes mellitus or hypoparathyroidism. That susceptibility to persisting infection indicates immunodeficiency is not in doubt but whether this deficiency is primary or secondary is not yet established.

Many patients with persistent candidiasis have a family history of it and they show a variety of clinical patterns (Wells et al, 1972). The mouth is usually involved and typical white plaques are seen on the tongue, buccal mucosa or palate. Infection of some of the nailbeds is common and the nail itself becomes thickened and deformed. Some of those patients whose infection dates back to early childhood also have involvement of the scalp and skin with granuloma formation. These individuals may also have an increased liability to lung infections, particularly by staphylococci.

Immunity function testing in patients with mucocutaneous candidiasis has revealed disparate abnormalities. This is particularly true of lymphocyte testing where there has been dissociation of the in vitro proliferative response to *Candida* antigen and the release of lymphocyte mediators. That some of these abnormalities have been corrected by iron treatment suggests that they may be secondary rather than primary defects.

Management. Despite the uncertain background three lines of treatment have had some success.

1. *Iron.* Iron is of major importance in the maintenance of a healthy epithelial barrier, so providing a non-specific defence mechanism. Clinical response to iron has been most consistently observed where previously low serum levels and marrow iron stores have been returned to normal by treatment. Remarkably this has also been followed by reversion of lymphocyte function tests to normal in some patients, (Wells et al, 1972).
2. *Transfer factor.* Independently of iron treatment some patients have shown clinical improvement following transfer factor injections. This has also been accompanied by a variable recovery of normal in vitro lymphocyte responses (Spitler, Levin and Fudenberg, 1972b).
3. *Grafts.* Success has followed the more heroic measure of bone marrow transplant from a compatible sibling. Thymus grafts have also been used.

Phagocyte Defects

Phagocytosis and intracellular digestion of microorganisms is the final common pathway for many specific and non-specific immunity mechanisms. Humoral immunity in particular often depends on the opsonisation of bacteria so polymorph defects enter the differential diagnosis of antibody deficiency syndromes. A wide variety of phagocyte defects has been reported and only a brief survey is possible here. The subject is reviewed by Baehner (1972).

Inherited neutropenia

A number of syndromes differing in severity and pattern of inheritance have been described. When there is severe neutropenia, as in infantile genetic agranulocytosis, the onset of multiple infections is early and death in the first years of life is usual. In the much milder familial benign neutropenia, the polymorph count is only moderately reduced; the inheritance is dominant and is compatible with a normal life span. Pancreatic insufficiency with neutropenia has symptomatology similar to fibrocystic disease with malabsorption and frequent lung infections. Several children with this condition have died suddenly with overwhelming virus infections.

Periodic neutropenia

In some family studies this condition has been inherited as an autosomal dominant. The polymorph count fluctuates on a cyclical basis and is severely depressed at approximately 21-day intervals. The neutropenia usually persists for three or four days and is accompanied by fever, skin infections and mouth ulceration. A monocytosis has been observed in those patients who escape infection during the episodes of neutropenia. The condition sometimes remits spontaneously after many years; favourable response to splenectomy has also been observed.

Myeloperoxidase deficiency

Leucocyte myeloperoxidase deficiency is rare. In one case it was associated with chronic *Candida* infection. Impaired in vitro killing of bacteria and especially *Candida* organisms has been found.

Glucose 6 phosphate dehydrogenase deficiency

A few patients with a deficiency of this enzyme in their leucocytes have been described. The leucocyte bactericidal capacity for staphylococci, *E. coli* and *Serratia* was impaired, perhaps because little hydrogen peroxide could be produced by hexose monophosphate shunt activity.

Job's syndrome

Only a few cases have been described. All the affected individuals have been girls and they have had fair skin and red hair. In some a familial trend has been noted. Clinically they have been liable to eczema and recurrent staphylococcal abscesses involving mainly the skin, subcutaneous tissue and lymph nodes. Typically these abscesses excite little inflammatory reaction.

Chédiak–Higashi syndrome

The granulocytes of these patients contain characteristic giant peroxidase-positive granules, and similar granules are found in some secretory cells of the pituitary and adrenals. The condition is transmitted as an autosomal recessive and is associated with partial oculocutaneous albinism. The patients are commonly neutropenic, and although the polymorphs are very active phagocytically, they respond poorly to chemotactic stimuli. Clinically they have an increased susceptibility to bacterial infections. Death in the second decade is usual and at autopsy a lymphocyte proliferation resembling lymphoma has been found.

Lazy leucocyte syndrome

Two unrelated children have been described both of whom had a history of recurrent coughs, gingivitis and stomatitis (Miller et al, 1968). Both were neutropenic and there was failure to mobilise polymorphs in response to adrenaline or pyrogen. In vitro, their polymorphs would phagocytose and kill ingested organisms normally but they failed to respond to serum chemotactic factors.

Other intrinsic defects of polymorphs in which these cells failed to respond by chemotaxis normally have been described; in one example there was also a defect of bacterial killing.

Combined macrophage-polymorph defect: chronic granulomatous disease

Although the phagocytes of children with this condition are capable of ingesting organisms, they are selectively deficient at killing some of them

(Holmes et al, 1968). The defect is present in both polymorphs and monocytes and, in vitro, affects predominantly their ability to destroy catalase-positive bacteria. The pathogenesis is related to defective peroxidase production by the phagocytic cells associated with reduced activity of the hexose monophosphate shunt. In vitro, this defect has been corrected by allowing the affected polymorphs to take up latex particles coated with glucose oxidase.

The condition is usually inherited as an X-linked trait and a proportion of the maternal polymorphs can be affected. In some cases abnormalities have also been observed in the fathers' polymorphs, suggesting an autosomal inheritance.

Presentation is usually in childhood and there is often a history of chronic skin and lymph node abscesses, which have required incision. Similar abscesses, which provoke a florid cellular reaction, can arise in the lung, bones, liver and gut. Despite the large amount of pus which can collect these children may experience relatively little malaise and the local signs are often slight. Diarrhoea is a common feature and may be accompanied by malabsorption of vitamin B_{12} (Ament and Ochs, 1973).

The diagnosis can often be made from the history. The nitroblue tetrazolium (NBT) test is a useful screening test as affected cells fail to reduce the tetrazolium dye. Qualitative abnormalities in the NBT test can be detected in carriers of the trait.

Management. Fully effective doses of antibiotics should be given when these children have evidence of local infection or if they become febrile. The antibiotic course should be prolonged as organisms within cells are protected. Abscesses commonly do form and they should be incised, following usual surgical principles. Wound closure is sometimes delayed and fistula formation following gut surgery has been observed.

Complement Deficiencies

Complement plays a major role in both specific and non-specific immunity mechanisms and an increasing variety of abnormalities is being recognised. The fragments C3a, C5a and $\overline{C567}$ which are released in the course of the complement cascade have chemotactic activity and are necessary for the induction of a normal inflammatory response. In addition, complement components are important in lymphocyte interactions, particularly the induction of cytotoxicity and cooperation in the production of antibody.

The mechanisms of complement activation by the classical or alternative pathways and their deficiencies have been reviewed recently (Ruddy, Gigli and Austen, 1972). Only those defects which have been demonstrated in man will be discussed here.

C1r deficiency

A deficiency, possibly genetically determined, has been described in two siblings who had a lupus-like syndrome. Low levels of complement components have been recognised in lupus erythematosus and are thought to be due to complement consumption by antigen–antibody complexes. It is unlikely that the C1r deficiency described was due to complement consumption as the levels of C3 and C4 were normal.

C2 deficiency

This was first recognised more than 10 years ago and an autosomal recessive inheritance has been documented. The original observations were in overtly healthy individuals but glomerulonephritis, lupus-like syndromes and Henoch–Schönlein purpura are now recognised as complications.

C3 deficiency

A partial C3 deficiency, apparently inherited as an autosomal dominant, has been detected in symptomless individuals. A more complete deficiency has been described in a girl, both of whose parents had approximately half normal C3 levels. She suffers from frequent bacterial infections similar to those experienced by patients with hypogammaglobulinaemia.

C3b-inhibitor deficiency

Only one such patient, a male with Klinefelter's syndrome, has been recorded. He suffers from repeated bacterial infections involving the respiratory tract.

Functional C5 deficiency

Three children with a clinical syndrome characterised by a failure to thrive, recurrent local and systemic infections, severe diarrhoea and a generalised seborrhoeic dermatitis have been described. The inheritance is not yet determined but functional abnormalities in the serum of the patients' relatives were observed in one family suggesting an autosomal dominant mode. In the second a recessive inheritance was postulated. In both families, a deficiency of a serum factor necessary for the phagocytosis of yeast by normal polymorphs has been found; the patients' own cells will phagocytose yeasts normally in the presence of normal serum. Although immunoreactive C5 was present in normal concentrations in the patients' serum, it was apparently functionally defective. This defect could be remedied in vitro by the addition of purified C5. These findings correlate well with the importance of C5a in chemotaxis in laboratory models. Particularly encouraging has been the response of some of these patients to infusion of fresh plasma (Miller and Nilsson, 1970).

Wider application of the opsonising test (by which functional C5 deficiency was recognised) suggests that abnormalities can be associated with various patterns of infection. It is likely that this test detects deficiencies other than C5 alone and some of these may involve alternative pathways for complement activation.

Secondary Immunodeficiency

Secondary immunodeficiency is common. Both humoral and cell-mediated immunity mechanisms can be depressed by a variety of conditions, often contributing significantly to the patient's clinical picture. It can be mediated by an impaired production of lymphocytes or antibody, or by excessive loss of either. In general, the clinical consequences parallel the comparable primary immunodeficiencies. Antibody deficiency is associated predominantly with increased susceptibility to bacterial infection, and defects in cell-mediated immunity result in liability to fungus and viral infections.

Some of the better recognised secondary immunodeficiencies are discussed below.

Loss of immunoglobulin or cells due to leakage

Depressed immunoglobulin levels are seen in patients with protein-losing enteropathy, nephrotic syndrome and exfoliative dermatitis, in each case due to a loss of protein from the body.

In intestinal lymphangiectasia there is a loss of lymph and lymphoid cells into the intestinal lumen and when this is severe it can result in hypoproteinaemia, oedema and lymphopenia. Impairment of the blood lymphocyte response to PHA is usual while the lymphocytes recovered from chylous effusions have a good response.

Low levels due to hypercatabolism

Hypercatabolism of proteins takes place in a number of syndromes. Usually several serum proteins are affected as in familial hypercatabolic hypoproteinaemia and the Wiskott–Aldrich syndrome; less commonly only a single protein is affected. IgG hypercatabolism can occur by itself and is also found in dystrophia myotonica where it is associated with low IgG levels. It is possible that multiple immunoglobulin classes have a reduced half-life in dystrophia myotonica and the isolated low IgG levels reflect inadequate compensation. Similar increased immunoglobulin turnover has been described in the collagen diseases and again the serum levels reflect the balance between increased synthesis and destruction.

Malnutrition

On a world-wide basis malnutrition must be one of the commonest causes of immunodeficiency. Although it is likely that both specific and non-specific immunity mechanisms can be impaired, it has, in man, been easiest to document defects in cell-mediated immunity. Most investigators have found normal immunoglobulin levels in children with protein–calorie malnutrition. However, this does not imply that antibody formation is normal. In a study of only mildly malnourished New Guinea children it was found that the antibody response to flagellin immunisation could be significantly improved by protein supplements. Much work remains to be done in this field, particularly on the effects of malnutrition on the quality of antibody produced.

Atrophy of the thymus, reduction in tonsil size and a lymphocyte depletion of the thymus-dependent areas of lymph nodes have been found in children with severe protein–calorie malnutrition. A functional in vitro correlate in these children was the depression of blood lymphocyte response to PHA. These changes underlie the well-recognised impairment of skin tests of delayed hypersensitivity in severely malnourished children. The clinical importance of these defects is confirmed by an increased liability to infection. Inflammatory responses are relatively poor: Gram-negative septicaemia and disseminated herpes simplex infections are particularly common.

Splenectomy

There has been an impression of an increased incidence of infection in children following splenectomy. It has, however, been difficult to control these observations with reference to a comparable population. In one review (Erickson, Burgert and Lynn, 1968) there was a 2·8 per cent incidence of severe infection in splenectomised children compared to an incidence of 0·7 per cent in children undergoing other abdominal operations. The major difference lay in the outcome of these infections as the mortality in splenectomised children who subsequently developed septicaemia was very high. The mechanism is unclear as, in addition to loss of the splenic phagocytic population, splenectomy may be associated with defects of specific immunity. Isolated low IgM levels are known to be associated with liability to septicaemia, and reduced IgM levels have been observed following splenectomy in children with thalassaemia.

One family with hereditary splenic hypoplasia has been described. Affected individuals developed severe recurrent infections and septicaemia despite normal immunoglobulin and antibody levels.

Secondary immunodeficiency complicating other conditions

Lymphoproliferative disorders. In general the lowest immunoglobulin levels are found in those conditions which have the most protracted course, such as giant follicular lymphoma and chronic lymphatic leukaemia. In these disorders IgM is the first immunoglobulin to be affected, followed by IgA and IgG. At the same time, there is a depression in the formation of antibody in response to antigen challenge. Delayed hypersensitivity is normal initially but can become impaired as the disease progresses. Blood lymphocyte culture can be difficult to interpret if there is an abnormal peripheral lymphocyte population. In chronic lymphatic leukaemia, for example, the PHA response is commonly impaired but, since the majority of circulating lymphocytes have surface IgM determinants, they are probably not thymus-derived. However, there is no intrinsic abnormality of the thymus-derived population as these cells can be selectively recovered and will respond normally to PHA.

Hodgkin's disease. These patients usually maintain normal immunoglobulin levels although their antibody responses may be depressed. Skin tests for delayed hypersensitivity are often impaired and the retention of foreign skin grafts is prolonged. In addition, injections of transfer factor fail to confer specific hypersensitivity, suggesting a lack of suitable receptor lymphocytes. In vitro, this correlates with a diminished lymphocyte proliferative response to antigen and PHA, although response in mixed lymphocyte culture can be selectively retained. Clinically patients with Hodgkin's disease are particularly liable to viral or fungus infections and their susceptibility to tuberculosis is well known.

Thymoma. A variety of syndromes such as red cell aplasia, myasthenia gravis and hypogammaglobulinaemia can complicate thymoma. In each case the mechanism is obscure and, in myasthenia, it is possibly not an immunological one. Clinical improvement in myasthenia following removal of the tumour has been reported sufficiently consistently to suggest that it has a causative role. Response in other syndromes following thymomectomy has been more variable. There have been few reports of immunity deficiencies in patients who have had their thymuses removed, even when they were studied many years after.

Multiple myeloma and macroglobulinaemia. Both these conditions are characterised by the synthesis of excessive amounts of a monoclonal immunoglobulin, and this is often associated with low concentrations of normal immunoglobulins. Two mechanisms can account for this reduction: one is a reduced rate of synthesis by normal plasma cells, and the other, which has only been demonstrated for IgG, is due to hypercatabolism. The reduction of normal immunoglobulin levels can be associated with impairment of antibody production and affected patients have an increased susceptibility to infection.

Down's syndrome. Death from respiratory tract infection is more common among children with mongolism than in a control population. The immunodeficiency is a complex one since they also have an increased rate of Australia antigenaemia, a high prevalence of antithyroid antibodies and an increased liability to acute myelocytic leukaemia. In vitro tests have shown impaired polymorph function and depressed lymphocyte responses to PHA.

Sarcoidosis. Patients with sarcoidosis are often Mantoux-negative and remain so following BCG immunisation. This anergy is different from that seen in Hodgkin's disease since they respond locally to injections of transfer factor. The serum immunoglobulins are often increased and this can be associated with an increase in the B-cell component of the peripheral lymphocyte population. Disappointingly little is known about the aetiology of sarcoidosis but many aspects of the pathology resemble an immunodeficient response to an infective agent.

Leprosy. In lepromatous leprosy an enormous load of antigen is present within macrophages but the patient shows little inflammatory response. A high titre of antibody to *Mycobacterium leprae* is detectable in serum, but there is no delayed hypersensitivity response to lepromin skin testing. Experimental correlates demonstrable in these patients include a depletion of lymphocytes in the thymus-dependent areas of lymph nodes and a lack of in vitro lymphocyte response to lepromin. The latter may be due to the presence of serum 'blocking' factors as positive responses have been reported following washing the lymphocytes and culture in heterologous serum. Lepromatous leprosy has a poorer prognosis than the tuberculoid type, and the lack of lymphocyte responsiveness underlies this difference. Administration of transfer factor from lepromin-positive patients can cause a flare-up of the skin lesions associated with the development of positive lepra skin tests.

Measles. That a tuberculin-positive individual could temporarily lose his sensitivity during an attack of measles was recognised by von Pirquet in 1908. Careful investigation of the Mantoux reactivity in children with tuberculosis has shown that the skin test can revert to negative as early as the beginning of the measles incubation period. Commonly, a positive response can be obtained by using a much larger dose of purified protein derivative (PPD). That measles virus can induce effective immunosuppression is also suggested by the occasional remission of nephrotic syndrome following infection.

Diffuse neoplastic disease. Liability to infection is a well-recognised hazard of advanced malignant disease, particularly lymphomas (see above). Local infection at the site of a carcinoma is common and is often due to disturbance of local non-specific defence mechanisms. Specific immunity function, particularly cell-mediated immunity, is often abnormal in patients with malignant tumours. This has been demonstrated in vivo with impaired delayed hypersensitivity skin tests and prolonged retention of skin homografts. Defective lymphocyte transformation in response to in vitro stimulation with PHA has been found in some studies. Primary defects in cell-mediated immunity are associated with an increase in some types of malignant disease so it is possible that in some cases the immunodeficiency precedes the development of neoplasia. This is discussed further below.

Drugs

Corticosteroids have a marked lympholytic effect and cause depletion of lymphocytes from the thymic cortex and the thymus-dependent areas of lymph nodes. The blood lymphocyte response to PHA is diminished and, in mice, there is evidence that this is due to sequestration of thymus-derived lymphocytes in the bone marrow. Similar findings have been reported in children on combination chemotherapy for acute lymphatic leukaemia. In high doses, steroids will also depress both primary and secondary antibody responses.

Immunosuppressive drugs, both alkylating agents and antimetabolites, have an immensely variable effect on immune responses depending mainly on the timing and dosage in which they are given. In general, cell-mediated immunity is most readily depressed and IgM antibody production is the most resistant.

Anticonvulsants. Anticonvulsants, particularly hydantoins, can produce lymphocytic reactions resembling lymphoma. There has been little systematic investigation of these drug effects but in one study the serum levels of IgA and C3 were depressed and sensitisation to DNCB could not be induced.

Associations of Immunodeficiency

Malignancy

Although adequate population studies are still lacking, there is a strong clinical association between malignant disease and immunodeficiency. It appears from sparse reports (Waldmann, Strober and Blaese, 1972) that the patients with primary immunodeficiency are mainly liable to lymphoproliferative disorders in contrast to the increased incidence of all types of neoplasm seen in immunosuppressed individuals. It is possible that some leukaemic reactions in immunodeficient individuals represent attempts at compensatory hyperplasia rather than neoplasia.

Up to 10 per cent of patients with X-linked hypogammaglobulinaemia have had leukaemia-like reactions at post-mortem. In the 'common variable' group of immunodeficiency about 10 per cent of patients have died from malignant disease, predominantly gastric cancers, sarcomas and lymphomas. Insufficient patients with DiGeorge syndrome have been studied to provide any information on liability to malignancy in isolated cell-mediated immunity deficiency. There is a similar lack of information in severe combined immunodeficiency, since survival in this condition tends to be short. In ataxia telangiectasia, a wide variety of malignancy has been reported, including leukaemia, lymphosarcoma, reticular cell sarcoma, Hodgkin's disease, medulloblastoma and epithelial tumours, again affecting some 10 per cent of cases in all. The incidence is similar in the Wiskott–Aldrich syndrome where lymphoreticular malignancy involving the brain has been described. This is interesting because it resembles the behaviour of lymphomas in immunosuppressed transplant recipients.

Allergic disorders

There is a strong clinical correlation between immunodeficiency and susceptibility to autoimmune disease. This is clearly indicated in family studies of patients with acquired hypogammaglobulinaemia, many of whose relatives have autoantibodies. Primary studies of atopic individuals have also shown abnormalities, such as a very high incidence of low IgA levels. The finding of raised IgE levels in individuals with symptomatic IgA deficiency emphasises the importance of immunoglobulin imbalance in the production of allergic disease.

Diagnosis in Immunodeficiency

Immunity function testing is still in its infancy and many of the tests employed on an empirical basis are incompletely understood. In particular, the range of normal responses is often poorly defined and it is not at present possible to exclude a diagnosis of immunodeficiency by laboratory tests.

The use of available tests on a rational basis related to the patients' clinical picture facilitates interpretation. The history is of paramount importance: it may for example suggest a local cause of recurrent infection rather than a generalised defect. The age at which symptoms started can distinguish such syndromes as prematurity associated with transient hypogammaglobulinaemia and the much later onset of primary acquired hypogammaglobulinaemia. Health in pregnancy is important too as intrauterine infection, particularly with rubella virus, can result in immunodeficiency.

The family history is important as defects in immunity often have a familial trend. The clinical value of such information is illustrated by severe combined immunodeficiency. Subsequent siblings of an affected individual can be screened at birth so that the diagnosis can be made within days, before infections become a problem. Inquiry should also be made of other clinical conditions associated with immunodeficiency, such as allergy or autoimmune disease.

Knowledge of past attempts at immunisation and any complications that arose is useful, and antigen-specific tests of humoral and cellular function can be planned.

The type of infection to which the patient has been susceptible usually gives good indication of the nature of the immunity defect. Deficiencies of polymorphs, complement or antibody are mainly associated with recurrent bacterial infections, while fungi and viruses are often dealt with normally. Conversely, susceptibility to *Candida* and viruses may point to a defect in cell-mediated immunity.

In addition to general examination, attention should be paid to any sites of recurrent infection as local defects may be present. Note should be made of the palpability of lymph nodes and the presence of tonsils; both typically absent in severe combined immunodeficiency. Lymphoid hyperplasia, on the other hand, is a feature of some cases of primary acquired hypogammaglobulinaemia. Splenomegaly, which also occurs in this condition, can itself cause neutropenia or lymphopenia. Skin signs include the multiple scars of old abscesses typical of antibody or polymorph defects; a variety of skin rashes has been seen where there is impairment of cell-mediated immunity.

Laboratory tests

Red cell count. Anaemia has been positively correlated with abnormal tests of cell-mediated immunity, and iron deficiency has been implicated in mucocutaneous candidiasis, though these patients are not always anaemic. Anaemia also occurs in chronically infected patients and may contribute to the severity of the clinical picture.

Polymorphonuclear leucocytes. The clinical consequences of agranulocytosis are well known. A low count is described in the lazy leucocyte syndrome and a normal count does not exclude other functional defects (as in chronic granulomatous disease).

An eosinophilia is a common feature of graft-versus-host disease and can be useful diagnostically. There is still little information available on the physiological function of eosinophils.

Lymphocytes. Abnormalities here may be of the total lymphocyte count or of specific subpopulations of cells. The functional heterogeneity of the cells morphologically described as lymphocytes is such that a normal blood count cannot exclude even severe combined immunodeficiency. More information is obtained from functional tests (see below).

Humoral immunity. Antibodies are gamma globulins and a gross deficiency of this protein class can be detected by the electrophoresis of serum. More information is obtained by immunoglobulin class-specific measurements and at present these are performed mainly by the Mancini procedure. Normal levels vary with age and the ranges with standard deviations have been well defined (Table 2.2). The serum immunoglobulin levels should be expressed as a percentage of a reference serum such as that provided by the WHO, as this reduces inter-laboratory variations. The presence of low molecular weight IgM may give rise to falsely high values when measured by conventional techniques. Such artefacts have been observed in ataxia telangiectasia and might also arise in other conditions. The Mancini technique is sufficiently sensitive to detect immunoglobulin in secretions such as saliva and tears, and these measurements can be quantitated with reference to the albumin concentration. Measurements of this sort are most useful in investigating defects of secretory IgA or IgM. Tests for serum immunoglobulin concentrations do not indicate the presence of useful antibody function. If the patient has been immunised in the past then specific antibody titrations are possible, or, as a simple in vivo approach, the Schick test may be appropriate. Exposure to streptococcal antigens is so common that most individuals have a detectable ASO titre. This test measures predominantly IgG antibody and positive results mean that the patient can mount an antibody response. IgM isohaemagglutinins do not depend on immunisation schedules and are normally detected in those over the age of three months, provided that their blood group is not AB. The absence of isohaemagglutinins has been shown to correlate better with susceptibility to meningitis than IgM measurements.

More detailed investigations of humoral immunodeficiency may necessitate estimation of other specific antibody responses. The WHO group recommended measurement of the antibody response to polysaccharide antigens as well as to tetanus, diphtheria and petussis proteins. Suitable polysaccharides

Table 2.2. Variation in immunoglobin concentration with age[a]

<table>
<tr><th>Age</th><th>IgA</th><th>IgG</th><th>IgM</th></tr>
<tr><td>0–2 weeks</td><td><1</td><td>50–95–180</td><td>1–7–21</td></tr>
<tr><td>2–4</td><td rowspan="2">1–2–8</td><td rowspan="2">39–72–131</td><td>6–15–30</td></tr>
<tr><td>4–6</td><td>10–22–52</td></tr>
<tr><td>6–12</td><td>3–8–20</td><td>21–40–78</td><td>15–35–72</td></tr>
<tr><td>3–6 months</td><td>5–12–30</td><td>24–46–89</td><td>20–50–91</td></tr>
<tr><td>6–9</td><td>8–15–36</td><td>30–52–90</td><td>35–70–150</td></tr>
<tr><td>9–12</td><td>12–20–38</td><td>31–58–110</td><td>45–90–200</td></tr>
<tr><td>1–2 years</td><td>15–35–66</td><td>31–65–139</td><td rowspan="6">40–90–170</td></tr>
<tr><td>2–3</td><td>17–42–71</td><td>37–70–158</td></tr>
<tr><td>3–6</td><td>20–50–110</td><td rowspan="4">54–100–170</td></tr>
<tr><td>6–9</td><td>28–62–125</td></tr>
<tr><td>9–12</td><td>34–72–130</td></tr>
<tr><td>12–15</td><td>40–88–150</td></tr>
<tr><td><15 (Adult)</td><td>45–100–172</td><td>54–100–170</td><td>50–100–180</td></tr>
</table>

(Modified from Hobbs, J. R., 1970, Association of Clinical Pathologists: Broadsheet 68.)

[a]Expressed as percentages of values for normal adult sera with range (lower limit–mean–upper limit).

are obtained from pneumococci, *Haemophilus influenzae* and *Neisseria meningitidis* but there is little information available on the range of normal results. The antibody titre obtained in serum one month after monomeric flagellin injection has been characterised and this test has been usefully applied in man. Special studies in immunodeficiency with the bacteriophage ϕX 174 have been described and although this antigen is a live virus no harmful effects have yet been recorded.

Complement. Total haemolytic complement is a crude estimate but reductions in titre occur in some cases of systemic lupus erythematosus and in acute glomerulonephritis. C4, C2, C3 and C5 can be measured by radial immunodiffusion but this technique detects immunoreactive rather than functional protein. The symptomatic C5 defect can only be demonstrated by an opsonisation test in which there is failure to phagocytose yeast.

Cell-mediated immunity

Skin tests. Delayed hypersensitivity is a manifestation of cell-mediated immunity and provides a simple functional test. A positive response means that the afferent, central and efferent components of the immune response are intact. It is preferable to choose an antigen to which the patient has already been exposed rather than attempt sensitisation. Two commonly used antigens are *Candida* extract and tuberculin (PPD). Most people are frequently exposed to *Candida* and so maintain a high level of cell-mediated immunity; the prevalence of tuberculosis is now so low that PPD skin tests are most informative when the subject has been immunised with BCG in the past.

Blood lymphocyte populations. The two major components of the blood lymphocyte population are thymus-derived (T) cells and B cells. T cells do not have easily detectable surface immunoglobulin but they do form rosettes with sheep erythrocytes (E rosettes) spontaneously when incubated in the cold

Table 2.3. Percentage of blood lymphocytes from normal donors with surface immunoglobulin detectable by immunofluorescence (mean and observed range)

No. studied	IgG	IgM	IgA	Source
36	17·3 (3·2–43)	8·9 (2·3–20)	5·5 (0·5–15·4)	Cooper, Lawton and Bockman, 1971
54	5 (2–7)	6 (3–12)	<1	Froland, Natvig and Berdal, 1971
10	14·5 (11–19)	8 (3–11)	5·5 (3–8)	Grey, Rabellino and Pirofsky, 1971
28	16 (11–23)	7 (4–10)	6 (4–10)	Papamichail, Brown and Holborow, 1971

(Jondal, Holm and Wigzell, 1971). B cells are characterised by the presence of surface immunoglobulins, readily detectable by immunofluorescence (Papamichail, Brown and Holborow, 1971). In healthy individuals most lymphocytes which do not form E rosettes do have surface immunoglobulin. This B-cell population can be further subdivided according to the heavy chain class of the immunoglobulin. Representative normal results for B and T cells are shown in Tables 2.3 and 2.4. Other lymphocyte markers have been described which are likely to be important in measuring lymphocyte subpopulations in patients with immunodeficiency. Most B lymphocytes can bind aggregated IgG (Dickler and Kunkel, 1972) and also have receptors for activated C3 products (Brain and Marston, 1973). Similar receptors are found on cells of the monocyte-macrophage series and these are a possible source of confusion in the identification of blood lymphocyte populations. Most boys with X-linked hypogammaglobulinaemia have lacked cells with surface immunoglobulin (Cooper and Lawton, 1972) although they have lymphocytes with complement and IgG(Fc) receptors. In primary acquired hypogammaglobulinaemia the counts of B cells may approach normal (Cooper,

Lawton and Bockman, 1971). It is likely that these tests will contribute to the classification of patients with hypogammaglobulinaemia and may allow a more accurate prognosis.

Lymphocyte culture

Lymphocytes can be stimulated in culture systems in vitro to react in a variety of ways which are thought to represent models of in vivo function. Response to antigens can be measured by proliferation, indicating that the afferent and central limbs of the immune response are intact; cytotoxicity and the production of humoral factors demonstrate effector mechanisms. Antigen-stimulated responses are specific in that they depend on the presence of lymphocytes sensitive to the antigen under test. In contrast, non-specific stimulants provoke a response by entire populations of cells, in the absence of previous experience of the stimulant.

The proliferative response to non-specific stimuli. The in vitro blastogenic response of thymus-derived lymphocytes to phytohaemagglutinins (PHA) is one of the most valuable tests in clinical immunology. A quantitative end-point measurement of tritiated thymidine uptake depends on the number of responding cells, and to achieve maximum sensitivity replicate cultures are stimulated with increasing amounts of PHA so that a dose-response curve can be drawn. The shape of this curve is abnormal when there is deficiency in the quantity or quality of mature T cells. Inhibitors of transformation are sometimes present in the patient's plasma and these can be tested for separately. A gross deficiency of the PHA response is a strong indication of defective cell-mediated immunity and would contraindicate immunisation with live organisms, or the administration of incompatible immunocompetent cells.

Table 2.4. Percentage of blood lymphocytes from normal adults forming spontaneous rosettes with sheep red cells

No. studied	Mean or range	Source
50	12 (4–40)	Wybran, Carr and Fudenberg, 1972
50	29	Papamichail et al, 1972
11	52–81	Jondal, Holm and Wigzell, 1972
3	69–75	Ross et al, 1973

Concanavallin A is generally similar to PHA in effect and stimulates T cells. There are some advantages associated with its use in experimental conditions but it is not widely used in clinical laboratories.

Pokeweed mitogen (PWM) has been shown in animal experiments to stimulate predominantly B cells in a non-specific manner. In man, it stimulates both T and B cells and can also result in immunoglobulin synthesis in vitro. The interaction of mitogens and lymphocytes has been extensively reviewed recently (*Transplantation Reviews*, 1972).

The proliferative response induced by antigens. With the exception of the mixed lymphocyte reaction these tests require prior sensitisation on the part of the subject, as do skin tests of delayed hypersensitivity. However, these in vivo and in vitro tests do not always run in parallel. Suitable antigens to which a normal individual's lymphocytes can be expected to show some response include *Candida* extract and streptodornase–streptokinase.

Mixed lymphocyte culture (MLC). The immunological significance of the mixed lymphocyte reaction is unclear but from a practical point of view a positive response provides useful evidence of recognition function by lymphocytes. Negative MLC results are found where there are gross defects of cell-mediated immunity, as in severe combined immunodeficiency; in the milder defects found in Hodgkin's disease, there may be dissociation of the MLC and PHA responses.

Cytotoxicity. Some activated lymphocytes are capable of lysing target cells following either specific or non-specific stimulation. Although this test is still mostly used as a research procedure, one patient with Hodgkin's disease has been reported in whom impaired cytotoxicity was associated with immunodeficiency.

Lymphocyte mediators. Activated lymphocytes release a variety of mediators, some of which can be measured in the laboratory. This subject has been extensively reviewed (Bloom and Glade, 1971). To date the most clinically useful results have been obtained with a migration-inhibition technique. Sensitive lymphocytes cultured with antigen release factors which inhibit the spontaneous migration of macrophages and, for convenience, heterologous macrophages can be used. Results in patients with immunodeficiency are at present sparse but it is likely that these techniques will provide further insight into isolated or partial defects of cell-mediated immunity.

Treatment in Immunodeficiency

Non-specific measures

The clinical response of some patients with mucocutaneous candidiasis to iron treatment is exciting because it offers a relatively safe form of therapy. Deficiency of dietary protein can impair antibody responses and it is likely that a wide variety of dietary deficiencies can result in different forms of reversible immunodeficiency.

Avoidance of microorganisms. An absolute avoidance of all potential pathogens is rarely possible. A few children thought to have severe combined immunodeficiency have been kept alive for more than a year in germ-free care and have shown normal physical development. In this respect they resemble the survival of immunologically deprived mice in germ-free conditions and confirm the importance of low-grade infection in the clinical syndrome. The techniques required for germ-free care are restricted to specialised centres and are of little practical help in most instances. Germ-free management could have an important place during the interval between the diagnosis of severe combined immunodeficiency and the selection of a suitable stem cell donor.

Isolation procedures which are less than absolutely rigorous are unfortunately of little use as severely immunodeficient patients are prone to such opportunists as *Candida* and *Pneumocystis carinii*, both of which are widely distributed in the environment. Attention can, however, be given to the carriage of virulent strains of bacteria whose antibiotic resistance would make infection difficult to treat. An example is the harbouring of tetracycline/methicillin resistant staphylococci in the noses of patients with chronic granulomatous disease and their attendants. These children are liable to severe and recurrent staphylococcal abscesses, the treatment of which require effective antibiotics. Obviously it is desirable that infection, when it occurs, should be by an antibiotic-sensitive strain so attempts should be made to reduce the carriage of drug-resistant organisms. A suitable regimen would include the use of Naseptin cream for the nose and antiseptic baths to reduce groin and axillary carriage. Systemic antibiotics should not be used to treat carriage of staphylococci as this is not only ineffective but may result in the emergence of further resistant strains.

Treatment of bacterial infections. In general this follows normal medical practice. Every effort should be made to isolate the organism to allow identification and determination of antibiotic sensitivity. Antibiotics should be administered in full doses but in many cases the course should be prolonged to two or three times the normal. This is necessary because patients with either a primary defect of phagocytes or defective opsonisation fail to make their own physiological contribution towards recovery. The improved response to prolonged treatment is seen most clearly in patients with chronic granulomatous disease.

Whenever possible bactericidal antibiotics should be used or, where bacteriological investigation has shown this to be appropriate, combinations of bacteriostatic agents which together have a bactericidal action.

Replacement therapy

Three lines of replacement are currently available: whole plasma, immunoglobulin and cells.

Whole plasma. Plasma, if obtained from a healthy adult, can be assumed to contain complement components and a population of antibodies which depend on the individual's sensitisation. Unless adequately centrifuged it may also contain platelets and lymphocytes. The principal clinical use of plasma in immunodeficiency states is in the management of complement deficiency, particularly for the C3b inactivator-deficient patient and some cases of C5 deficiency (Miller and Nilsson, 1970). In neither case is there sufficient experience to recommend a dosage.

Plasma is in general an inconvenient means for administering immunoglobulin, large volumes are required, it may transmit hepatitis and account must be taken of isohaemagglutinins. Although the concentration of immunoglobulin is small, it does contain IgM and IgA.

Immunoglobulin injections. Immunoglobulin replacement therapy has been shown to be of statistically significant value in the protection of patients with hypogammaglobulinaemia. The material used is prepared from human plasma and contains mainly IgG. This has practical advantages as the injection of isohaemagglutinins is avoided, and, in addition, the immunoglobulin preparation is free of hepatitis virus. Doses found to confer significant protection against infection, such as 25 mg per kilogram body weight per week, do not raise the patient's serum immunoglobulin levels to normal so the half-life of injected immunoglobulin may be prolonged.

The initial recommended dose is 25 mg/kg/week and most patients with hypogammaglobulinaemia are kept reasonably free of infection by this. Some patients require 50 mg/kg/week or more to achieve the same degree of protection. Whole immunoglobulin preparations must be given intramuscularly as intravenous injection can be followed by severe systemic reactions. These develop within minutes or hours of injection and are characterised by hypotension and impaired consciousness; such episodes may be fatal. It is possible that these reactions are caused by the presence of immunoglobulin aggregates in the injected material which activate complement. Sensitisation to the injections has not been demonstrated and some groups of patients are significantly spared, such as boys with affected male relatives and patients with leukaemia.

Transfer factors

Transfer factor (TF) is a lymphocyte extract which can transfer a specific antigen sensitivity from one individual to another (Lawrence, 1969). It is neither antigen nor antibody and has, so far, only been demonstrated in man and certain primates. The lack of a suitable laboratory model has hindered characterisation of transfer factor but it has a small molecular size (mol. wt 4000) so that it can be dialysed. For clinical use TF is most often prepared from the separated leucocytes of a unit of blood. The cells are lysed by freezing and thawing, and are then placed in a dialysis sac. The dialysate is concentrated, sterilised by filtration and can be injected.

Clinical usefulness of transfer factor has been demonstrated in a proportion of patients with chronic mucocutaneous candidiasis (CMC) or with Wiskott–Aldrich syndrome. In CMC it is predominantly the patients with the granulomatous form of the disease who have benefited most (Valdimarsson et al, 1972) but they usually require concomitant antifungal treatment. This may act by reducing the antigenic 'load' on the patient so that there is relatively less for the lymphocytes to deal with.

In Wiskott–Aldrich syndrome it has been the patients who lacked monocytes with receptors of IgG who showed the best response to TF (Spitler et al, 1972a). Interestingly, the tendency to bleed has remitted after treatment and this is associated with a rise in the proportion of peripheral lymphocytes making E rosettes.

Thymus grafts

Human fetal thymuses have been implanted in a variety of cases of immunodeficiency and clinical evidence of benefit has followed in the DiGeorge syndrome (August et al, 1968). The mechanism of this immunological reconstitution is unclear. Where the thymus derived pool is absent one would anticipate that it would take some weeks to regain it. However, in both the cases of DiGeorge syndrome treated by fetal thymic grafts there was recovery of the PHA response within days. The case for thymus grafts in DiGeorge syndrome is not complete as some untreated children slowly recover spontaneously (Rosen, 1972).

One case of chronic mucocutaneous candidiasis in a 17-year-old boy which was resistant to TF treatment has responded to fetal thymus transplant (Levy et al, 1971).

Fetal material was chosen by early workers in this field in the hope that it would be immunologically tolerant of the recipient. Burnet originally proposed that such tolerance to self antigens was acquired during an immunological null period of fetal life and this prediction was apparently born out by Medawar's early transplantation experiments. There is, however, now an extensive amount of information available on the immunological maturity of human fetal thymus. These cells respond to PHA and their capacity to recognise tissue antigens is shown by positive MLC responses. The occasional observation of graft-versus-host disease following fetal thymus transplant (Kay, 1972) suggests that such treatment is not entirely without hazard.

Stem cell grafts

Fetal liver. The fetal liver contains haemopoietic stem cells which have been shown to protect mice after lethal doses of irradiation. Liver cell preparations from human fetuses of less than about 14 weeks' gestation do not respond to PHA and do not form E rosettes: presumably they do not contain mature T lymphocytes. Such preparations can be administered by intraperitoneal injection and they have been recommended for the treatment of SCID where no suitable marrow donor is available. Experience with such grafts is limited; favourable results have been obtained in two infants, but in another a fatal graft-versus-host disease ensued.

Marrow grafts. Complete immunological reconstitution of infants with SCID has been achieved on several occasions by the grafting of histocompatible sibling marrow (Van Bekkum, 1972). These dramatic successes contrast with the numerous failures where either the marrow has failed to take, or where graft-versus-host (GVH) disease has followed. There are several factors in determining the success of a marrow graft. In the first place there must be a physical 'space' which the engrafted cells can colonise and a sufficient number of marrow cells must be given, although numbers at present can only be extrapolated from results in other primates. More cells are required if an intraperitoneal route is chosen than an intravenous one. Most critical of all is the tissue matching. Many recipients of HL-A identical sibling marrow have experienced mild to severe GVH reactions and a fatal outcome is usual where the donor is non-identical (Bortin, 1970). In fact, HL-A identity may be difficult to determine as children with SCID can demonstrate multiple extraneous HL-A specificities on serological testing, a finding which may also account for the transient disease. Some children who have recovered from this phase have factors present in their serum which can, in vitro, block cytoxicity of the donor lymphocytes to recipient fibroblast layers (Jose et al, 1971).

Immunological recovery can be rapid; in one case a positive *Candida* skin test developed two weeks after engraftment and two weeks later serum immunoglobulins increased in level. These had the Gm markers of the marrow donor, and chromosome studies of blood lymphocytes confirmed chimaerism.

Iatrogenic Hazards

Hospitalisation. Pathogenic organisms, particularly drug-resistant strains, are much more common within a hospital environment than outside it, so the decision to admit a patient for the investigation of suspected immunodeficiency should be considered seriously. Fortunately, most of the available tests can be undertaken with equal speed on an outpatient basis. When admission for treatment is required, efforts should be made to avoid exposure of the patient to further pathogens.

Blood transfusion. Fatal GVH disease has followed the transfusion of blood into patients with severely impaired cell-mediated immunity. Lymphocytes are known to survive in stored blood for some weeks so special precautions, such as irradiation, are required to limit their competence. Van Bekkum (1972) has recommended that a unit of well-oxygenated blood should be given 1500 rads, and for sealed bottles or transfusion packs this should be increased to 3000 rads. A cobalt source is ideal to assure adequate radiation penetration.

Vaccination. The administration of live organisms such as BCG or the attenuated viruses of poliomyelitis and vaccinia should be avoided in patients with suspected immunodeficiency. In antibody deficiency prolonged excretion of vaccine strains of poliovirus following oral immunisation has been observed, and in one case it is possible that the virus regained potential pathogenicity. With severe defects of cell-mediated immunity the danger is greater; progressive vaccinia and progressive BCG infections have been observed. It is likely that the use of killed organisms is less hazardous. Endotoxin shock has, however, been observed following the injection of typhoid vaccine into an individual with hypogammaglobulinaemia, possibly following direct complement activation by the alternative pathway.

References

Ament, M. E. & Ochs, H. D. (1973) Gastrointestinal manifestations of chronic granulomatous disease. *New England Journal of Medicine*, **288,** 382–387.

August, C. S., Rosen, F. S., Filler, R. M., Janeway, C. A., Markowski, B. & Kay, H. E. M. (1968) Implantation of a fetal thymus, restoring immunological competence in a patient with thymic aplasia (DiGeorge's syndrome). *Lancet*, **ii,** 1210–1211.

Baehner, R. L. (1972) Disorders of leukocytes leading to recurrent infection. *Pediatric Clinics of North America*, **19,** 935–956.

Bloom, B. R. & Glade, P. R. (1971) *In Vitro Methods in Cell Mediated Immunity*. London: Academic Press.

Bortin, M. M. (1970) A compendium of reported human bone marrow transplants. *Transplantation*, **9,** 571–587.

Brain, P. & Marston, R. H. (1973) Rosette formation by human T and B lymphocytes. *European Journal of Immunology*, **3,** 6.

Bruton, O. C. (1952) Agammaglobulinaemia. *Pediatrics*, **9,** 722–728.

Buckley, R. H. & Durham, N. C. (1972) Plasma therapy in immunodeficiency diseases. *American Journal of Diseases of Children*, **124,** 376–381.

Cooper, M. D. & Lawton, A. R. (1972) Circulating B lymphocytes in patients with immunodeficiency. *American Journal of Pathology*, **69,** 513–528.

Cooper, M. D., Chase, H. P., Lowman, J. T., Krivit, W. & Good, R. A. (1968) Wiskott-Aldrich Syndrome. *American Journal of Medicine*, **44,** 499–513.

Cooper, M. D., Lawton, A. R. & Bockman, D. E. (1971) Agammaglobulinaemia with B lymphocytes. *Lancet*, **ii,** 791–794.

de Vaal, O. M. & Seynahaeve, V. (1959) Reticular dysgenesia. *Lancet*, **ii,** 1123–1125.

Dickler, H. B. & Kunkel, H. G. (1972) Interaction of aggregated γ globulin with B lymphocytes. *Journal of Experimental Medicine*, **136,** 191–196.

DiGeorge, A. M., Lischner, H. W., Dacou, C. & Arey, J. B. (1967) Correspondence, *Lancet*, **i,** 1387.

Erickson, W. D., Burgert, E. O. & Lynn, H. B. (1968) The hazard of infection following splenectomy in children. *American Journal of Diseases of Children*, **116,** 1–12.

Froland, S., Natvig, J. B. & Berdal, P. (1971) Surface bound immunoglobulin as a marker for B lymphocytes in man. *Nature New Biology*, **234,** 251–252.

Fudenberg, H. H., Good, R. A., Goodman, H. C., Hitzig, W., Kunkel, H. G., Roitt, I. M., Rosen, F. S., Rowe, D. S., Seligmann, M. & Soothill, J. F. (1971) Primary immunodeficiencies. Report of a World Health Organisation Committee. *Pediatrics*, **47,** 927–946.

Gitlin, D., Vawter, G. & Craig, J. M. (1964) Thymic alymphoplasia and congenital aleukocytosis. *Pediatrics*, **33,** 184–192.

Grey, H. M., Rabellino, E. & Pirofsky, B. (1971) Immunoglobulins on the surface of lymphocytes. IV. Distribution in hypogammaglobulinaemia, cellular immune deficiency and chronic lymphatic leukaemia. *Journal of Clinical Investigation*, **50,** 2368–2375.

Hitzig, W. H., Barandun, S. & Cottier, H. (1968) Die Schweizerische form der Agammaglobulinamie. *Ergebnisse der inneren Medizin und Kinderheilkunde*, **27,** 79.

Holmes, B., Page, A. R., Windhorst, D. B., Quie, P. G., White, I. G. & Good, R. A. (1968) Fatal granulomatous disease: a genetic defect of phagocytic function. In *Immunologic Deficiency Diseases in Man*, ed. Bergsma & Good. New York: National Foundation.

Jondal, M., Holm, G. & Wigzell, H. (1972) Surface markers on T and B lymphocytes. *Journal of Experimental Medicine*, **136,** 207–215.

Jose, D. G., Choi, Y. S., Gatti, R. A., Kersey, J. H., Biggar, W. D. & Good, R. A. (1971) Humoral antagonism of cellular immunity in children with immune-deficiency disease reconstituted by bone-marrow transplantation. *Lancet*, **ii,** 841–843.

Kay, H. E. M. (1972) Fetal thymus transplants in man. In *Ontogeny of Acquired Immunity*, Ciba Foundation Symposium, p. 249. London: Elsevier.

Lawrence, H. S. (1969) Transfer factor. *Advances in Immunology*, **11,** 196–267.

Lawrence, J. S. (1971) *Hypogammaglobulinaemia in the United Kingdom*, Ch. 4. London: H.M.S.O.

Levy, R. L., Bach, M. L., Huang, S. W., Bach, F. M., Hong, R., Ammann, A. J., Bortin, M. & Kay, H. E. M. (1971) Thymic transplantation in a case of chronic mucocutaneous candidiasis. *Lancet*, **ii,** 898–900.

McFarlin, D. E., Strober, W. & Waldmann, T. A. (1972) Ataxia telangiectasia. *Medicine (Baltimore)*, **51,** 281–314.

Miller, M. E., Seals, J., Kaye, R. & Levitzky, L. C. (1968) A familial, plasma associated defect of phagocytosis. A new cause of recurrent bacterial infections. *Lancet*, **ii,** 60–63.

Miller, M. E. & Nilsson, U. R. (1970) A familial deficiency of the phagocytosis enhancing activity of serum related to a dysfunction of the fifth component of complement (C5). *New England Journal of Medicine*, **282,** 354–358.

M.R.C. Report. Working Party on Hypogammaglobulinaemia (1971) *Special Report Series*, **310.**

Nezelov, C., Jammey, M. L., Lortholary, S., Labrune, B. & Lamy, M. (1964) L'hypoplasie hereditaire du thymus. *Archives francaises de pediatrie*, **21,** 897–920.

Papamichail, M., Brown, J. C. & Holborow, E. J. (1971) Immunoglobulins on the surface of human lymphocytes. *Lancet*, **ii,** 850–852.

Papamichail, M., Holborow, E. J., Keith, H. & Currey, H. L. F. (1972) Subpopulations of human peripheral blood lymphocytes distinguished by combined rosette formation and immunofluorescence. *Lancet*, **ii,** 64.

Perlmann, P., Perlmann, H. & Wigzell, H. (1972) Lymphocyte mediated cytotoxicity in vitro induction and inhibition by humoral antibody and nature of effector cells. *Transplantation Reviews*, **13**, 19–114.

Peterson, R. D. A. & Good, R. H. (1968) Ataxia telangiectasia. In *Immunologic Deficiency Diseases of Man*, ed. Bergsma Good, New York: National Foundation.

Rosen, S. F. (1972) Human immunological defects (discussion, p. 218). In *Ontogency of Acquired Immunity*, Ciba Foundation, Symposium London: Elsevier.

Ross, G. D., Rabellino, E. M., Polley, M. J. & Grey, H. M. (1973) Combined studies of complement receptor and surface immunoglobulin bearing cells and sheep erythrocyte rosette-forming cells in normal and leukaemic human lymphocytes. *Journal of Clinical Investigation*, **52**, 377–385.

Ruddy, S., Gigli, I. & Austen, K. F. (1972) The complement system of man. *New England Journal of Medicine*, **287**, 489–495.

Spitler, L. E., Levin, A. S., Fudenberg, H. H. & Huber, H. (1972a) Prediction of results of transfer factor therapy in the Wiskott Aldrich-Syndrome by monocyte IgG receptors. A preliminary report. In *Proceedings of the Sixth Leucocyte Culture Conference*, ed. Schwartz, M. R. London: Academic Press.

Spitler, L. E., Levin, A. S. & Fudenberg, H. H. (1972b) Human lymphocyte transfer factor. In *Methods in Cancer Research*, ed. Busch, H. New York: Academic Press.

Steele, R. W., Limas, Catherine, Thurman, G. B., Schuelein, M., Bauer, H. & Bellanti, J. A. (1972) Familial thymic aplasia. (Attempted reconstitution with fetal thymus in a millipore diffusion chamber). *New England Journal of Medicine*, **287**, 787–790.

Tomasi, T. B. (1972) Secretory Immunoglobulins. *New England Journal of Medicine*, **287**, 500–506.

Transplantation Reviews (1972) II: Lymphocyte activation by mitogens.

Valdimarsson, H., Wood, C. B. S., Hobbs, J. R. & Holt, P. J. L. (1972) Immunological features in a case of chronic granulomatous candidiasis and its treatment with transfer factor. *Clinical and Experimental Immunology*, **11**, 151–163.

Van Bekkum, D. W. (1972) In Lymphoid cell replacement therapy. *Transplantation Reviews*, **9**, pp. 3–53. Copenhagen: Munksgaard.

Waldmann, T. A., Strober, W. & Blaese, R. M. (1972) Immunodeficiency disease and malignancy. *Annals of Internal Medicine*, **77**, 605–628.

Wells, R. S., Higgs, J. M., Macdonald, A., Valdimarsson, H. & Holt, P. J. L. (1972) Familial chronic muco-cutaneous candidiasis. *Journal of Medical Genetics*, **9**, 302–311.

Wybran, J., Carr, M. C. & Fudenberg, H. H. (1972) The human rosette forming cell as a marker of a population of thymus derived cells. *Journal of Clinical Investigation*, **51**, 2537–2543.

3. Paraproteinaemia

HYLTON McFARLANE

The immunoglobulins (Ig) represent a class of proteins with widely different characteristics. Some of these differences greatly influence the effects produced when increased concentrations exist in the body. During the past decade or so, several reviews on immunoglobulin structure and function have been published; therefore in this chapter emphasis will be placed on those aspects of immunoglobulin structure and function which bear some relationship to the effects produced by abnormally high concentrations as in paraproteinaemia.

PHYSICOCHEMICAL PROPERTIES OF THE IMMUNOGLOBULINS

The broad zone of serum proteins which migrate in the slowest region on electrophoresis is now known to consist of at least five different major classes of immunoglobulins—IgG, IgA, IgM, IgD and IgE—present in serum in decreasing order of concentration with IgG having the highest and IgE the lowest concentration in human serum.

All classes of immunoglobulins have a common basic structure of two light chains and two heavy chains, as shown in Figure 3.1. The light (L) chains, of which there are two types, kappa (κ) and lambda (λ), are common to all the immunoglobulin classes but the heavy chains are specific for each immunoglobulin class (Table 3.1).

The light chains

Each has a molecular weight of about 22 000 and, commencing from the N-terminal end of the L chains, the first 107 amino acid residues constitute the variable (VL) region, whereas the second 107 amino acids constitute the constant (CL) region, providing a total of 214 amino acids in each light chain.

In the V portion of each κ chain, three subgroups have been identified: VκI; VκII; and VκIII. On the other hand there are five subgroups of the λ variable region: VλI; VλII; VλIII; VλIV; and VλV.

Ropartz, Lenoir and Rivat (1961) observed that the immunoglobulin from a patient, N.V., possessed a factor capable of inhibiting a typing system which they were using at the time. This factor (Inv) was subsequently shown to be

Table 3.1. Some properties of the immunoglobulins

Property	IgG	IgA	IgM	IgD	IgE
Mol. weight	160 000	170 000–390 000	850 000–1 000 000	186 000	190 000
Heavy chain	γ	α	μ	δ	ϵ
S_{20}	7	7, 10, 11	19, 29, 38	7	8
% intravascular	40	40	80	75	amount not known
% carbohydrate	3·1	8	11·5	12	10
Normal range mg/100 ml	600–1800	150–350	50–150	1–5	0·01–0·05
Placental transfer	Yes	No	No	No	No
Complement activation	Yes	Yes, the 11 S only	Yes	?	No
Antibody activity	Yes, bacteria, virus toxins secondary response	Yes, especially at mucosal surfaces	Yes, particulate antigens primary response	Yes, insulin penicillin diphtheria	Yes, reagins

confined to the κ, and not present on the λ L chains. There are now three types of Inv allotypes: Inv (1); Inv (2); and Inv (3). Both the Inv (1) and (2) allotypes are associated with leucine amino acid residue at position 191 of the κ chain whereas the Inv (3) is associated with valine at this position.

In approximately corresponding positions on the λ light chain, between positions 191 and 154, an alternation of arginine with lysine amino acid residue

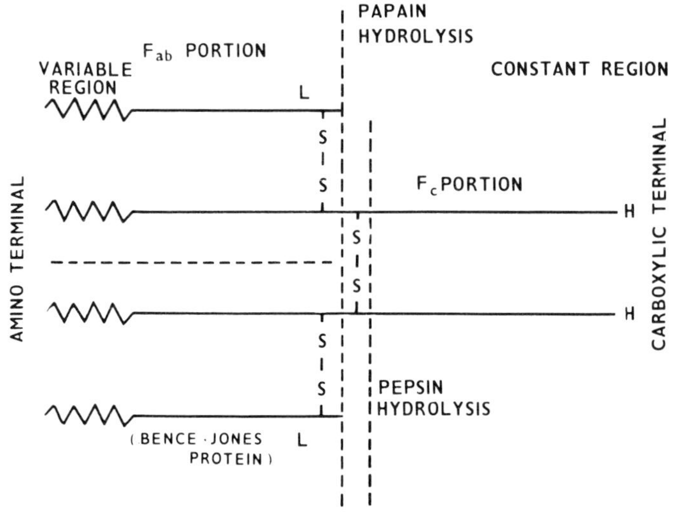

Figure 3.1. Basic structure of the immunoglobulin molecule showing the various regions of the heavy and light chains.

was discovered and when Ein and Fahey (1967) produced a rabbit antiserum to λ light chains, they found that this antiserum could distinguish between two genetic polymorphic forms of λ light chains—Oz (+) and Oz (−).

The heavy (H) chains

Each heavy chain has a molecular weight of 55 000 and is specific for individual immunoglobulin classes. The heavy chains are primarily responsible for antibody activity although both VH and the VL chains are required for full antibody activity. In fact most of the secondary biological activity of the immunoglobulin molecule is determined by the H chains. For instance, passage across the human placenta is confined to the IgG immunoglobulin and not all the immunoglobulin classes are able to fix complement or take part in passive cutaneous anaphylaxis (PCA) reactions; these are because of H chain differences.

Each chain consists of about 446 amino acid residues, and the variable (V) portion of the H chain (VH) is confined to the first 121 amino acid residues, whereas the remaining 325 amino acids constitute the constant (C) region which has three equal homologous regions—CH1, CH2 and CH3.

IgG

This immunoglobulin accounts for 75 to 80 per cent of the total serum immunoglobulin and is responsible for a considerable part of the antibody activity in both the intravascular and extravascular spaces. In the intravascular

Table 3.2. Characteristics of metabolisms of the Igs

	IgG	(7S) IgA	IgM	IgD	IgE
Synthetic rate mg/kg/day	36	30	7	0·4	7
Half life $T\frac{1}{2}$ days	23	6	7	3	3
% catabolised/day	3	12	14	33	?
FCR% intravascular pool	7	40	36	37	15·8

space the concentration of IgG ranges between 500 and 1800 mg/100 ml in normal adults. Although external secretions contain some IgG it is IgA which there predominates. In the secondary response to most antigens the main antibody is that of the IgG class. Some unique characteristics of IgG include the high rate of synthesis (Table 3.2) long half-life and low catabolic rate, it being the only immunoglobulin to cross the human placenta, and having four known subclasses, some of which are associated with Gm allotopic determinant and one (IgG 4) which may be associated with reaginic activity (Stanworth and Smith, 1972).

Subclasses of IgG

There are four subclasses of IgG and their percentage composition of the total IgG is as follows: IgG 1, 75 per cent; IgG 2, 11 per cent; IgG 3 10 per cent; and IgG 4, 4 per cent.

With the exception of IgG 4, all the other three IgG subclasses are capable of fixing complement, in the order of IgG 3 having greater complement binding activity than IgG 1 which has a greater binding affinity than IgG 2 (Augener et al, 1971).

The catabolic rate of the various subclasses of IgG differ widely: IgG 2 and IgG 4 have T$\frac{1}{2}$ of 20 to 21 days; IgG 1, T$\frac{1}{2}$ of 11 to 12 days and IgG 3, T$\frac{1}{2}$ of 5 days.

Genetic markers of the γ H chains are found in IgG 1, 2 and 3, but not in IgG 4 subclasses.

Wang et al (1970) reported that the degree of placental transfer of IgG 1, IgG 3 and IgG 4 resulted in concentrations in cord blood similar to those of the mother whereas IgG 2 reached somewhat lower concentrations in cord blood. These results have been confirmed by Virella, Nunes and Tamagnini (1972) who observed that all four subclasses of IgG were transferred across the placenta but IgG 2 and IgG 4 had a slightly less efficient transfer than IgG 1 and IgG 3.

IgG 1, IgG 2 and IgG 4, but not IgG 3, have the capacity to interact with staphylococcal A protein (Kronwall and Williams, 1969) whereas only IgG 1 and IgG 3 are capable of binding macrophage receptors. Natvig and Kunkel (1973) stated that IgG 1, IgG 3 and IgG 4, but not IgG 2, are capable of transferring PCA reaction to heterologous skin.

IgA

This immunoglobulin is present in both serum, as the monomer 7 S form, and in external secretions as the dimer 11 S form. The 11 S IgA, also known as SIgA because of the presence of the secretory component, is the chief immunoglobulin of the external secretions and is found in relatively high concentrations in colostrum (150 mg/100 ml); saliva (20 mg/100 ml); tears (70 mg/100 ml). Nasal, bronchial, gastrointestinal, seminal and vaginal secretions also contain high concentrations of SIgA.

Table 3.3. Some properties of IgA components

	IgA	SIgA	J chain	SC	H chain	L chain
Mol. weight	186 000	390 000	26 000	60 000	55 000	22 000
% carbohydrate	8	11	10	3·1	8	
S 20	7	11	?3	4·5	4·5	?3
Complement activation	Nil	Yes	Nil	Nil	Nil	Nil

Two distinct antigenic determinants, A1 and A2, have been described in association with IgA forming two IgA subclasses (Feinstein and Franklin, 1966). When subjected to electrophoresis in 8M urea in starch gel IgA 1 proteins which have the interchain disulphide bonds linking H and L chains remain intact whereas IgA 2, which lacks the disulphide link, is dissociated. IgA 1 accounts for 90 per cent of normal IgA in serum whereas 50 per cent of salivary IgA contain the IgA 2 molecules. An allotypic determinant on IgA, designated Am 2, is associated with the non-disulphide linked IgA 2 immunoglobulin and is located in the Cα 2 region, whereas the Am 2 (—) determinant is associated with the IgA 1 disulphide-linked molecule.

About 90 per cent of the serum IgA is of the monomeric 7 S form, whilst the other 10 per cent is of the dimeric and polymeric forms. The IgG–IgA ratio in most external secretions is several-fold less than that in serum, and in the gut wall there are about 20 times more IgA secreting plasma cells than IgG secreting cells. The majority of SIgA is synthesised by plasma cells in the submucosa of the respiratory and gastrointestinal tracts. At this site too, the joining chain is synthesised and becomes attached to some of the IgA molecules giving rise to the dimeric 10 S IgA. Some IgA molecules synthesised at this site do not become attached to the joining chain, but reach the systemic circulation via the lymphatic–venous circulation as 7 S IgA. The joining (J) chain has a molecular weight of about 20 000 and is attached to the IgA and IgM polymers by disulphide linkage.

On the other hand the 10 S IgA, by a process of pinocytosis, finds its way to the epithelial cells of the mucous membrane and at this site, where the secretory component SC is synthesised, the 10 S IgA becomes attached to the SC and thereupon is secreted into the lumen as 11 S secretory IgA. The attachment of the SC to the IgA molecule apparently renders it resistant to proteolysis by gut enzymes. Some physico-chemical properties of the various IgA molecules are summarised in Table 3.3. Isolated human IgA fractions have been found associated with anticholera, antidiphtheria, antibrucella, anti-insulin, anti-influenza and other enterovirus and antibacterial antibodies.

IgM

As summarised in Table 3.1, about 80 per cent of this Ig is found mainly in the intravascular space. It is the chief antibody of the primary immune response and is probably evolutionarily the earliest antibody. About 10 per cent of IgM is found in the external secretions where the SC secretory component becomes attached to it. In certain gut diseases such as Crohn's disease, coeliac disease, ulcerative colitis and maybe tropical sprue, IgA producing cells in the lamina propria may be replaced by IgM producing cells. It is interesting that only the IgA and IgM dimers and polymers have been known to be associated with the J chain. Presence of 7 S IgM in human serum suggests that synthesis of the J chain may be defective. The high fractional catabolic rate (FCR) of 36 per cent with a daily turnover of 0·4 g probably accounts for the relatively low serum levels of IgM range of 50 to 150 mg/100 ml. Pentameric and hexameric IgM are much more efficient antibodies than IgG, for whereas it requires one IgM molecule to activate complement to lyse a cell it requires two or more IgG molecules. Particulate foreign antigens entering into the blood stream must be efficiently and rapidly destroyed and from our present knowledge of IgM structure, it is apparent that it is eminently suited to this function.

IgD

We are on less certain ground about the antibody function of this Ig. Davey et al (1970) found IgD insulin antibodies in three out of six diabetics; Colwell, Bernier and Fife (1971) reported high levels of IgD in malarious

Vietnamese subjects. These authors also reported that patients with penicillin-induced haemolytic anaemia had IgD receptors on their erythrocyte surfaces, and that sera from subjects allergic to penicillin G were found to have IgD antibodies specific for some penicillin antigenic determinants. Marasmic children had elevated IgD levels in their serum (Rowe et al, 1968) and Michaux (1966) found it difficult to explain the low or absent levels of IgD from the serum of those patients who had trypanosome infection.

IgE

Because of the extremely low concentration of the IgE in human sera our present knowledge about its usefulness as a measure of the severity of allergic diseases in particular has been severely limited. Apart from the high levels found in patients with various forms of allergic diseases, high levels have also been found in African children with helminth infections by Johansson, Mellbin and Vahlquist (1968).

MALIGNANT DISEASES ASSOCIATED WITH ABNORMAL PRODUCTION OF IMMUNOGLOBULINS

Purposeless proliferation of a single clone of plasma cells or other lymphoid cells in patients with a variety of malignancies is frequently characterised by a corresponding increased synthesis of a monoclonal type of protein. The commonest among these malignancies are those which are classified as the paraproteinaemias, of which there are several types.

Paraproteinaemia is found in diseases such as multiple myelomatosis, Waldenström macroglobulinaemia, soft tissue plasmacytoma, cryoglobulinaemia, heavy chain disease, amyloidosis, lymphomas, sarcomas, leukaemia, diseases of the gastrointestinal tract associated with malignancies and occasionally endocrine abnormalities and chronic infections.

MULTIPLE MYELOMATOSIS

Incidence

Multiple myelomatosis is primarily a disease of the above-50-year age groups and rarely occurs under the age of 30. In a total of 200 patients with multiple myelomatosis the majority had ages ranging between 50 and 70 years with a mean of 61 years. The disease affects both males and females alike and has been reported in most races.

The disease is characterised by a marked proliferation of a single clone of plasma cells which produces usually a single type of monoclonal paraprotein although di- and polyclonal paraproteins have been described. Osteolytic change in the skeleton occurs in over 60 per cent of the patients and hypercalcaemia is a common finding. Paraproteins, especially those belonging to the IgG 3 subclass, when present in excessive concentrations in the serum may give rise to manifestations of hyperviscosity and occasionally to bleeding diathesis. Over 80 per cent of the patients have a detectable paraprotein in the serum but in the remaining 20 per cent the urine may contain the bulk of the paraprotein in the form of a single isolated light chain type. Prolonged excretion of light chains, especially those of the λ type, eventually may lead to myeloma kidney frequently encountered in the disease. Hypogammaglobulinaemia of the non-myeloma immunoglobulins is a constant finding. Antibody production to specific antigenic challenge may be markedly reduced and, both in vivo and in vitro tests of cell-mediated immunity, are often impaired. The reduced concentration of normal immunoglobulins and some components of complement, the subnormal production of antibody and the impaired cell-mediated immunity are responsible for the high frequency of both pulmonary and renal infections found in patients with multiple myelomatosis.

Methods of diagnosis

(1) Radiological evidence of diffuse or discrete osteolytic lesions, vertebral collapse or pathological fractures in the absence of other known causes; (2) presence of excess plasma cells in the bone marrow biopsy; (3) serum and/or urine containing paraprotein identified by both cellulose acetate electrophoresis and immunochemical analysis. At least two of the above criteria should be positive before a firm diagnosis of multiple myelomatosis is made and before treatment with cytotoxic drugs is commenced. Nevertheless a solitary isolated tumour may be missed by either or both marrow biopsy examination and radiological examination. In such patients a search for the abnormal protein in both the serum and urine may provide the only clue to the diagnosis, whereupon the bone marrow and radiological investigations should be repeated. Cellulose acetate electrophoresis is capable of detecting about 200 mg/100 ml of a paraprotein band, and Salmon (1973) has shown that this is equivalent to a tumour mass of about 2×10^{10} cells or 20 g tumour. However, unless such a tumour cell mass was localised it would be impossible to make an early diagnosis. Here it ought to be emphasised that immunochemical analysis is several-fold more sensitive than cellulose acetate and if applied in the routine screening of suspected cases, should make it possible to detect multiple myelomatosis in patients even in the early pre-clinical stage.

Salmon (1973) observed that there is an enormous *'pre-clinical iceberg'* in monoclonal disorders with extensive tumour proliferation occurring asymptomatically. Furthermore, patients who have less than 1×10^{12} myeloma cells, equivalent to less than 10 per cent of myeloma cells in marrow aspirates, usually had no weight loss or widespread osteolytic lesions, although they may have some osteoporosis with few isolated osteolytic lesions. However, those patients with an excess of 2×10^{12} myeloma cells equivalent to about 1 kg of tumour in the body usually have evidence of widespread myelomatosis with generalised osteolytic lesions, heavy Bence Jones proteinuria, hypocalcaemia, fractures and a shorter life expectancy because of a poor response to therapy.

The average doubling time of plasma cells of an IgA myeloma was estimated to be about 6·3 months with a natural history of 20 years (Hobbs, 1969), and Salmon and Smith (1970) confirmed this by showing that the average tumour doubling time of IgG myelomas was about six months during the clinical phase of the disease. However, there was a marked decrease in doubling rate when the tumour became well established, from an initial rapid rate of one to three days, and accounting for a natural history of only one to two years rather than sixteen to twenty years as had previously been speculated. Salmon (1973) found that human myeloma tumour growth behaved similarly to animal tumour growth which Laird (1964) and (1965) had earlier calculated was an excellent fit for the Gompertz equation. In support of the Gompertzian type of tumour cell growth first proposed by Laird (1964), Salmon (1973) observed that production of a monoclonal protein after initial antigenic stimulation such as bone marrow transplant, required not more than four weeks. Furthermore, on treatment of myeloma patients with chemotherapy, the tumour regressed rapidly at first then slowed down until it reached a plateau similar to the Gompertz growth curve. Consequently, by use of the Gompertz equation, it should be possible in the near future to predict which combination or schedules of chemotherapy with multiple alkylating agents such as melphalan cyclophosphamide and bischloroethylnitrosourea can 'break the log jam' and initiate further tumour cell reduction after plateau.

Bence Jones (BJ) proteins

BJ protein was first described by H. Bence Jones in 1847, after he had examined a specimen of urine sent to him by Dr. Watson from a patient who had fractured two ribs. He reported that the specimen contained a protein substance that was distinguishable from albumin by its solubility in nitric acid and lack of heat coagulability. After the protein was separated by precipitation with alcohol, it still retained its characteristic of solubility in cold water but increased solubility in boiling, coagulation with continued boiling, and return to solubility by even further boiling! This discovery paved the way for further intensive work on the investigation of paraprotein in malignancies.

Apart from the qualitative test, it should be borne in mind that quantitation of BJ proteins as a guide to the efficacy of chemotherapy is a very worthwhile investigation. It must, however, be emphasised that on account of the idiotypic nature of each BJ protein, their quantitation by immunochemical methods may not be very accurate and therefore densitometric scanning of the urine electrophoretic strip should be favoured. The half life ($T\frac{1}{2}$) of BJ protein in serum is extremely short—$T\frac{1}{2} = 8$ to 12 hours in comparison to $T\frac{1}{2}$ for IgG of 15 to 20 days; in which case a significant reduction in BJ protein concentration in urine usually occurs much sooner after effective chemotherapy than any decrease of abnormal serum paraprotein (Farhangi and Osserman, 1973).

About 60 per cent of patients with myelomatosis usually excrete increased quantities of Bence Jones protein light chains into the urine. The concentration varies enormously from patient to patient and values may range from 5 mg to 3 g/24 hours.

With the development of more recent techniques the classical heat test for Bence Jones is now largely replaced by more sensitive electrophoresis and immunochemical methods. However, the importance of simple screening of the suspected patient's urine for proteins should not be overlooked. In a patient suspected of having myelomatosis such screening results should be confirmed by further careful investigations on both the serum and urine (McFarlane, 1966).

Several rapid and simple methods are now available for concentrating urine specimens for electrophoresis (McFarlane, 1964) and the presence of a single band of protein in the gamma-globulin region on the electrophoretic strip is virtually diagnostic of Bence Jones proteins. Frequently, however, in the later stages of the disease, the BJ protein in the urine may be accompanied by albumin excretion in which case two bands will appear on the cellulose acetate strip, the BJ protein in the gamma-globulin region being usually the predominant band, since it is of lowest molecular weight, escaping through the kidneys more rapidly.

It should be noted that although multiple myelomatosis is the commonest disease in which Bence Jones proteins are excreted, there are several other diseases in which they may also be found. Therefore the presence of BJ protein in the urine of a patient should not be regarded as pathognomonic for multiple myelomatosis and additional investigations should be conducted.

Detection of paraproteinaemia

Ideally both the serum and the urine of the patient under investigation should be simultaneously examined. When paraproteinaemia exists over 60 per cent of patients show a distinct prominent homogenous band of protein in both the serum and urine with approximately similar mobilities on cellulose acetate electrophoresis.

Quantitation of the three main immunoglobulins in the serum of suspected patients is a very useful method for diagnosis of malignant paraproteinaemia. In well over 70 per cent of such patients there exists a very marked increase in the concentration of one of the immunoglobulin classes often with a decrease of other immunoglobulin classes.

Abnormalities of the concentration of Ig in the serum and of the light chains in the urine can be detected by immunoelectrophoretic typing of the serum and urine against monospecific heavy and light chain antisera. When no abnormalities are detected in the immunoprecipitin lines against a good panel of monospecific antisera then the presence of a malignant paraproteinaemia can be almost ruled out. When, however, abnormal precipitin lines are detected, as shown in Figure 3.2 they should be interpreted in conjunction with those of the radiological and bone marrow results.

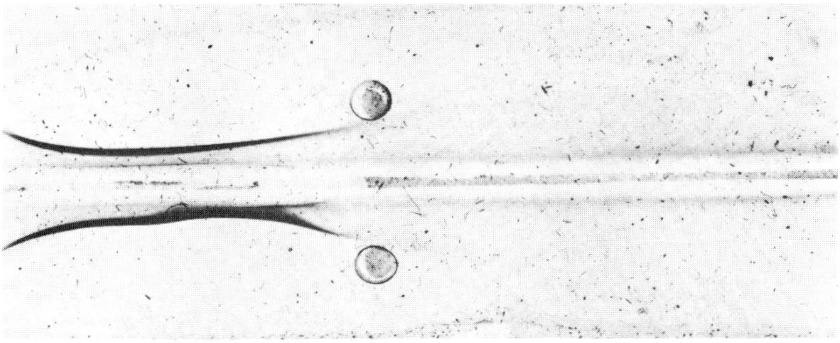

Figure 3.2. Typical immunoelectrophoretic pattern to show an IgG paraprotein. The top well contained normal serum, the bottom well serum from a patient with IgG myelomatosis. Note the 'double' curvature of the IgG line with thickening and spur formation.

Patients with IgG λ type multiple myelomatosis have been reported to have a graver prognosis than those with κ type myelomatosis. Indeed Galton (1971), in a series of 276 patients with myelomatosis, reported that twice as many patients with IgG λ than κ had more than 100mg/100ml of Bence Jones proteins in their urine, the mean concentration being 291 mg compared with 64 mg/100 ml for the IgG κ cases. This suggests either more active or more widely disseminated disease in those patients with λ type. In addition more patients with λ type paraproteinaemia tended to be associated with higher blood urea levels, and their survival was rather worse than those with the κ type paraprotein. These results are contrary to: (1) the observation of the most recent report by the M.R.C. Working Party on the First Myelomatosis Trial, 1973, when it was observed that those patients with κ type myelomatosis fared slightly worse than those of the λ type; and (2) to studies in the author's laboratory where, of 150 patients with multiple myelomatosis, it was found that there was no difference in incidence of patients with κ light chain type of myeloma either in those who survived or in those who died. It would seem, then, that there are a number of variables which influence the survival of patients with myelomatosis and some of these must include age of the patient at the time of diagnosis, nutritional status and method of therapy.

Subclasses of IgG myeloma

Of the various types, the IgG κ myeloma is the most frequent and usually belongs to only one of the subclasses IgG 1 or IgG 2 or IgG 3 or IgG 4; IgG 1 being the commonest and IgG 4 the rarest. Virella (1971) reported that IgG 3 paraproteins increase the viscosity of serum at a much lower concentration than the other IgG subclasses, probably because IgG 3 proteins tend to form concentration dependent aggregates which may give rise to cryoglobulins in the serum of the affected patient. This propensity of IgG 3 to aggregate has also been ascribed to the higher molecular weight of 61 000 of the γ 3 heavy chains than the molecular weight of 54 200 for γ 1, γ 2 and γ 4 H chains. Further, the higher sensitivity of IgG 3 proteins to proteolytic cleavage may also promote this aggregation tendency (Virella and Parkhouse, 1972). After isolation of IgG 3 proteins from 14 patients with IgG 3 multiple myelomatosis, Capra and Kunkel (1970) observed that hyperviscosity syndrome may develop when the IgG 3 protein reached a concentration of 4 g/100 ml which was far below the expected concentration for other IgG subclasses.

A patient with IgG type myelomatosis usually has a marked elevation of the serum IgG concentration frequently above 2000 mg/100 ml, simultaneously with a significant reduction of one, or all of the other serum immunoglobulin concentrations. Immunoelectrophoretic typing of the serum and urine against monospecific antisera against γ heavy chain as well as against κ and λ light chains should confirm the presence of a paraprotein. Besides carrying the antigenic specificity of only one of the four γ chain subtypes, IgG myeloma proteins are associated with single genetic units of Gm allotypes, and the light chains of myeloma proteins also belong to either the κ or λ chains but very rarely both. Absence of an abnormal band from the serum of a suspected patient should be confirmed by careful analysis of the urine, since in over 20 per cent of patients with myelomatosis no paraprotein is detectable in the serum but may be found only in the urine.

IgA paraproteinaemia

IgA myelomatosis is rarer than the IgG type. Usually about 76 per cent of any series of patients with myelomatosis belong to the IgG type and about 20 per cent to the IgA type. There are unconfirmed reports that the survival rates of patients with IgA myeloma are less than those of IgG myeloma but this needs further investigation.

Infiltration of the liver with myeloma cells is a not uncommon finding in patients with IgA type myelomatosis and when this occurs jaundice and abnormal liver function tests are found in such patients. Laurell (1968) observed that irrespective of the paraprotein type, a paraprotein concentration above 2 g/100 ml was associated with a poor prognosis. For patients with paraprotein concentrations between one and two g/100 ml the prognosis was better when they were IgG than when they were IgA. Patients with IgA myelomatosis on first presentation frequently have IgA paraprotein concentration above 2 g/100 ml and hypogammaglobulinaemia of the non-myeloma immunoglobulins. Bence Jones proteins have been observed to be just as common as in those with IgG myelomatosis.

The intrinsic ability of IgA to form complexes both with itself as well as with alpha 1-antitrysin, haptoglobin, beta-lipoprotein, albumin and anti-haemophilic factor are probably responsible for the hyperviscosity syndrome frequently found in association with patients with IgA myelomatosis.

IgM myelomas have been reported and their clinical appearances are distinct from those of true Waldenström macroglobulinaemia but resemble those of the IgG or IgA type with multiple osteolytic lesions, plasma cell infiltration into the bone marrow and, rarely, bleeding diathesis. The occurrence of IgM myeloma is much less frequent than either those of IgG and IgA (Kjeldsen and Asfeldt, 1963).

IgD and IgE myelomas occur even less frequently than IgM myelomas and so far about six cases of IgE myeloma have been detected.

Waldenström macroglobulinaemia

This disease was first described by Waldenström in 1944. It affects both males and females although the incidence is higher in males. The age incidence is lower than that of multiple myelomatosis and it may be found in persons of twenty years of age and above. Typical clinical features include fatigue, weakness, retinal haemorrhages, epistaxis, bleeding gums, anaemia, marked elevation of the erythrocyte sedimentation rate, splenomegaly and lymphadenopathy.

Kok, Whitmore and Ainsworth (1963) reported that the tendency of red blood cells of patients with Waldenström macroglobulinaemia to aggregation combined with the viscosity effects of the high concentration of 19 S macroglobulins give rise to blood sludging which is sometimes accentuated by reduced temperatures. Spontaneous haemorrhages in the patient may also occur from the respiratory, alimentary and urinary tracts which are probably related to the protein–protein interaction of high concentration of IgM coating the platelets and causing an inhibition of the release of factor III essential for clotting. Some patients with Waldenström macroglobulinaemia may possess red cell auto-antibodies. Such IgM blood group antibodies may, in part, account for the haemolytic jaundice and anaemia which is sometimes seen in patients with Waldenström macroglobulinaemia.

The osteolytic changes frequently encountered in patients with multiple myelomatosis are absent from patients with Waldenström macroglobulinaemia; however, the bone marrow and lymph nodes of affected patients are usually infiltrated with small lymphocytes, plasmacytoid-lymphocytes and mast cells. Periodic acid-Schiff positive staining intranuclear inclusions of the plasmacytoid lymphocytes are frequent observations in patients with Waldenström macroglobulinaemia (Harrison, 1972), although it should be noted that these inclusion bodies may also be found in the nuclei of the plasma cells from patients with multiple myelomatosis which are also known to elaborate large quantities of periodic acid-Schiff positive staining glycoproteins (Brittin, Tanaka and Brecher, 1963).

A clinical diagnosis of Waldenström macroglobulinaemia should be confirmed by the following laboratory observations:

1. Serum total protein above 7·5 g/100 ml.
2. Serum IgM above 500 mg/100 ml.
3. An abnormal homogenous band of paraprotein in the gamma globulin region.
4. Massive increase of doubly curved immunoprecipitin line in agar gel after the patient's serum has been allowed to react with monospecific anti μ serum.
5. Abnormal immunoprecipitin line of the patient's serum in agar against antiserum to κ or λ light chain type and
6. The presence of Bence Jones protein of one light chain type in the urine of the patient.

Invariably present in the serum of most patients with Waldenström macroglobulinaemia is a zone of spontaneous precipitation of protein in the agar gel on electrophoresis. This zone of spontaneous precipitation is most likely due to IgM complexes and/or cryoglobulins which are not removable even after extensive washing of the agar gel plates for several days.

Frequently the concentrations of the other serum immunoglobulins, especially the IgG and IgA, are markedly reduced. Bence Jones proteinuria occurs in patients with Waldenström macroglobulinaemia with equal frequency as it does in patients with myelomatosis, the difference here being that about 95 per cent of the patients with Waldenström macroglobulinaemia have κ type Bence Jones proteins whereas 50 to 60 per cent of patients with myelomatosis have κ type, the rest being λ. Additional laboratory tests for macroglobulinaemia include the Sia test which is largely non-specific, analytical ultracentrifugation for the presence of large quantities of 19 S macroglobulins, frequently with a mixture of higher sedimenting IgM aggregates of 28 to 35 S. Occasionally the IgM in some patients with Waldenström macroglobulinaemia may have a sedimentation coefficient of 7 S, a defect which is probably due to imbalance of synthesis of H and L chains and/or defect of synthesis of the J chain which is responsible for joining monomers of IgM into dimers and pentamers.

The survival of patients with Waldenström macroglobulinaemia is usually much longer than for patients with myelomatosis. Most, but not all, patients with Waldenström macroglobulinaemia respond to cytotoxic drugs such as cyclophosphamide, melphalan and prednisolone in various combinations. However, plasmaphoresis for the rapid removal of the increased macroglobulin from the plasma of the patients usually provides quick symptomatic relief, with rapid lowering of the plasma viscosity, improvement in the circulatory system, cessation of bleeding and decreased severity of retinopathy. Oral administration of penicillamine, a thiol reducing agent as well as a cytotoxic agent, is known to provide substantial reduction of plasma viscosity and a decrease of the serum macroglobulin concentration.

Ratcliff, Soothill and Stanworth (1963) reported that below a concentration of 5 g of protein of IgM or IgG/100 ml, there was no distinction between their relative viscosity, but above this concentration the macroglobulinaemic serum does show higher viscosity than serum containing similar concentrations of 7 S gamma globulins. The relative viscosity at 20°C of normal serum ranges from 1·54 to 1·80, of myeloma serum from 1·76 to 3·82 and for patients with Waldenström macroglobulinaemia from 2·40 to 15·80. Steel (1963) observed that treatment in vitro of macroglobulinaemic serum with 2-mercaptoethanol lowered its viscosity to a minimum within thirty minutes, although the mercaptoethanol had no effect whatever on normal serum, myeloma serum or nephrotic serum. Rivanol (6,9 diamino-2 ethoxyacridine lactate) added to serum in a five to one ratio causes complete disappearance of the macroglobulin peak, but has little or no effect on 7 S myeloma proteins (Saifer, 1964). Both mercaptoethanol and rivanol can therefore be used in any clinical laboratory as simple tests to distinguish between 7 S myeloma globulin and 19 S macroglobulin.

Unlike IgG whose synthesis is subject to a concentration-dependent negative feedback, the metabolism of IgM is independent of its concentration. Thus Wilkinson, Davidson and Sommaripa (1966) observed that in patients with Waldenström macroglobulinaemia there was little variation in the plasma half-life and fractional catabolic rate of ^{131} I-labelled normal or abnormal IgM. This property of IgM plus its high molecular weight and polymeric structure are likely to be contributory factors to the high frequency of cryoglobulinaemia and hyperviscosity syndrome in patients with Waldenström macroglobulinaemia.

HEAVY CHAIN DISEASES (HCD)

First described by Franklin et al (1964), heavy chain disease is apparently a variant of a paraprotein type. Both γ, μ and α heavy chain diseases have been described (Frangione and Franklin, 1973). Unlike multiple myelomatosis, x-ray of the skeleton rarely shows osteolytic changes although the lymph nodes and the bone marrow usually show infiltration with atypical and immature plasma cells. The clinical features of HCD usually include leucopenia and thrombocytopenia, lymphadenopathy, splenomegaly and swelling of the soft palate.

Gamma heavy chain disease (γ HCD)

The majority of the patients so far reported with γ HCD belonged to the γ 1 subclass type and, of 26 patients with γ HCD, twenty belonged to γ 1; four were γ 3 and one each belonged to γ 2 and γ 4. The disease appears to be much more common in males than in females and is more frequent in the over-forty-year age group. The disease may not be fatal and many of the patients have survived longer than five years.

The paraprotein band on electrophoresis is of the broad type rather than the narrow type and immunochemically it reacts with antiserum produced to the γ chain, but not with that produced to the Fab portion of the molecule. About 60 per cent of the patients have the same protein in both the serum and urine, although the serum γ HC concentration is frequently above 2 g/100ml. It would appear that four types of abnormal γ HC may exist:

Type I. A partial deletion of Fd fragment and resumption of normal synthesis at position 216 amino acid residue from the amino terminal end of the γ chain.

Type II. Deletion of 15 amino acid residues from the hinge region between positions 216 and 232.

Type III. Partial deletion of the Fd fragment and hinge region and normal synthesis after position 230.

Type IV. This appears to be enzymatically derived and the γ H chain appears to commence at a portion of the chain 100 residues from the N-terminal end which is known to be sensitive to a large number of proteolytic enzymes.

Alpha heavy chain disease (α HCD)

This disease was originally thought to be restricted to Arabs and Jews and for this reason was referred to as Mediterranean lymphoma, but it has now been detected in several other races. In 1968, Seligmann et al first described the presence of an IgA protein in a young Arab patient which was devoid of L chains and which was found in the urine, serum and saliva of the patient. Since then about 25 such patients have been described in the literature.

The predominant clinical features of the patients with α HCD include varying infiltration of the lamina propria of the entire length of the gut and lymph nodes with lymphocytes, plasma cells and reticulum cells, flattening of the intestinal villi, profuse diarrhoea which may reach up to ten litres per day, extensive loss of fluid and electrolytes, giving rise to hypocalcaemia and hypokalaemia and marked dehydration. It would appear that the malabsorption, steatorrhoea and diarrhoea precedes the development of the malignant lymphoma and indeed, Ramot, Shahin and Bubis (1965) observed that thirteen patients (Arabs and Jews) gave a history of bulky diarrhoea up to four years prior to admission with malignant lymphoma of the gut.

Unlike patients with multiple myelomatosis or even those with γ HCD, α HCD is a disease affecting mainly young individuals between the ages of fifteen and thirty years and it is the commonest occurring HCD.

Cellulose acetate electrophoresis of the serum may reveal a broad rather than narrow band of protein which on immunochemical analysis belongs to α 1 heavy chain subclass. The abnormal protein invariably shows a distinctly extended, fast-moving, abnormal α chain precipitin line, although a normal immunochemical reaction against light chain antiserum (Zlotnick and Levy, 1971).

Further work is necessary to elucidate the structural abnormality of the α chain which occurs in α HCD but preliminary studies have shown normal Fc fragment and intact hinge region. Probably because of its high carbohydrate content and tendency to polymerise, difficulties have been encountered with the structural analysis of the Fd N-terminal region of the α chain. Seligmann, Mihaeseo and Frangione (1971) stated that depending upon the concentration of the abnormal α chain protein and on its electrophoretic mobility, when the normal serum IgA precipitin line either forms a spur over or may be seen inside the abnormal α HC precipitin line and closer to the antibody trough, then such a pattern is highly suggestive of α HCD.

Stoop et al (1971) described α chain disease in an eight-year old girl of pure Dutch extraction who had no gastrointestinal abnormality, but had infiltrative pulmonary changes with marked eosinophilia, and enlarged mediastinal lymph nodes. The abnormal IgA component was not particularly high but was detected in both the serum and urine of the patient in follow-up studies.

Since a considerable portion of total body IgA is synthesised locally by plasma cells in the mucosa of both the respiratory tract and gastrointestinal tract, it is perhaps not surprising therefore to discover that α chain disease is not only associated with lymphoma of the gut but also with respiratory tract malignancies. Furthermore, now that we have a better understanding of the metabolism of the IgA system, and monospecific antisera to its different component parts have become available, one may expect to find more diseases of the mucosal surfaces of the body being associated with different abnormalities of the alpha chain, the secretory component and the J chain of the IgA system.

Mu heavy chain disease (μ HCD)

So far only three patients with this rare abnormality of HCD have been reported (Josephson, Price and Biro, 1969; Ballard et al, 1970; Franklin, Frangione and Cooper, 1971). In all three patients the μ HCD was associated with hepato-splenomegaly, excess plasma cells in the bone marrow, chronic lymphocytic leukaemia and the production of increased amount of μ chain fragments of molecular weight 55 000. Although it has a molecular weight less than that of albumin, the μ chain does not necessarily appear in the urine of affected patients, indicating that the μ fragments may exist in the serum as dimers or higher polymers too large to pass through the glomerular filtration apparatus.

In patients with μ HCD, the cellulose acetate pattern of the serum protein is usually normal, and the abnormal protein can only be detected by careful immunochemical analysis of the serum, which frequently reveals a rather rapidly migrating μ precipitin line.

As in patients with multiple myelomatosis, skeletal changes may be found in the patients with μ HCD. It would appear that an imbalance of synthesis of H and L chains, and/or failure of assembly of these chains, may account for some structural abnormality in this disease. Intact Fc fragment is known to occur and the suggestion has been made that there might also be some deletion of a portion of the Fd region of the μ chain.

Finally, HCD is now thought to be due to a combination of all of or one of: (1) mispairing of DNA strands during cell division; (2) deletion of a section of a gene and recombination with another gene; and/or (3) DNA breakage at a branched point. However, regardless of the genetic origin of the defect, it is clear that HCD represents a gross abnormality of a clone of malignant cells which produce a monoclonal protein having an imbalance of H and L chains which cannot be assembled in the normal manner.

DI- AND POLYCLONAL PARAPROTEINAEMIA

The occurrence of two or more separate bands of homogenous serum paraproteins on an electrophoretic strip is a relatively unusual finding. This finding raises the question of whether each of the paraproteins is synthesised by a single clone of malignant plasma cells or represents in vivo or in vitro complexes of different molecules or fragments. Various suggestions have been made that transitional forms between multiple myelomatosis and primary macroglobulinaemia may have evolved from the same clone of cells and, indeed, in 1962 Waldenström reported such transitions between chronic lymphatic leukaemia and lympho- or reticulum cell sarcoma.

Paraproteinaemia is quite rare in patients with chronic lymphatic leukaemia, but a few patients with this disease have been reported with markedly elevated levels of IgM. However, the combination of increased serum macroglobulinaemia with the clinical picture of lympho-sarcoma is not so rare and several such cases have been reported in the literature. Similarly, the occurrence of multiple myelomatosis and plasma cell leukaemia have been described in a number of patients. Among 300 patients with paraproteinaemia, Waldenström (1962) reported two instances where there was a combination of the clinical and laboratory findings of both multiple myelomatosis and Waldenström macroglobulinaemia. Waldenström macroglobulinaemia has also been reported concomitantly in patients with reticulum cell sarcoma and frequently in patients with rheumatoid arthritis (Svartz, Liljamma and Ericsson, 1962; Gothoni, Wasastjerna and Jeglinsky, 1965; McFarlane and Nwokolo, 1966).

Waldenström (1962) reported the interesting combination of multiple myelomatosis, chronic lymphatic leukaemia and reticulum cell sarcoma in the same patient. A year later Kjeldsen and Asfeldt (1963) described an unusual case of paraproteinaemia where the patient's serum at the same time contained two paraprotein bands; one a macroglobulin with sedimentation constant of 18 to 19 S, and the other a γ myeloma protein of 7 S, and suggested for the first time that the transitional forms between multiple myelomatosis and primary Waldenström macroglobulinaemia might have evolved from the same clone of cells.

It would appear that in patients with di- or polyclonal paraproteinaemia the general clinical features seem to correlate with the identity of the predominant immunoglobulin abnormality. In the majority of the patients so far described and in the author's own experience, the predominant diclonal proteins frequently belong to IgA and IgG, although one patient with coexisting IgG and IgD myeloma was reported by Fahey et al (1968). Sanders et al (1969) described three patients with lymphoproliferative disorders—one of whom had three abnormal paraproteins in the serum consisting of IgG myeloma—770 mg/100 ml; IgA myeloma—810 mg/100 ml plus Bence Jones proteins in the urine. The light chain belonged to the κ type in each of the proteins. This patient suffered from recurrent bouts of respiratory tract infection as well as cold intolerance, nose bleeding and arthralgia. Their two other patients had both G myeloma proteins between 900 and 1000 mg/100 ml and Waldenström macroglobulinaemia of 700 and 2100 mg/100 ml respectively, with clinical features of typical macroglobulinaemia. Biosynthetic studies in each case indicated that a single clone of cells was capable of synthesising the several abnormal immunoglobulins seen in each patient's serum.

Structural studies on the relationship between diclonal paraproteins were carried out on both their heavy and light chains by Fudenberg et al (1971) in a patient who had both an IgG 2κ and IgM κ paraproteinaemia. The light chains of the two paraproteins were identical and contained the same amino acid residues in the hypervariable region of the light chain. Furthermore, although the constant Fc region of the two paraproteins differed in amino acid sequences, the variable portion of the H chains of both the γ and μ proteins were the same. Therefore it was postulated that on first exposure to a hypothetical antigen the plasma cell was first stimulated to produce IgM as in a primary response followed by IgG synthesis in the same cell. Rudders and Buell (1971) also suggested that a single clone of tumour plasma cell line synthesising two paraproteins of different immunoglobulin classes may represent different stages of differentiation in a cell line manifesting a genetic switch over in immunoglobulin heavy chain synthesis.

CRYOGLOBULINAEMIA

Cryoglobulins may occur in a wide variety of both malignant and benign diseases such as Waldenström macroglobulinaemia, multiple myelomatosis, cold agglutinin syndrome, cirrhosis, rheumatoid arthritis, parasitic infections, tuberculosis, chronic lymphatic leukaemia, systemic lupus erythematosus and occasionally in nephritis.

Cryoglobulin-related symptoms include Raynaud's phenomenon, cold sensitivity, cold urticaria, vascular occlusions and gangrene following exposure to cold and, occasionally, impairment in the central nervous system due to increased plasma viscosity which, in turn, may produce transient deafness, cerebral haemorrhages and coma paraproteinaemia.

Protein–protein interaction with the formation of immune complexes between cryoglobulins, notably IgM and blood coagulation factors such as factor V and VII, fibrinogen and prothrombin, may contribute to the bleeding tendencies often seen in patients with cryoglobulinaemia. Activation of the complement system through activation of C1q by IgM cryoglobulin complexes may be involved in the haemolytic jaundice and/or nephritis which sometimes occur in cryoglobulinaemia.

Grey and Kohler (1973) summarised the different types of cryoglobulinaemia as follows:

1. Monoclonal type, where only a single immunoglobulin is involved. About 25 per cent of all cryoglobulins belong to this class and the cryoglobulin concentration is invariably above 1 mg/ml (IgG or IgA or IgM or IgD types are known).
2. Mixed type, in which two or more immunoglobulins are involved, i.e. IgM—IgG complexes with IgM being the antibody to the antigen—a type of autoimmune process. About 14 per cent of all cryoglobulins belong to this type with cryoglobulin concentration $>$1 mg/ml.
3. Polyclonal type. Unlike the other two types, no monoclonal proteins are associated with the polyclonal type of cryoglobulinaemia and 61 per cent of all cryoglobulins belong to this type with cryoprecipitate frequently less than 1 mg/ml.

The formation of cryoglobulins depends upon a large number of factors, chief of which appear to be the concentration of the offending protein in the circulation. Normal serum does contain some cryoglobulins which range in concentration between 10 and 80 μg/ml. Temperature, pH, ionic strength and size of the complexes formed also appear to influence the development of cryoglobulinaemia. Storage of serum may or may not affect its formation, and in the author's laboratory, when a monoclonal cryoglobulin was kept at 37°C for one year, no loss of the reformation of copious cryoprecipitate was observed even after the serum was intermittently removed from the incubator and kept either at room temperature or at 4°C. However, Grey and Kohler (1973) reported that prolonged storage and handling of some forms of cryoglobulin may result in proteolytic breakdown with loss of cryoprecipitability.

Removal of sialic acid and other carbohydrate moieties from cryoimmunoglobulins decreases their solubility and Zinneman, Levi and Seal (1968) have shown that the IgG portion of a mixed IgM–IgG cryoglobulin lacked sialic acid and when an IgM rheumatoid factor was mixed with normal IgG, the formation of precipitates of cryoglobulins was greatly enhanced if the normal IgG previously had its sialic acid removed. Apart from the solubilising properties of carbohydrate in the formation of cryoprecipitates the presence of an increased number of hydrophobic amino acids appears to contribute to the formation of cryoglobulins. Both the heavy and the light chains of the immunoglobulins may form cryoglobulins and Saha et al (1969) have shown that the fragment of the immunoglobulin F $(ab)^2$ had a greater tendency to form cryoprecipitates than either the Fab or Fc fragments, indicating that the variable portion of the H and L chains must be important elements in the formation of cryoglobulins.

Most of the various classes of the immunoglobulins may form cryoglobulins but IgG and IgM are by far the commonest. The majority of the IgM cryoglobulins belong to the κ light chain type, whereas those of the IgG belong to the λ light chain type. We are as yet uncertain why the IgG 3 subclass has a greater tendency to form cryoglobulins than the rest of the IgG subclasses although it has been suggested that this increased tendency of IgG 3 to form aggregates in vivo is responsible for its much shorter half-life than the other IgG subclasses. Cream, Howard and Virella (1972) observed four patients with cryoglobulins in which IgG 3 was the predominating immunoglobulin subclass. It is likely that the ease with which IgG 3 subclass immunoglobulin is degraded by proteolytic enzymes into its $F(ab)^2$ fragment and the relative molecular weight of the IgG 3 H chain may be contributory factors to its increased tendency to form cryoglobulins.

Finally, it should be emphasised that the chief limiting factor in detecting cryoglobulins lies in the method of collection of the blood. Ideally the patient should be kept in a warm room at 37°C for 30 minutes before blood is withdrawn into a warm syringe. The blood should then be allowed to clot in an incubator at 37°C, then centrifuged at the same temperature. The cryoglobulin concentration in such a specimen of blood can then be readily determined by calculating the total protein concentration before and after the serum sample was kept at 4°C. In addition, cryofibrinogens may occur with the same frequency as cryoglobulins and this should be borne in mind when tests are carried out for the presence of cryoglobulins.

AMYLOIDOSIS

The earliest account of this disease is that given by Rokitansky in 1842, when he observed that patients with long-standing inflammatory disease, especially tuberculosis of the lungs, bones or joints, often showed certain characteristic changes in their viscera at post mortem. Rokitansky thereupon coined the term lardaceous disease on account of the translucent greasiness of the affected organs. Virchow (1860) renamed this waxy lardaceous deposit 'amyloid' (starch-like) because of the positive staining colour reaction it gave with iodine followed by sulphuric acid. Soon after this it was observed that amyloid deposits consisted largely of abnormal proteins rather than of carbohydrate or fats. Lachmann (1968) reported C3 components of complement in amyloid deposits, an association which strengthened the view of the close relationship of amyloid with immunoglobulins.

With the development of more sophisticated techniques for the identification of specific proteins, it soon became clear that amyloid deposits could be detected in a large number of diseases. These include: multiple myelomatosis, Waldenström macroglobulinaemia, Hodgkin's disease, tuberculosis, various carcinomas and diabetes mellitus. In these diseases amyloid deposits may be found in almost all organs of the body, but it would appear that the kidneys, the spleen, the liver, the heart, the lungs, the tongue and salivary glands, the bone marrow and the endocrine glands are the organs most frequently affected.

Because of the association with paraproteinaemia, it soon became clear that amyloidosis must be due to some form of plasma cell dyscrasia.

The clinical symptoms associated with amyloidosis may include: haemorrhagic diathesis, purpura, macroglossia, carpal tunnel syndrome, weight loss, lymphadenopathy, jaundice, glomerulonephritis and chronic infections.

The original method used for confirming the presence of amyloid consisted of staining with Congo Red with resulting birefringence and dicroisms and the demonstration of a pale green fluorescence in ultraviolet light after staining with thioflavine-T (Azzopardi and Lehner, 1966). Since it is known that amyloidosis is intimately associated with plasma cell dyscrasia, tests for its presence usually included the search for plasmacytosis and abnormal proteins. In a very large series of 8758 necropsies, Azzopardi and Lehner (1966) showed that the incidence of secondary amyloidosis in multiple myelomatosis was at least 10 per cent, but it was considerably higher in patients with Waldenström macroglobulinaemia, whereas in patients with Hodgkin's disease the incidence of amyloidosis was about 4 per cent. Furthermore, over 15 per cent of all patients dying with amyloid had some form of malignancy and renal carcinoma accounted for at least 25 per cent of all carcinomas associated with systemic amyloidosis. The disease may occur in any age group but it is particularly common in the elderly.

Barth et el (1969) stated that despite the presence of significant plasmacytosis in fifteen patients with primary amyloidosis, immunoglobulin synthesis was decreased and severe hypogammaglobulinaemia was common among all the patients. The marked hypogammaglobulinaemia seems to be due to a decreased synthetic rate of immunoglobulins and a defect of assembly of H and L chains, thus producing an increased deposition in many tissues of the body as well as excretion of Bence Jones proteins into the urine. Indeed, 40 per cent of their patients with primary amyloidosis had detectable Bence Jones proteinuria either of a single light chain type or consisting of both κ and λ light chains. Consequently, immunoelectrophoresis rather than routine serum electrophoresis was the chief means of detecting abnormalities in the serum since the paraprotein was either completely absent or not markedly elevated. In the author's own laboratory all six patients with primary amyloidosis had no detectably paraprotein band by electrophoresis, but immunoelectrophoresis of both serum and urine revealed the abnormal serum protein and excess of light chains in the urines.

Protracted stimulation of the reticuloendothelial system may result in amyloidosis and in experimental animals; Cohen (1965) and Sriram, Glenner and De Lillies (1971) were able to induce amyloid deposits in animals by hyperimmunisation with Freund's adjuvant, thus supporting the early clinical observations of Rokitansky, over a hundred years earlier, of the frequency of amyloidosis in his patients with long-standing inflammatory diseases.

When cleavage with pepsin experiments were carried out on several λ and κ Bence Jones proteins to produce variable and constant region fragments, the precipitate so formed had characteristics indistinguishable from amyloid fibrils. Also x-ray crystallography showed that these fragments contained typical β-pleated sheets as formed by authentic amyloid fibrils. Details of structural composition of amyloid fibrils have been well documented and reviewed by Glenner, Terry and Isersky (1973). They showed that about 70 per cent of the major protein of amyloid fibrils is derived from the variable portion of the amino terminal half of the light and heavy chain of immunoglobulin, although some amyloid fibrils are known to contain only non-immunoglobulin protein which show some of the same β-pleated antiparallel sheet structure as the immunoglobulins; furthermore that inherent in the structure of the variable region, especially that of the λ light chain, was the capacity to form antiparallel β-pleated sheet fibrils when this region was cleaved from the intact light chain, hence the greater frequency of λ type amyloidosis. Glenner, Terry and Isersky (1973) postulated that in vivo endocytosis of light polypeptide chains by intralysosomal proteolytic enzymes of phagocytic cells caused partial hydrolysis producing VL fragments which were responsible for the formation of amyloid fibrils

Osserman (1971) suggested that amyloidogenic light chains have greater affinity for tissues than non-amyloidogenic light chains.

Using fluorescence labelling and circular dichroism studies, Pollet, Rossi and Edelhoch (1972) showed that Bence Jones proteins may be classified into λ and κ types depending upon the presence or absence of the β structure. Furthermore, both x-ray crystallography and infra red spectroscopy have confirmed that amyloid fibrils consisted primarily of anti-parallel β-pleated sheet. In addition, when the standard thermal reaction for Bence Jones proteins was applied the κ light chains acquired, while the λ light chains maintained a β conformation prior to precipitation. Glenner, Terry and Isersky (1973) have stated the thermal characteristics of BJ proteins are confined to the VL region and furthermore that the thermal properties of BJ proteins depend upon their β conformation which is normally present in λ light chains or can be induced thermally in the variable region of the κ light chain. The original description of the thermal physico-chemical properties of light chains by Professor Bence Jones is probably related to the fact that on further heating of certain types of Bence Jones proteins to 100°C, all the Bence Jones protein precipitate is dissolved—a property which is shared by amyloid fibrils.

BENIGN PARAPROTEINAEMIA

In any survey of paraproteinaemia there usually occur about five to ten per cent of patients who show no evidence of any malignant condition. This is especially true in elderly subjects in whom up to 30 per cent may have a benign paraproteinaemia and in persons living in areas where parasitic infections are endemic. Usually patients with benign paraproteinaemia are symptomless and have no detectable Bence Jones proteins for periods of longer than five years. In addition, in the majority but certainly not in all of them, the other serum immunoglobulin concentrations are not so markedly reduced as they are in patients with malignant paraproteinaemia and their blood urea and serum calcium concentrations are within the normal ranges.

Acknowledgement

I am particularly grateful to the British Cancer Research Campaign for a grant for our studies on Paraproteins in Malignancies.

References

Augener, W., Grey, H. M., Cooper, N. R. & Müller-Eberhard, H. J. (1971) The reaction of monomeric and aggregated immunoglobulins with C_1. *Immunochemistry*, **8**, 1011–1020.

Azzopardi, J. G. & Lehner, T. (1966) Systemic amyloidosis and malignant diseases. *Journal of Clinical Pathology*, **19**, 539–548.

Ballard, H. S., Hamilton, L. M., Marcus, S. J. & Illes, C. H. (1970) A new variant of heavy chain disease: μ-chain disease. *New England Journal of Medicine*, **282**, 1060–1062.

Barth, W. F., Willerson J. T., Waldmann, T. A. & Decker, J. L. (1969) Primary amyloidosis. Clinical, immunochemical and immunoglobulin metabolism in fifteen patients. *American Journal of Medicine*, **47,** 259–273.

Brittin, G. M., Tanaka, Y. & Brecher, G. (1963) Intranuclear inclusions in multiple myeloma and macroglobulinaemia. *Blood*, **27,** 335–351.

Capra, J. D. & Kunkel, H. G. (1970) Aggregation of γG 3 proteins, relevance to the hyperviscosity syndrome. *Journal of Clinical Investigation*, **49,** 610–621.

Cohen, A. S. (1965) The constitution and genesis of amyloid. *International Review of Experimental Pathology*, **4,** 159–165.

Colwell, E. J., Bernier, G. M. & Fife, E. H. (1971) Serum immunoglobulins and malarial antibodies in South Vietnamese residents. *Transaction of the Royal Society of Tropical Medicine and Hygiene*, **65,** 310–314.

Cream, J. J., Howard, A. & Virella, G. (1972) IgG heavy chain subclasses in mixed cryoglobulins. *Immunology*, **23,** 405–411.

Davey, M., Carter, D., Sanderson C. J. & Coombs, R. R. A. (1970) IgD antibody to insulin. *Lancet*, **ii,** 1280–1282.

Ein, D. & Fahey, J. L. (1967) Two types of polypeptide chains in human immunoglobulins. *Science*, **156,** 947–948.

Fahey, J. L., Carbone, P. P., Rowe, D. S. & Bachmann, R. (1968) Plasma cell myeloma with D-myeloma proteins. IgD myeloma. *American Journal of Medicine*, **45,** 373–380.

Farhangi, M. & Osserman, E. F. (1973) The treatment of multiple myeloma. *Seminars in Haematology*, **10,** 149–161.

Feinstein, D. & Franklin, E. C. (1966) Two antigenically distinguishable subclasses of human myeloma proteins differing in their heavy chains. *Nature, London*, **212,** 1496–1498.

Frangione, B. & Franklin, E. C. (1973) Heavy chain disease: clinical features and molecular significance of the disordered immunoglobulin structure. *Seminars in Haematology*, X, 53–64.

Franklin, E. C., Lowenstein, J., Bigelow, B. & Meltzer, M. (1964) Heavy chain disease—a new disorder of serum γ-globulins. Report of the first case. *American Journal of Medicine*, **37,** 332–373.

Franklin, E. C., Frangione, B. & Cooper, S. (1971) Heavy chain disease. *Annals of the New York Academy of Sciences*, **190,** 457–466.

Fudenberg, H. H., Wang, A. C., Pink, J. R. L. & Levin, A. S. (1971) Studies of an unusual biclonal gammopathy. Implications with regard to genetic control of normal immunoglobulin synthesis. *Annals of the New York Academy of Sciences*, **190,** 501–506.

Galton, D. A. G. (1971) Treatment of myelomatosis—M. R. C. Trial. *British Medical Journal*, **ii,** 323–324.

Glenner, G. G., Terry, W. D. & Isersky, C. (1973) Amyloidosis. Its nature and pathogenesis. *Seminars in Haematology*, **10,** 65–86.

Gothoni, G., Wasastjerna, C. & Jeglinsky, B. (1965) Macroglobulinaemia: primary (Waldenström) and symptomatic in rheumatoid arthritis. *Acta Medica Scandinavia*, **17,** 263–273.

Grey, H. M. & Kohler, P. F. (1973) Cryoimmunoglobulins. *Seminars in Haematology*, **X,** 87–112.

Harrison, C. V. (1972) The morphology of the lymph node in the macroglobulinaemia of Waldenström. *Journal of Clinical Pathology*, **25,** 12–16.

Hobbs, J. R. (1969) Growth rates and responses to treatment in human myelomatosis. *British Journal of Haematology*, **16,** 607–617.

Johansson, S. G. O., Mellbin, T. & Vahlquist, B. S. (1968) Immunoglobulin levels in Ethiopian pre-school children with special reference to high concentrations of immunoglobulin E IgND. *Lancet*, **i,** 1119–1121.

Jones, H. Bence (1847) Papers on chemical pathology lecture III. *Lancet*, **ii,** 88–92.

Josephson, A. S., Price, E. & Biro, L. (1969) A low molecular weight fragment related to IgM in the serum of a patient with an IgA plasma cell dyscrasia. *Clinical Research*, **17,** 604–606.

Kjeldsen, K. & Asfeldt, V. H. (1963) Macroglobulinaemia or multiple myeloma. *Acta Medica Scandinavica*, **174,** 407–413.

Kok, D. A., Whitmore, D. N. & Ainsworth, R. W. (1963) Four cases of Waldenström macroglobulinaemia. *Journal of Clinical Pathology*, **16**, 351–361.

Kronwall, G. & Williams, R. C. (1969) Differences in anti-protein activity amongst IgG subclasses. *Journal of Immunology*, **103**, 828–833.

Lachmann, P. J. (1968) *Complement in Clinical Aspects of Immunology* (Ed.) P. G. H. Gell & R. R. A. Coombs. pp. 384–419. Oxford: Blackwell.

Laird, A. K. (1964) Dynamics of tumour growth. *British Journal of Cancer*, **18**, 490–502.

Laird, A. K. (1965) Dynamics of tumour growth. Comparison of growth rates and extrapolation of growth curve to one cell. *British Journal of Cancer*, **19**, 278–291.

Laurell, C. B. (1968) The diagnostic significance of immunoglobulin M-components in clinical work. *Scandinavian Journal of Clinical and Laboratory Investigation*, **22**, 83–86.

McFarlane, H. (1964) A simple rapid method for concentrating urine for protein electrophoresis. *Clinica Chemica Acta*, **9**, 376–380.

McFarlane, H. (1966) Comparative quantitation of immunglobulins in Nigerians. *West African Medical Journal*, **17**, 149–152.

McFarlane, H. & Nwoloko, C. (1966) Waldenström macroglobulinaemia in a Nigerian with rheumatoid arthritis. *Journal of Clinical Pathology*, **19**, 603–605.

Michaux, J. L. (1966) *Les Immunoglobulines des Bantous a l'État Normal et Pathologie.* Thèse en vue de l'obtention de Grade d'alagrègre de l'enseignement superieur, Université Louvanium Kinshasa and Université Catholique de Louvain.

Murray, W. D. & Cook, I. A. (1968) Primary acquired hypogamma globulinaemia and amyloidosis. *Journal of Clinical Pathology*, **21**, 32–34.

Natvig, J. B. & Kunkel, H. G. (1973) Human immunoglobulin classes, subclasses, genetic variants and idiotypes. *Advances in Immunology*, **16**, 1–59.

Osserman, E. F. (1971) Plasma cell dyscrasia. In Beeson, P. B. & McDermott, W. (Ed) *Cecil-Loeb Text Book of Medicine*, 13th edition. pp. 1101–1116. Philadelphia: W. B. Saunders.

Pollet, R., Rossi, G. & Edelhoch, H. (1972) Fluorescence and circular dicroism of Bence Jones proteins at high temperature. *Journal of Biological Chemistry*, **247**, 5921–5927.

Ramot, B., Shahin, N. & Bubis, J. J. (1965) Malabsorption syndrome in lymphoma of small intestine. A study of thirteen cases. *Israel Journal of Medical Science*, **1**, 221–226.

Ratcliff, P., Soothill, J. F. & Stanworth, D. R. (1963) Physicochemical and immunological studies of pathological serum macroglobulins. *Clinica Chemica Acta*, **8**, 91–108.

Rokitansky, C. (1942) *Handbuch de Speciellen pathologischen Anatomie*, Vienna: Vol. 3, p. 311. Braumüller & Seidel. Quoted by Payling Wright, G. in *An Introduction to Pathology*, 3rd edition. Longmans (1958) pp. 259–260.

Ropartz, C., Lenoir, J. & Rivat, L. (1961) A new inheritable property of human sera: the Inv factor. *Nature, London*, **189**, 586 inclusive.

Rowe, D. S., McGregor, I. A., Smith, S. J., Hall, P. & Williams, K. (1968) Plasma immunoglobulin concentration in a West African Gambian community and in a group of healthy British adults. *Clinical and Experimental Immunology*, **3**, 63–79.

Rudders, R. A. & Buell, D. N. (1971) Multiple myeloma with IgG (λ) and IgA (λ) serum components: immunohistologic studies. *Journal of Laboratory and Clinical Medicine*, **78,** 847–849.

Saha, A., Sambury, S., Smart, K., Heiner, D. C., Sargent, A. U. & Rose, B. (1969) Studies on cryoprecipitation. II. Immunochemical characterisation of a human cryoglobulin. *Journal of Immunology*, **102**, 476–484.

Saifer, A. (1964) A simple chemical test for distinguishing myeloma globulins from macroglobulins. *Journal of Laboratory and Clinical Medicine*, **63**, 1054–1060.

Salmon, S. E. (1973) Immunoglobulin synthesis and tumour kinetics of multiple myeloma. *Seminars in Haematology*, **10**, 135–148.

Salmon, S. E. & Smith, B. A. (1970) Immunoglobulin synthesis and total body tumour cell number in IgG multiple myeloma. *Journal of Clinical Investigation*, **49**, 1114–1121.

Sanders, J. H., Fahey, J. L., Finegold, I., Ein, D., Reisfield, R. & Berard, C. (1969) Multiple anomalous immunoglobulins. *American Journal of Medicine*, **47**, 43–59.

Seligmann, M., Danon, E., Harez, D., Mihaeseo, E. & Preud'Homme, J. L. (1968) Alpha chain disease. A new immunoglobulin abnormality. *Science*, **162**, 1396–1397.

Seligmann, M., Mihaeseo, E. & Frangione, B. (1971) Studies of alpha chain disease. *Annals of the New York Academy of Sciences*, **190,** 487–500.

Sriram, J., Glenner, G. G. & De Lillies, R. A. (1971) Amyloid, 1. Use of Freunds adjuvant in experimental amyloidosis. *Proceedings of the Society of Experimental Biology and Medicine*, **127,** 854–856.

Stanworth, D. R. & Smith, A. K. (1972) Human IgG subclass with primate skin binding activity. *Lancet*, **ii,** 491.

Steel, A. E. (1963) The laboratory diagnosis of macroglobulinaemia by viscometry. *Clinica Chemica Acta*, **8,** 86–90.

Stoop, J. W., Ballieux, R. E., Hijmans, W. & Zegers, B. J. M. (1971) Alpha-chain disease with involvement of the respiratory tract in a Dutch child. *Clinical and Experimental Immunology*, **9,** 625–635.

Svartz, N., Liljamma, J. & Ericsson, B. (1962) Amino acid analysis of the rheumatoid factor macroglobulin. Preliminary Report. *Acta Medica Scandinavica*, **172,** 767–768.

Virchow, R. (1860) *Cellular Pathology*. (English Translation, London) p. 372. Quoted by Payling Wright, G. in *An Introduction to Pathology*. 3rd edition (1957). Longmans, pp. 259–260.

Virella, G. (1971) Relaciones entre las subclases de IgG humana, hiperviscosidad y crioprecipitación. *Sangre*, **16,** 329–336.

Virella, G., Nunes, A. S. & Tamagnini, G. (1972) Placental transfer of human IgG subclasses. *Clinical and Experimental Immunology*, **10,** 475–478.

Virella, G. & Parkhouse, R. M. E. (1972) Determination of the molecular weight of gamma-3 chains by polyacrylamide gel electrophoresis in the presence of sodium dodecyl sulphate. *Immunology*, **23,** 857–860.

Waldenström, J. (1944) Incipient myelomatosis or 'essential' hyperglobulinaemia with fibrinogenopenia. New syndrome. *Acta Medica Scandinavica*, **117,** 216–247.

Waldenström, J. (1962) Hypergammaglobulinaemia as a clinical haematological problem: Study in the gammopathies. *Progress in Haematology*, **3,** 266–280.

Wang, A. C., Faulk, W. P., Stuckley, M. A. & Fudenberg, H. H. (1970) Chemical differences of adult foetal and hypogammaglobulinaemic IgG immunoglobulins. *Immunochemistry*, **7,** 703–708.

Wilkinson, P., Davidson, W. & Sommaripa, (1966) Turnover of ^{131} I-labelled autologous macroglobulin in Waldenström's macroglobulinaemia. Report of a case studied during treatment with phenylalanine mustard. *Annals of Internal Medicine*, **65,** 308–316.

Zinneman, H. H., Levi, D. & Seal, U. S. (1968) On the nature of cryoglobulins. *Journal of Immunology*, **100,** 594–603.

Zlotnick, A. & Levy, M. (1971) α-heavy chain disease. *Archives of Internal Medicine*, **128,** 432–436.

4. Immunology of Connective Tissue Diseases

RODNEY BLUESTONE

The group of clinical syndromes referred to as connective tissue or rheumatic diseases are generally characterised by various immune aberrations. Whether these abnormalities are primary events in an immune-mediated disease or merely secondary markers of ongoing generalised tissue injury remains speculative. Whatever the case, detection and measurement of these immune aberrations provide valuable diagnostic tools in many rheumatic diseases, and sometimes permit objective means of following the disease course.

Two main immunological events provide a basis for both the investigation and understanding of rheumatic disorders. One is autoantibody formation. An increased production of inappropriate humoral antibodies with reactivity for autologous or homologous tissue antigens appears to be a hallmark of some connective tissue diseases. This abnormal humoral antibody response frequently lacks specificity and its biological role in the disease pathogenesis may not be apparent. Furthermore, it is quite likely that a cellular immune response to normal or altered autologous tissues accompanies the humoral autoantibody response. Investigations along this approach are indeed interesting but, as yet, constitute research tools rather than diagnostic tests in the clinical setting. The detection and assay of humoral autoantibodies as hallmarks of disease are of real clinical value if interpreted with caution and in light of the whole clinical picture.

The second, possibly consequent, immunological event in these diseases is the formation of immune complexes localised at the site of tissue damage. The classic models of serum sickness in rabbits (Dixon, Feldman and Vazquez, 1961), and the chronic viral syndromes of mice (Oldstone and Dixon, 1969, 1970) and mink (Norton, 1970), have focussed attention onto the concept of human immune complex-mediated disease. It appears that the deposition of antigen–antibody complexes in the presence of antigen excess and their subsequent fixation of complement in vivo can, to some extent, be monitored by measuring the complex components. Their qualitative or quantitative measurement, whether in biological fluids or at the site of tissue damage, can facilitate the diagnosis and treatment of the disease. In certain states such as systemic lupus nephritis, immune complexes located on the glomerular capillary basement membrane appear to play a key role in the generation of disease. In other situations such as the rheumatoid synovial space, immune complex components can be identified but their pathogenic role is less certain.

The diseases to be discussed in this chapter have, for the most part, their own distinguishing features and can usually be diagnosed one from the other by astute clinical evaluation (Boyle and Buchanan, 1971). Nevertheless, certain patients manifest their disease in less classical form and may present with clinical features common to more than one well-recognised syndrome. Moreover, many of the immunological tests to be described reveal abnormalities in more than one type of connective tissue disease. For the purposes of this chapter, the main rheumatic disorders under discussion are grouped according to their clinical presentation regardless of pathogenetic mechanisms they may or may not have in common.

Systemic Lupus Erythematosus (SLE)

The clinical syndrome of systemic lupus erythematosus is characterised by striking immune aberrations which constitute important diagnostic features of the disease (Miescher, Rothfield and Miescher, 1966). These aberrations indicate two main processes—immune hyperreactivity with autoantibody formation, together with humoral and tissue evidence of in vivo immune complex deposition.

A moderate to severe degree of hypergammaglobulinaemia is usual during disease activity. This is manifest as a diffuse increase in the gamma globulin region on plasma protein electrophoresis and contrasts sharply with the depressed albumin level in patients with gross proteinuria. However, there should be no evidence of a monoclonal (paraprotein) spike with sharply restricted electrophoretic mobility as the hypergammaglobulinaemia of SLE is due to an overall increase in production of normal (polyclonal) immunoglobulins. Consequently, quantitative serum immunoglobulin assays may reveal increased levels of IgG and IgM, although rarely the extreme elevation of a single class of immunoglobulin seen in patients with paraproteinaemia. Further, the excess serum and urinary free light-chains in SLE are of both κ and λ type, thus differing from homogeneous Bence Jones protein.

The immune hyperreactivity of SLE is reflected in the appearance of various serum autoantibodies characterising the disease.

Antinuclear antibody (ANA)

The demonstration of circulating antibody with specificity for cell nuclei is a cardinal diagnostic feature of SLE and sometimes typifies other autoimmune diseases. The pathogenic significance of antibody to nuclear antigens is unclear although it is noteworthy that immunoglobulin with ANA activity can be recovered from the renal glomeruli of patients with lupus nephritis.

The precise definition of the numerous nuclear antigens for which ANA may have specificity have been only partly elucidated. These include deoxyribonucleic acid (DNA), ribonucleic acid (RNA), nucleohistone, a phosphate-extractable antigen and nucleolar material. Most, but not all, antinuclear antibodies are IgG or IgM proteins and are characterised by their reactivity with autologous, homologous or even heterologous cell nuclei in vitro. Regardless of the ANA immunoglobulin class or the source of reactive nuclear antigens, the methods for demonstrating the autoantibody follow the same basic principle (Friou, 1967).

To detect ANA in biological fluids (usually serum) a source of cell nuclear antigen must be provided. This usually consists either of a human peripheral

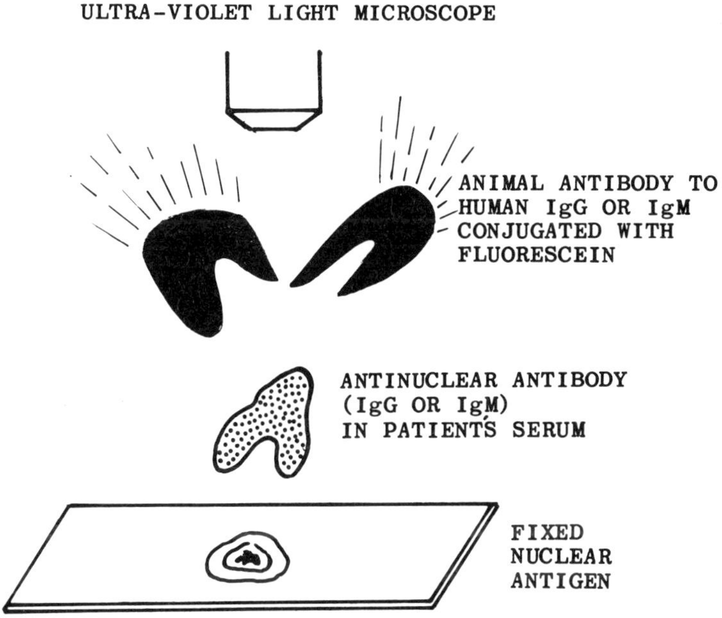

Figure 4.1. Schematic representation of antinuclear antibody detected by indirect immunofluorescence. The source of nuclear antigen may be human polymorphonuclear leucocytes in a blood smear or cryostat-cut sections of rat or mouse liver. The antibody (IgG or IgM) in the patient's serum fixes to the nuclear antigens. After washing, the fixed antibody is demonstrated by a fluorescein-conjugated antiserum monospecific for human IgG or IgM viewed by ultraviolet microscopy.

blood buffy coat smear (i.e. polymorphonuclear leucocyte nuclei) or cryostat-cut thin sections of rat liver or kidney (hepatic or tubular cell nuclei). If a patients' serum containing ANA is layered onto the antigen substrate the antibody reacts with, and sticks onto, the nuclear antigen. After washing, the antigen-fixed ANA can then be demonstrated by immunofluorescence by applying a second layer of antiserum which is monospecific for human IgG or IgM and is conjugated with a fluorescent dye (fluorescein or rhodamine). Reaction between the conjugated antiserum and antigen-fixed ANA is manifest as nuclear fluorescence when viewed under ultraviolet light (Figure 4.1). Thereby, according to the specificity of the conjugated antiserum, the ANA immunoglobulin class is ascertained.

Considerable significance was once attached to the actual pattern of nuclear

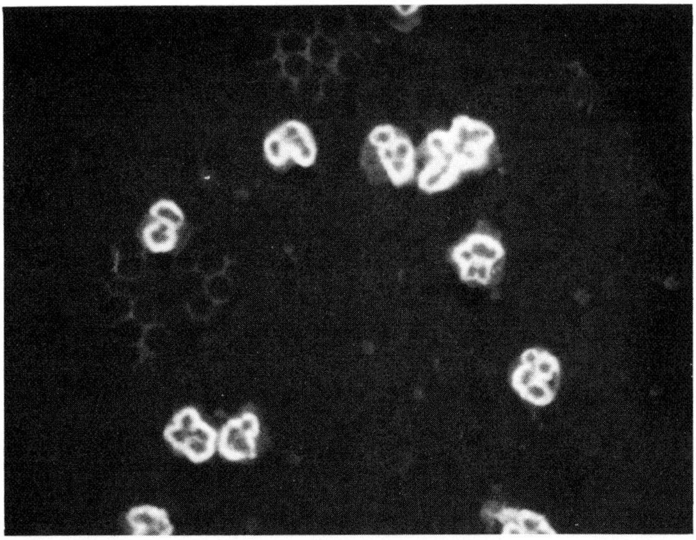

(a)

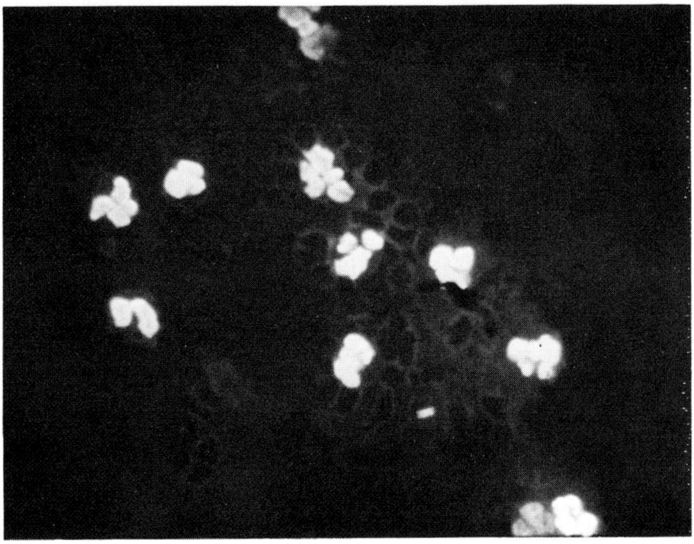

(b)

Figure 4.2. Antinuclear antibody demonstrated by indirect immunofluorescence of polymorph nuclei using fluoroscein-conjugated antiserum to human IgG (× 500). (a) Patient's serum tested undiluted showing typical nuclear rim ('shaggy') pattern of fluorescence. (b) Same serum tested at a dilution of 1:16 evoking a homogeneous pattern.

fluorescence seen, both for differential diagnosis and prognosis. Further, attempts were made to identify the specifically reacting nuclear antigen by the type of staining pattern evoked. However, absolute categorisation of immunofluorescent patterns is not possible. Indeed, the same serum containing

ANA may give marked nuclear rim staining when tested undiluted, yet show homogeneous nuclear fluorescence when tested at a dilution (Figure 4.2). Nevertheless, the pattern of nuclear fluorescent staining may appear predominantly as one of several types and the clinician may glean some help from the pattern in certain situations. Thus, a speckled pattern of fluorescence usually indicates systemic sclerosis, systemic lupus or other connective tissue disease and may result from antibodies reactive with ribonucleoprotein or other phosphate-extractable nuclear antigens. A similar staining pattern appears to be common in Africans residing in malarious zones. Nuclear rim staining ('shaggy' pattern) probably represents ANA reactivity with DNA or nucleoprotein, may correlate with DNA binding (see later), and is very suggestive of SLE. Homogeneous nuclear staining is most often associated with antibody to nucleoprotein; nucleolar fluorescence may be more common in systemic sclerosis or Sjögren's syndrome although this awaits confirmation. In summary, it is becoming abundantly clear that many nuclear antigen–antibody systems are operative in SLE. Moreover, the ANA specificity may be but one factor influencing the pattern of nuclear fluorescent staining. When studied in depth every patient with SLE probably has her own profile of nuclear antigen–antibody systems.

Nonetheless, positive staining of cell nuclei indicates the presence of ANA whatever the pattern of fluorescence. If undiluted serum evokes staining a titre is obtained by diluting the serum with saline and testing the serial dilutions for ANA activity. However, the clinician should be aware of the many pitfalls inherent in immunofluorescent techniques. The antigen substrates must be carefully prepared and preserved. The antihuman immunoglobulin antisera should be highly specific and well conjugated, containing no excess free fluorescein. Positive and negative control sera should be included in all assays. Even with all precautions doubtful fluorescence may be seen and false positives frequently arise depending on the care and experience of the observer. Non-specific staining may be due to unbound fluorescein, denatured antiserum, foreign proteins or normal inadvertent serum antibodies. Indeed, many laboratories disregard solid tissue-substrate nuclear fluorescence evoked with undiluted serum if staining is not confirmed at serial dilutions. It follows that a high-titre positive ANA (e.g. $>$ 1:64) is much more suggestive of SLE than low titres. However, the test is highly sensitive and with good laboratory facilities it is difficult to diagnose SLE without a positive ANA test. The usual exception to this rule is if the patient is on corticosteroid therapy. Prednisone in a dose of 40 to 60 mg per day may effectively suppress the formation of ANA.

A haemagglutinating antibody to an extractable nuclear antigen (ENA) containing protein and ribonucleic acid has been described in the serum of certain patients with 'mixed connective tissue disease' (Sharp, 1971). Such patients may manifest characteristic features of SLE, polymyositis and systemic sclerosis, have high-titre ANA producing speckled fluorescence, normal complement levels and DNA binding, no renal lesion, and a good prognosis. If confirmed, the detection of haemagglutinating antibody to ENA in selected patients might be important since this reputed clinicopathological syndrome appears to be steroid-responsive.

Lupus erythematosus cells (LE cells)

Recognition and characterisation of the LE cell phenomenon has played a major role in the clinical and laboratory investigation of SLE (Hargraves, 1969). The detection of LE cells indicates the presence of an 'LE factor' now recognised to be a humoral antibody to the deoxyribonucleoprotein component of cell nuclei. This antibody is usually IgM, but may occasionally be IgG or IgA.

The basis of the LE cell test is the detection of anti-deoxyribonucleoprotein antibody in the patient's serum in vitro. This is done in a remarkable and indirect way (Figure 4.3). The antibody does not appear to be cytotoxic to

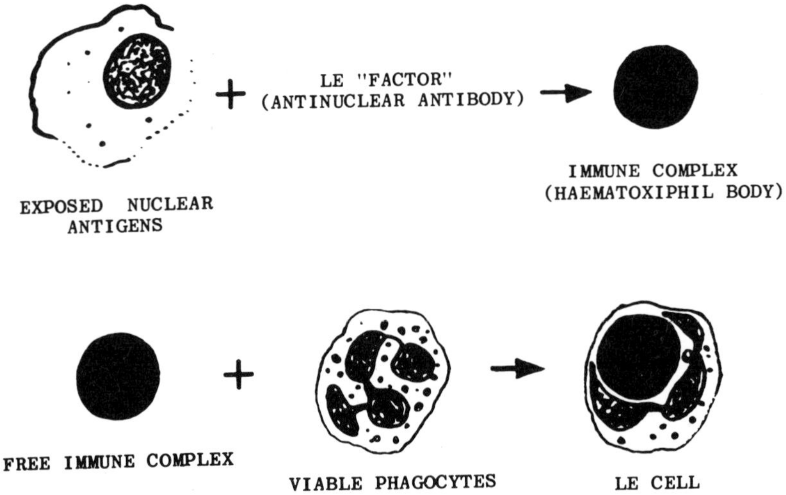

Figure 4.3. Schematic representation of method used for detecting LE cells. The source of nuclear antigen may be autologous, homologous or heterologous polymorphonuclear leucocytes incompletely traumatised to expose cellular contents. The addition of a serum containing 'LE factor' (anti-deoxyribonucleoprotein) results in the formation of immune complexes which may be phagocytosed by non-traumatised, viable polymorphs. The characteristic staining and morphological appearance of a polymorph almost filled by an ingested complex which displaces the normal nucleus towards the cell margin, constitutes the LE cell (see Figure 4.4).

intact cells, but if damaged cells, and therefore nuclear material, are exposed to serum containing the 'LE factor' certain events occur. The anti-deoxyribonucleoprotein forms immune complexes with its antigen resulting in gross derangement of the exposed nuclei which become large, pale, purple-pink staining homogeneous masses lacking the normal dense nuclear chromatin pattern, i.e. quite different to normal phagocytic inclusions. As the damaged cells further deteriorate, these masses are released into the serum where they may be phagocytosed by other viable polymorphonuclear leucocytes. The effect of ingestion by the normal, undamaged phagocyte results in the 'LE cell'—a large polymorph almost filled with the ingested homogeneous mass and its own intact nucleus displaced and compressed to the cell margin

(Figure 4.4). Thus, three components are necessary to demonstrate LE cells: a patient's serum containing antibody to deoxyribonucleoprotein, damaged cells exposing deoxyribonucleoprotein antigen and viable phagocytic neutrophils.

In practice, the source of damaged cells or normal phagocytes is not critical and most clinical laboratories follow a single perfected routine. Either the patient's serum or plasma may be used and the type of anticoagulant is not critical—although heparin in concentrations of greater than 5 units/ml inhibits LE cell formation. Widely used methods include taking the patient's

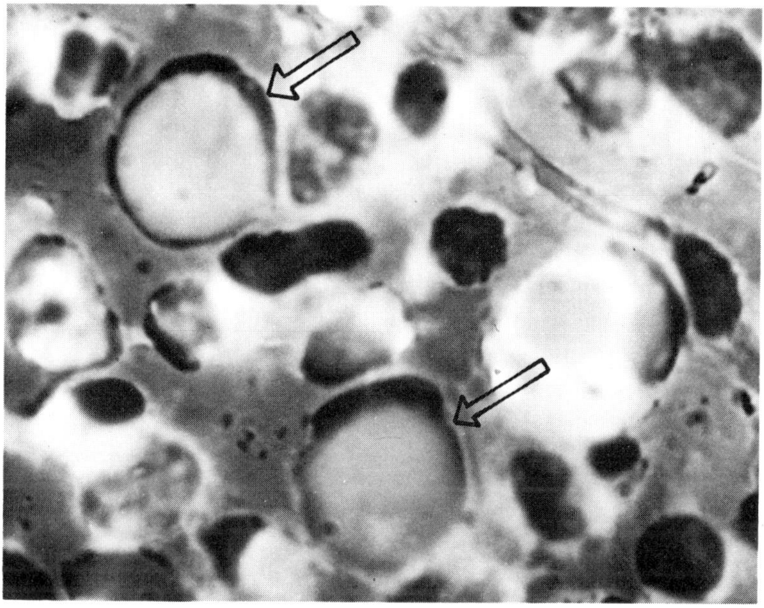

Figure 4.4. Positive LE cell preparation (× 1800). Two typical LE cells are shown (arrows). Using Wright's stain the cells appear to be almost filled by pale, purple-pink homogeneous masses. The darker intact nuclei are compressed and flattened to the cell margins.

whole blood into a container with glass beads. Mixing the blood with the beads defibrinates it and, at the same time, traumatises a proportion of the polymorphs. Following defibrination and incubation, a buffy coat suspension can be obtained. This buffy coat contains fragmented white cells which have been exposed to any 'LE factor' present in the patient's plasma, together with some viable leucocytes. A stained smear preparation of the cells and debris is then examined for LE cells. Another popular method of performing this test is to use the patient's whole clotted blood. This is forced through a wide-mesh filter, the effect of which is to traumatise some polymorphs thereby exposing nuclear antigen. The filtered clotted blood is incubated, centrifuged, the buffy coat removed and examined as above. Other methods incorporate preparation of room-air-dried homologous white cells as the source of nuclear antigen; even heterologous nuclear antigen (e.g. mouse leucocytes) appear to be satisfactory.

The all-important last stage of the test—reading the stained slide—determines the accuracy and reliability of this classical investigation. Generally speaking the more traumatised the source of nuclear material the more LE cells produced. Clearly, high titres of anti-deoxyribonucleoprotein antibody are more likely to give strongly positive LE cell tests than low ones. Deficiency of phagocytosis by intact polymorphs will result in a negative test, even in the presence of high titres of antibody. However, with optimum cellular fragmentation, adequate antibody and active phagocytosis the time and care spent reading the preparation finally determines its usefulness. Sparse LE cells may be missed if inadequate scrutiny is applied. Conversely, overzealous cell fragmentation often results in much non-specific cell debris in the system which becomes phagocytosed. This results in 'tart' cells which should not be confused with specific-appearing LE cells. Occasionally, differention of LE cells from 'tart' cells is difficult and may be facilitated by staining with Feulgen reagent which stains deoxyribonucleoprotein brown and thereby distinguishes true LE cells. Even with the most scrupulous inspection of well-prepared cell preparations, negative results may be obtained in patients with positive antinuclear antibody detected by immunofluorescence and DNA-binding.

The relative insensitivity of the LE cell test, its heavy dependence on careful prolonged microscopy, and its suppression by modest doses of corticosteroids are considerable disadvantages. Moreover, although LE cells are quite specific they are not titratable. Indeed, the greatest sensitivity of immunofluorescent techniques together with the high specificity of DNA-binding (see later), render LE cell preparations less important in the diagnosis of SLE. However, the demonstration of LE cells in synovial fluid may be quite helpful in the differential diagnosis of early lupus arthritis.

Attempts at a direct assay of antibody to deoxyribonucleoprotein have proved rather unsatisfactory. The LE rapid slide test incorporates latex particles coated with deoxyribonucleoprotein which agglutinate in the presence of serum containing antibody to nucleoprotein (i.e. LE factor). Positive and negative control serums are used for comparison and macroscopic agglutination read within minutes. The assay is insensitive and has little more attraction than a simple, inaccurate screening test.

DNA-binding

One of the main nuclear components identifiable as an antigen in SLE is deoxyribonucleic acid (DNA). Although the source of the native nuclear antigen in vivo is unclear, evidence suggests a central role for DNA–antiDNA complexes in the pathogenesis of lupus nephritis (Koffler and Kunkel, 1968). This despite the fact that DNA alone is a poor immunogen when used in laboratory animals. Reactivity of serum antibody with DNA probably accounts for nuclear rim staining on immunofluorescence; and in some instances the antibody can be demonstrated by a precipitin reaction in agarose gel between the patient's serum and calf thymus DNA. Interestingly, it appears that almost all patients with active SLE have heterogeneous serum antibodies that can bind in vitro with 'native' (undenatured) DNA from any source. Moreover, this DNA-binding activity would appear to be quite specific for SLE, being only occasionally seen in other rheumatic diseases. Thus, DNA-binding provides a valuable diagnostic test and, used in conjunction with immunofluorescent tests for ANA, facilitates a clearer distinction between SLE and other systemic disorders (Pincus et al, 1969).

The basic principle underlying the DNA-binding assay is the insolubility of immune complexes in 50 per cent saturated ammonium sulphate (Figure 4.5). Hence, DNA antigen–antibody complexes precipitate in this strength ammonium sulphate whereas free DNA remains in solution. Due to the cross-reactivity of DNA antibodies almost any source of radioactive DNA can be used in the test system. ^{3}H-thymidine-labelled calf thymus 'native' DNA is adequate for most purposes. Various investigators use different DNA sources,

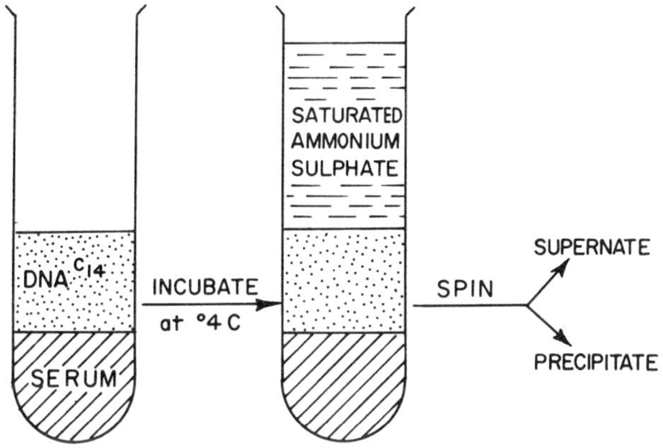

Figure 4.5. Method for measuring DNA-binding activity. A radioactive form of native DNA is added to the test serum. Any DNA–antiDNA complexes are then precipitated with ammonium sulphate. The percentage binding activity of the serum is expressed as

$$\frac{\text{radioactive counts/minute (cpm) of precipitate}}{\text{cpm of supernate} + \text{cpm of precipitate}} \times 100$$

e.g. ^{14}C-DNA derived from tissue-cultured cells or microorganisms grown in medium containing ^{14}C-thymidine. The important property of the DNA is a high specific activity easily measurable by liquid scintillation spectrometry. If serum containing DNA-binding activity is added to the radioactive DNA source and incubated, DNA–antiDNA immune complexes form. The addition of 50 per cent saturated ammonium sulphate results in precipitation of all immunoglobulins including those bound to antigen. The amount of radioactivity in the centrifuged precipitate is then a measure of the antiDNA antibody activity of the serum. Conventionally, the results are expressed as a percentage binding activity, calculated as radioactive counts per minute in the precipitate divided by the total count of the supernate plus precipitate, multiplied by 100. In practice, a small amount of unbound radioactive DNA precipitates out with normal sera. Hence, only binding activities greater than 20 per cent are considered significant. Binding values up to 100 per cent may be found in patients with active SLE while normal binding in patients with proven SLE usually indicates quiescent disease.

The advantages of the DNA-binding test are its relative simplicity, high sensitivity and reputed specificity. This test is of particular value in supporting a diagnosis when the ANA test is only doubtfully positive in a patient with suspected or atypical lupus. Certainly, most patients with a positive LE cell preparation have a greater than 50 per cent DNA-binding. Moreover, there is evidence to suggest that significant DNA-binding may be predictive of in vivo immune complex formation before the overt signs of active lupus nephritis appear. This interesting assay may become one of the more definitive tests available in the investigation of patients with rheumatic disorders. Nevertheless, the precise interpretation and significance of DNA-binding by serum proteins is complicated. Finally, refinement and standardisation of the assay is difficult and has barely been achieved amongst various laboratories.

Humoral antibodies to nuclear antigens are a cardinal diagnostic feature of SLE. They are best detected and titred by the immunofluorescent technique which, in reliable hands, is positive in almost every patient with active disease. The actual ANA titre can be a useful indicator of disease activity although there is not always close correlation. The formation of LE cells in vitro, although classical and useful, is a less satisfactory way of demonstrating ANA. Although the LE cell test is probably positive at some time in most patients with SLE, it is not as sensitive as the immunofluorescent assay. Hence, it is not uncommon to see patients with definite SLE, ANA titres of less than 1:16 and negative LE cell preparations. The DNA-binding test, on the other hand, promises to become a useful assay for serum antibodies with specific reactivity for nuclear antigen. In some laboratories it is reputed to be highly specific for SLE, even to the extent of being negative (less than 20 per cent binding) in patients with drug-induced lupus syndrome. In addition, the degree of DNA-binding might be an objective and useful index of in vivo disease activity.

Other autoantibodies

Various other autoantibodies are frequently found in patients with SLE Rheumatoid factor (see later) is present in the serum and synovial fluid of 50 to 60 per cent of patients. It appears to possess all the characteristics of antiglobulin detected in patients with rheumatoid arthritis and may be present in very high titre. Conceivably the reaction between IgG antinuclear antibodies and nuclear antigens in vivo alters IgG and renders it immunogenic, thereby stimulating rheumatoid factor production.

It is well recognised that sera from patients with SLE, but without treponemal infection, may give positive serological tests for syphilis (Moore and Lutz, 1955). Apparently, antibodies evoked by the autologous tissue damage in SLE cross-react with certain non-treponemal cytoplasmic antigens such as cardiolipin-lecithin. Consequently such patients have positive Venereal Disease Research Laboratory (VDRL) slide tests or Wassermann reactions (WR) without having syphilis and are said to be 'chronic biological false reactors'. This phenomenon is noted in about 5 to 10 per cent of patients with active lupus, sometimes presenting as the first serological manifestation of the disease. Other tests for syphilis utilise the specific organism *Treponema pallidum* as antigen, either in a fluorescent treponemal-antibody-absorption test (FTA-ABS) or in a treponemal immobilisation test (TPI). The organisms used may have small breaks in their cell walls exposing nuclear antigens which may then show cross-specificity with humoral antiDNA antibodies. Consequently false-positive FTA-ABS test results may be obtained in patients with SLE (Kraus et al, 1971). However, instead of being uniform, the pattern of false-positive treponemal fluorescence often has a beaded appearance. Although the TPI is perhaps even more specific for syphilis a few false-positive results have likewise been demonstrated in patients with SLE. Notwithstanding, the majority of chronic false-positive reactors demonstrate positive serological tests (utilising non-treponemal antigen) and negative or atypical treponemal tests.

Sera containing ANA may also give false-positive indirect fluorescent antibody (IFA) tests for toxoplasmosis (Araujo et al, 1971). The IFA test in this disease is a useful supplement to the Sabin–Feldman dye test. However, it appears the *Toxoplasma* organisms contain antigens indistinguishable by conventional immunological techniques from some of those found in polymorph nuclei or calf thymus DNA. Thus the majority of patients with serum ANA show positive *Toxoplasma* IFA tests with an immunofluorescent appearance indistinguishable from that obtained in patients with proven toxoplasmosis.

Autoantibodies directed against peripheral blood elements may be of great clinical significance in patients with SLE (Dubois, 1966). Anti-red cell antibodies are manifest usually as a positive direct Coombs' test; occasionally both the direct and indirect Coombs' test may be positive. Antibodies reactive with human and animal polymorphonuclear leucocytes have been detected by leucoagglutination tests; and anti-platelet antibodies can be detected by a difficult and sensitive platelet aggregation assay. The detection of anti-white cell or platelet antibodies is very difficult and at present constitute research procedures. However, profound Coombs-positive haemolytic anaemia, immune thrombocytopenia or leucopenia may sometimes complicate SLE and titration of the harmful antibody then becomes desirable. In addition to thrombocytopenic purpura, occasional patients have profound clotting and bleeding abnormalities due to a circulating antibody reactive with factor VIII and/or factor IX.

The immune overactivity in SLE is exemplified by the recent recognition of yet another type of anti-blood cell antibody associated with the disease—lymphocytotoxins (Terasaki, Mottironi and Barnett, 1970). These are antibodies directed against cell-membrane histocompatibility antigens and were once thought to be restricted to patients immunised by pregnancy, multiple transfusions or organ transplantation. It is now apparent that lymphocytotoxins may appear during acute viral infections (whether naturally acquired or by vaccination) or accompany connective tissue diseases. They are detected by the orthodox microcytotoxicity technique used for tissue typing, and are present in the serum of most patients with active SLE, correlating with the ANA activity. However, unlike lymphocytotoxins resulting from allogeneic immunisation, the autoantibody in SLE is predominantly IgM with maximum activity in vitro at a temperature of 15°C. Furthermore, the antibody in SLE is frequently cytotoxic to autologous lymphocytes. Although their pathogenic significance is uncertain, lymphocytotoxins in patients with SLE may represent another example of breakdown in immunological self-tolerance.

A better understanding of pathogenetic mechanisms operative in SLE and allied syndromes has evolved as a result of methods for the clinical detection of in vivo immune complex deposition. These methods are indirect since, as yet, there are no certain ways to detect easily and characterise circulating immune complexes. However, by measuring serum complement levels and studying tissue localisation of immune complex components much valuable information can be obtained.

Complement determinations

The formation of immune complexes in vivo may result in the fixation and consumption of complement. This is certainly true for experimental immune complex disease in animals and appears to apply equally to those human disorders where antigen–antibody reaction in vivo is a commensurate feature of the disease (Cochrane and Dixon, 1969). In particular, some connective tissue diseases feature immune complexes detectable at the site of tissue damage (Christian, 1969). Complement components can be identified in those complexes, and determination of serum complement may provide a guide as to the extent of immune complex formation and deposition in that individual thereby indicating disease activity. For this reason complement determinations in serum and synovial fluid are interesting and important. The complement system is complex and its activation and role in inflammary processes, including its regulation by homeostatic mechanisms, are all pertinent considerations (Cooper, Polley and Müller-Eberhard, 1971). However, for practical purposes a description of the complement system and its activation is outside the scope of this chapter. The precise measurement of various complement components in biological fluids is of great investigational and experimental interest but highly specialised, hard to interpret and not widely available. For most clinical purposes measurement of the total serum complement or its third and major component (C3) provides valuable information.

Complement determinations necessitate that serum be separated from the whole blood within one hour and kept frozen until assayed. Heating of any biological sample at 56°C for a short while inactivates and destroys complement activity. Total haemolytic complement is a gross measure of the interaction of all nine known complement components and their activators. It is estimated as the smallest amount of fresh serum which produces lysis of a specified proportion of sensitised red blood cells, i.e. cells coated with antibody (Kabat and Mayer, 1971). For technical reasons, 50 per cent haemolysis is the optimum end-point. A 50 per cent haemolytic unit of complement is designated $C\,H_{50}$ and is defined as the quantity of complement which lyses $2{\cdot}5 \times 10^8$ of optimally sensitised red blood cells out of a total of 5×10^8 cells in the presence of optimal Ca^{2+} and Mg^{2+}, at an ionic strength of 0·147, in one hour's incubation at 37°C and in a total volume of 7·5 ml. This is an arbitrary unit and clearly depends on many variable factors. However, by standardising the number of sheep red cells used, the quality of coating antibody and the physical and chemical properties of the medium, 50 per cent haemolysis of sensitised cells can be accurately and reproducibly determined by analysing the release of oxyhaemoglobulin by spectrophotometry. The haemolytic complement titre can then be expressed as the number of haemolytic units ($C\ H_{50}$) contained in 1 ml of undiluted serum. Normal values for total haemolytic complement vary somewhat according to the laboratory but are approximately from 70 to 140 haemolytic units. Clearly, this range is rather wide but profound lowering of the total haemolytic complement levels is regarded as significant.

Commercial assay plates for the measurement of total complement have recently become available. Although less accurate than the conventional assay, they appear to be adequate. The plate contains standardised sensitised sheep cells in a buffered gel medium and precision wells for receiving test specimens are cut into the gel. Reaction between the cells and active complement in the test specimens produces lysis of the cells, and a cleared zone. The zone diameter is directly proportional to the concentration of complement activity in the test sample and can be measured against zones produced by a reference serum containing a known concentration of complement.

A similar principle of radial immunodiffusion is used for the assay of C3. A monospecific antiserum to this component of complement is incorporated into agar. Samples and serum standards are applied to the wells and precipitin ring diameters are measured in the same way as for quantitative immunoglobulin determinations. The level of C3 in the serum of normal adults ranges from 120 to 200 mg/100 ml.

Immunoconglutinins

Immunoconglutinins (I-K) are IgM antibodies to hidden antigenic determinants located predominantly within the third and fourth components of complement molecules (Lachmann and Coombs, 1965). The antigens become exposed naturally when complement is adsorbed onto an antigen–antibody complex thereby stimulating I-K formation. Hence, I-K measurement may provide yet another index of immune complex disease activity since their appearance in human serum possibly indicates excessive fixation of complement in vivo. Their detection requires a sensitive resuspension technique using whole horse complement or purified complement components. The presence of I-K has been reported in many rheumatic diseases, notably SLE, acute gout and in patients with Sjögren's syndrome. This unusual antibody also frequently accompanies chronic bacterial infections as well as acute post-streptococcal nephritis. However, as an index of in vivo disease activity, serum complement levels (total haemolytic and C3) are far easier to measure and interpret. Moreover, to date the clinical significance of raised I-K levels is far from clear.

Persistent in vivo immune complex deposition in SLE results in excessive activation and consumption of complement. If complement consumption exceeds production a resultant fall in serum complement level ensues. This process can best be detected as a lowering of total haemolytic complement and/or C3. The complement level appears to be a fairly sensitive indicator of disease activity, response to therapy and impending clinical relapse. This is particularly so in following the progress of lupus nephritis (Figure 4.6). Low complement levels are found in the synovial fluid of SLE joint effusions, while selective lowering of the fourth component of complement (C4) in cerebrospinal fluid is reputed to be diagnostic of cerebral lupus (Petz et al, 1971). Interestingly, an over-utilisation and turnover of serum complement

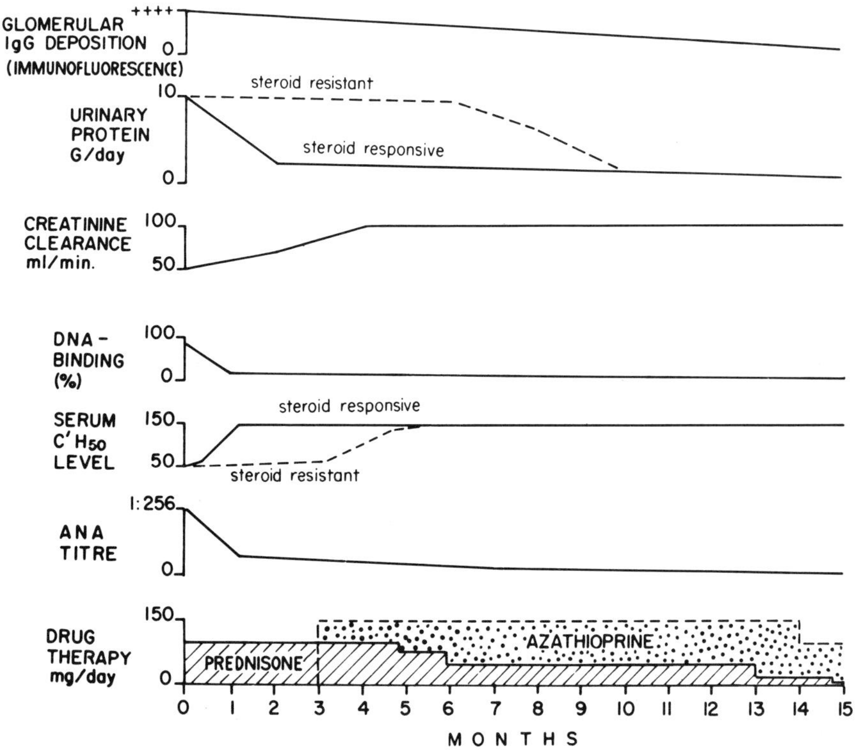

Figure 4.6. Composite chart depicting useful laboratory indices in a patient with lupus nephritis, and their alteration with treatment. Note that the fall in ANA titre and DNA-binding, and the rise in serum complement may occur before obvious clinical improvement. Following commencement of azathioprine in a steroid-resistant patient the decrease in proteinuria may lag behind other indices of improvement by several months. The renal glomerular immunoglobulin deposition, although only a semiquantitative index, usually shows definite reduction by 12 months. In most cases steroid-resistant and steroid-responsive disease indicates diffuse and focal glomerulonephritis respectively.

may be masked by increased complement production. Consequently, normal serum complement levels may occasionally mask active immune complex deposition, including serious lupus nephritis.

Immunofluorescent tests

Kidney. One of the major manifestations of SLE is a proliferative glomerulonephritis. A characteristic feature of the glomerular lesion is the deposition of immune complexes on the capillary endothelial basement membrane. The composition of the complexes has been carefully studied and

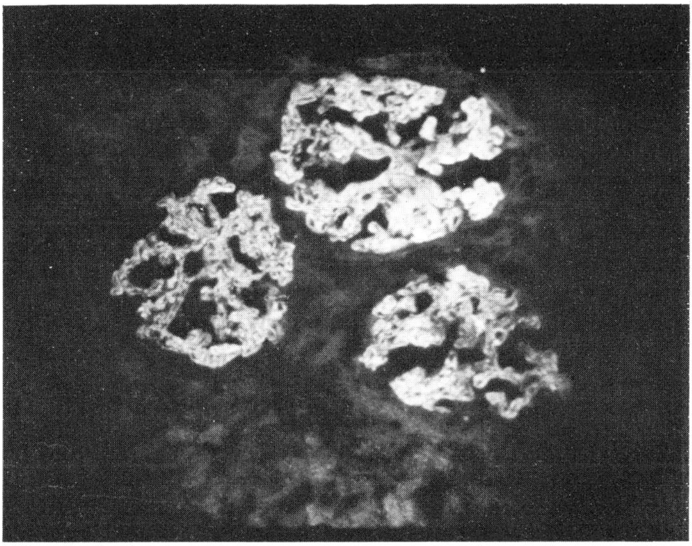

(a)

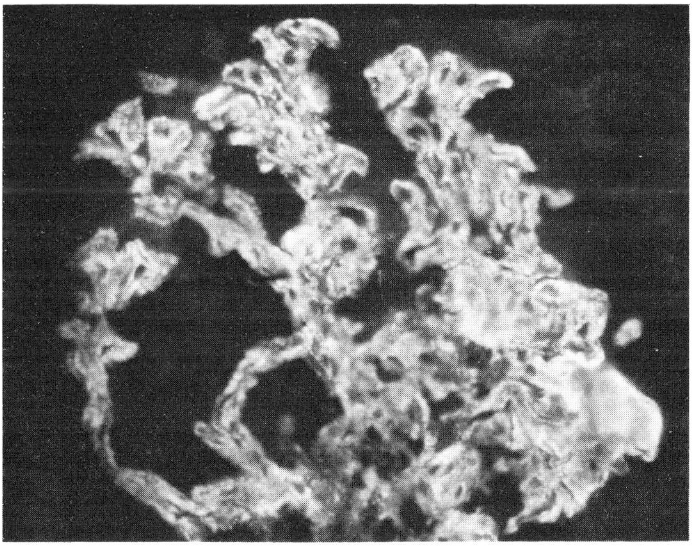

(b)

Figure 4.7. Renal biopsy from patient with SLE stained with fluoroscein-conjugated antiserum to (a) human C3 (× 125), and (b) human IgG (× 500). Note the widespread and irregular deposition of complement within all the glomeruli, and the 'lumpy-bumpy' appearance of IgG deposition on the glomerular basement membrane.

shown to contain native DNA antigen, IgG (with ANA activity) and complement (Koffler and Kunkel, 1968). In addition, IgM rheumatoid factor may be present in the complex, presumably secondary to the denatured IgG.

For routine diagnostic immunopathology, fresh-frozen renal tissue is studied by direct immunofluorescence using fluorescein-conjugated antiserum to IgG or C3. Deposition of gamma globulin or complement within the glomerular tufts together with the precise site and pattern of fluorescence may be evident (Figure 4.7). The presence of IgG and C3, or occasionally C3 alone, on the glomerular endothelial basement membrane is thought to indicate renal immune complex disease in vivo. Characteristically, the immune deposits of SLE appear as irregular, granular or nodular fluorescent clumps widespread along the basement membranes—the 'lumpy-bumpy' appearance of lupus nephritis (Koffler, Schur and Kunkel, 1967). However, linear deposits may sometimes be seen. Immunofluorescent examination appears to be quite a sensitive test of disease activity revealing significant glomerular immune

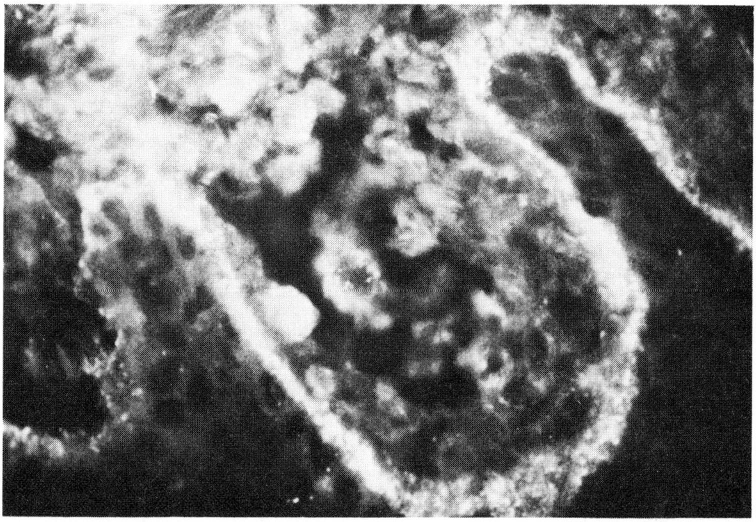

Figure 4.8. Skin biopsy from patient with systemic lupus, stained with fluoroscein-conjugated antiserum to human IgG (× 405). Note the linear band of IgG deposited along the dermal-epidermal junction.

complex deposition in some patients with mild clinical manifestations. Like most immunofluorescent techniques its interpretation requires considerable experience.

Skin. The detection of immune complex components at the dermal-epidermal junctional zone of the skin provides another interesting diagnostic test in patients with suspected SLE (Burnham and Fine, 1971). If a biopsy from an active lupus skin lesion is examined by immunofluorescence an uneven band of immunoglobulin (mainly IgG and IgM) can be identified in the immediate subepidermal zone adjacent to the basal cells (Figure 4.8). Complement components can similarly be identified, suggesting the presence of immune complexes like those seen in lupus nephritis. The subepidermal localisation of gamma globulin is fairly specific, and has so far been described in SLE, discoid lupus and bullous pemphigoid. Further, it is detected in the clinically uninvolved skin of some patients with SLE, but not discoid lupus, whether or not the patient has an active lupus rash elsewhere. Thus, skin immunofluorescence provides useful diagnostic data in patients with early disease and helps to distinguish between the cutaneous lesion of systemic and discoid lupus. Like all tissue immunofluorescence, care must be taken with non-specific staining. Finally, the real specificity and significance of dermal-epidermal junction immune deposits awaits further clarification.

Cryoglobulins

Cryoproteins are plasma proteins that precipitate in the cold (Ritzmann and Levin, 1961). Cold precipitable fibrinogen (cryofibrinogen) may be detected if plasma is allowed to stand at 4°C for 24 hours. This appears to be a common physical phenomenon in normal plasma, although in some instances cryofibrinogens may be disease-associated. Serum cryoglobulins may be detected if serum from blood, drawn and separated at 37°C, is allowed to stand at 4°C for 24 to 48 hours; on rewarming the serum the cryoprecipitate redissolves. The amount of cryoglobulin in a specimen is expressed as the cryocrit. This is best measured as the percentage volume of cryoglobulin precipitated from a tube of whole serum after standing for 42 to 72 hours at 4°C. The cryoglobulin consists of an identifiable immunoglobulin or a mixture of immunoglobulins ('mixed cryoglobulins') and can be characterised in agar gel immunodiffusion or immunoelectrophoresis conducted in the warm.

Cryoglobulinaemia may be associated with many different diseases, notably paraproteinaemia (where the cryoglobulin usually consists entirely of monoclonal immunoglobulin), acute viral infections such as infectious mononucleosis, and chronic infections such as syphilis and leprosy. Small amounts of serum cryoglobulin containing IgG and IgM antiglobulin are a fairly frequent finding in active SLE (Barnett et al, 1970). Moreover, these mixed cryoglobulins frequently contain DNA and complement components. Hence, they appear to represent a cold-insoluble immune complex and, as such, may reflect the circulating and tissue-deposited immune complexes thought to play a pathogenic role in SLE.

Lupus-like Syndromes

Drug-induced lupus

It is known that exposure of some individuals to certain drugs results in, or uncovers a predisposition to, a syndrome clinically identical to SLE—'drug-induced lupus'. The best recognised of the many drugs associated with this syndrome are hydrallazine and procainamide (Alarcon-Segovia, 1969). The serological changes accompanying the illness may be similar to those in spontaneous SLE, although evidence for an immune complex-mediated nephritis is most unusual and increased DNA-binding or profound lowering of serum complement is rarely found. Usually the clinical manifestations of the illness regress following withdrawal of the precipitating agent. However, the positive ANA may persist for up to two years after drug withdrawal and complete clinical remission. It should also be remembered that a drug-related partial lupus-like syndrome may manifest solely as a positive ANA test.

Essential (mixed) cryoglobulinaemia

This disease is characterised by arthritis, purpura, vasculitis and glomerulonephritis in the presence of gross cryoglobulinaemia (Figure 4.9), with cryocrits of up to 50 per cent being recorded (Meltzer and Franklin, 1966). The mixed nature of the cryoglobulin complex—polyclonal IgG with monoclonal IgM antiglobulin (i.e. IgM rheumatoid factor)—would appear to reflect the presence of an immune complex disease in vivo. Further, DNA and

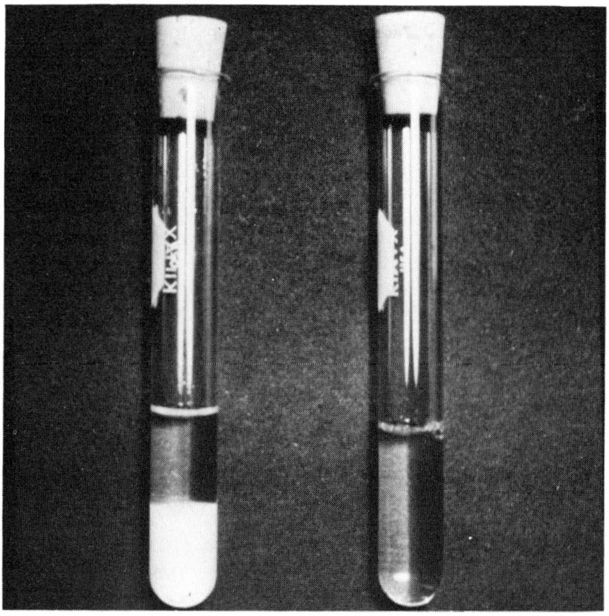

Patient Normal

Figure 4.9. Serum from a patient with recurrent skin purpura, lymphadenopathy and arthralgia who later developed immunofluorescent-positive glomerulonephritis. The cryocrit of 50 per cent was apparent after standing his serum for 48 hours at 4°C. Immunodiffusion analysis of the cryoglobulin precipitate revealed monoclonal IgM antiglobulin, IgG and C3.

complement components have been demonstrated in the cryoglobulin complex. These patients have high rheumatoid factor titres and may have positive ANA tests. Like patients with active SLE their serum complement levels may be depressed, DNA-binding is increased and sparse renal biopsy studies suggest the presence of immune complexes on the glomerular endothelial basement membrane. Hence, in many ways, this illness resembles SLE and may in fact result from similar, if not identical, pathogenetic mechanisms. In treating the disease the absolute cryocrit, autoantibody titres and complement levels appear to be useful indicators of in vivo tissue damage.

Viral hepatitis arthritis

With the increasing incidence and better recognition of serum hepatitis it is now clear that a transient polyarthritis may precede, and occasionally accompany, the icteric phase of the disease (Alpert, Isselbacher and Schur, 1971). Most patients with hepatitis-associated arthritis are seronegative with respect to rheumatoid factor and ANA. However, in some patients the temporal relationship between the synovitis, Australia antigenaemia, circulating antibody to Australia antigen and decreased complement levels (both in serum and synovial fluid), suggests an immune-mediated mechanism for the arthritis. Hence, the arthritis has been observed during the period of Australia antigen excess (preicteric phase) and has subsided with the appearance of demonstrable antibody (icteric phase). However, not all patients with hepatitis-associated arthritis are Australia antigen positive and some have normal complement levels. Moreover, demonstration of Australia antigen complexed to antibody and fixing complement within the inflamed synovial membrane has not yet been proven. Nevertheless, the suggestive evidence for Australia antigen–antibody complex-mediated synovial inflammation is attractive.

Chronic active hepatitis ('lupoid hepatitis')

The serological alterations characterising SLE are frequently present in patients with chronic active hepatitis (Mackay, 1968). Thus, extreme hypergammaglobulinaemia, LE cells, ANA and antiglobulins commonly accompany this chronic hepatic disease. Moreover, the preponderance of chronic active hepatitis in young women often associated with fever, polyarthritis and a therapeutic response to corticosteroids or immunosuppressives, has suggested a link between SLE and the hepatic disease. However, many other features of chronic active hepatitis indicate that the disease is best considered a primary hepatic disorder and not a variant of the rheumatic diseases.

Lupus Variants

Systemic sclerosis (scleroderma)

In contrast to SLE there is but scanty evidence of an immune pathogenesis underlying systemic sclerosis (SS). Nonetheless, patients with this disorder frequently demonstrate aberrations of humoral immunity. Furthermore, clinical features may develop in certain patients which make the absolute differentiation of SS from SLE quite difficult, if not impossible (Dubois et al, 1971).

Hypergammaglobulinaemia due to modest elevations of serum immunoglobulin levels is sometimes seen in patients with SS. Antinuclear antibodies, usually of IgG class, are detected in 40 to 70 per cent of such patients, often producing a speckled pattern of nuclear fluorescence. Nucleolar immunofluorescence is seen in some patients with SS especially when associated with Sjögren's syndrome. Despite the presence of high-titre ANA, DNA-binding is reputed to be normal. Positive LE cell tests are less frequent, with a reported incidence of about 5 per cent in patients with well-defined SS. Rheumatoid factor is present in about 40 per cent of patients although high titres are unusual. False-positive serological tests for syphilis are sometimes found and Coombs-positive haemolytic anaemia has been reported. The detection of serum antimitochondrial antibodies in about 8 per cent of patients with SS (compared to 0·5 per cent in normal control subjects) is of interest. This antibody might indicate autoimmune liver disease, and the coexistence of SS with primary biliary cirrhosis has been noted. In summary, serological abnormalities more typical of SLE or severe rheumatoid arthritis may accompany classical SS.

However, only rarely will clinical features more suggestive of a lupus or rheumatoid-like syndrome lead to diagnostic difficulties. Moreover, the immunological abnormalities in SS rarely indicate the presence of in vivo immune complex deposition. Thus, immunofluorescent studies on skin and kidney are, in the main, unrevealing; and serum complement levels are normal. Consequently, the development of glomerular basement membrane immune complex deposition, low serum complement and increased DNA-binding in a patient previously thought to have atypical SS, might indicate an SLE-like illness and greatly influence therapy and prognosis.

Polymyositis (dermatomyositis)

There is growing experimental evidence to suggest that polymyositis (with or without skin involvement) is a cell-mediated immune disease (Currie et al, 1971). However, the clinical investigation of this disorder reveals little in the way of diagnostic humoral immune features. Non-specific findings in some patients include elevated serum gamma globulin levels together with rheumatoid factor and ANA. Circulating antimyosin antibodies would appear to be relatively non-specific and their demonstration at present is best regarded as a research procedure. Occasionally other well-defined connective tissue diseases such as SLE or SS may feature severe muscle involvement. In such patients the immunological investigations reflect the underlying disorder.

Polyarteritis

The pathogenesis of acute polyarteritis is a complete mystery. Although immune complex deposition has been proposed as the cause of vasculitis in serum sickness, rheumatoid arthritis and SLE, there is little evidence to suggest a similar mechanism in patients with idiopathic polyarteritis in its many and various forms. Hence, the clinical immunology of this disease is largely undefined although rheumatoid factor or ANA may be demonstrated in a variable percentage of patients. Of great current interest is the finding of Australia antigenaemia in some patients with classical polyarteritis nodosa. In some, the antigen has been localised by immunofluorescence within the vascular lesion. However, this is by no means a universal relationship and certainly does not yet rank as a realistic diagnostic test.

Adult Rheumatoid Arthritis

There are no pathognomonic serological features of rheumatoid arthritis (RA). However, various well-defined immunological events in the serum and synovial space frequently characterise the disease and may be helpful in differential diagnosis.

Serum immunoglobulin levels may be elevated although extreme elevations of IgG or IgM are unusual. Paraproteinaemia, with a monoclonal immunoglobulin evident on serum electrophoresis, is never a usual feature of RA, and excess urinary free light-chains are polyclonal in type. Occasionally, however, so much serum antiglobulin may be present that circulating macromolecular immune aggregates form resulting in a hyperviscosity syndrome similar to that characterising advanced Waldenström's disease. Since the synovial fluid in RA is an exudate, it contains significant amounts of plasma proteins, including gamma globulins. Rarely, however, do synovial immunoglobulin levels match the serum values. Occasionally, patients with congenital agammaglobulinaemia or familial absence of serum IgA develop RA. In such patients the profound immunoglobulin deficiency usually persists, despite the development of the rheumatoid state.

Rheumatoid factor

Tests for rheumatoid factor (RF) provide some of the most useful and widely-used investigations in patients with acute or chronic arthritis (Rheumatoid Factors: Conference Proceedings, 1969). Basically, RF is a circulating

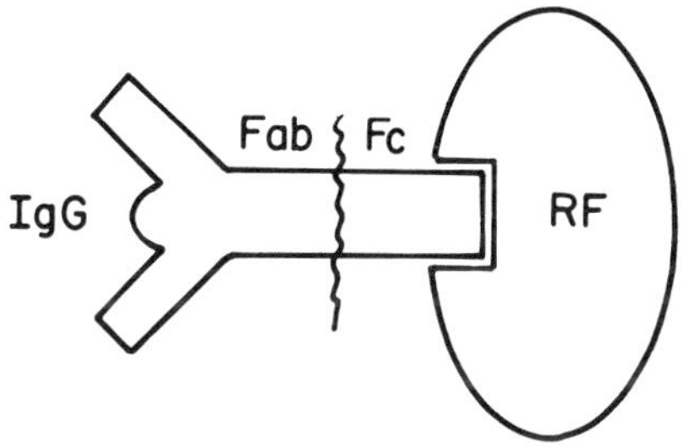

Figure 4.10. Schematic representation of rheumatoid factor interaction with IgG. The IgG antigenic sites (human or rabbit) reside on the Fc portion of the molecule. The rheumatoid factor is usually IgM but may be IgG, IgA or low-molecular weight (7S) IgM.

autoantibody directed against the Fc fragment of the patient's own IgG, i.e. an 'antiglobulin' (Figure 4.10). Invariably, RF specificity is not limited to autologous IgG but reacts with homologous, and frequently heterologous, antigen. Most detectable RF reacts with IgG in vitro only when the antigen is denatured and a similar prerequisite is thought to operate in vivo. However, the sera and synovial fluid of some patients with RA contain antiglobulin which appears to be directed mainly against native (undenatured) IgG.

The pathogenic significance of RF is unknown and its biological role as a by-product or mediator of disease is speculative (Hollander and Rawson, 1968). Whether or not the in vivo reaction of this autoantibody with its antigen can generate immune complex-mediated tissue damage is unclear. Indeed, RF production may be an entirely secondary event, subsequent to a prolonged immune stimulus and generated only after local tissue damage alters host IgG rendering it autoantigenic. Nevertheless, regardless of its actual role in the disease process, RF can be detected in the serum and synovial fluid of most patients with RA.

RF is usually an IgM class of antibody. However, it is evident that antiglobulin activity can reside in other immunoglobulin classes. Thus, IgG and IgA molecules may possess RF activity with typical antibody specificity for denatured IgG. Further, another type of RF—possessing most of the chemical properties of conventional heavy molecular weight serum IgM but having qualitative ultracentrifugal characteristics typifying the lighter molecular weight immunoglobulins (7S IgM)—has been identified. Hence, in any individual, RF may consist of a population of antiglobulin molecules heterogeneous with respect to class, molecular weight, avidity and specificity. Notwithstanding, for most practical clinical purposes in vitro assays are used

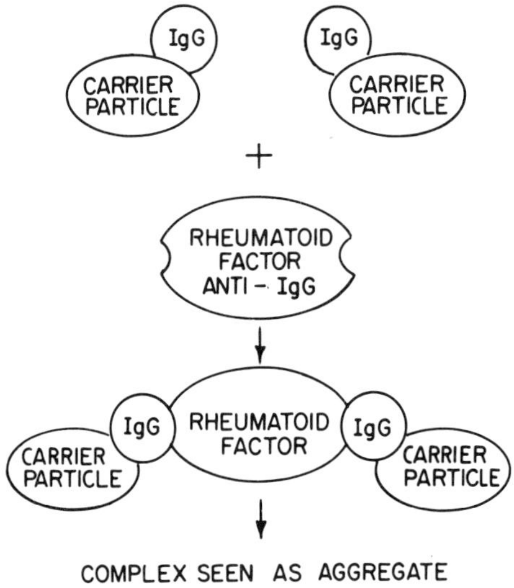

Figure 4.11. Schematic representation of a rheumatoid factor assay. The carrier particle may be latex or bentonite particles, fresh or tanned sheep red blood cells, or human group O positive red cells. The IgG antigen may be human or rabbit protein, grossly or minimally denatured. The attachment of IgG to the carrier particle may be non-specific (physico-chemical) or specific (immunological). The IgG-coated particle alone appears as a fine suspension; when reacted with rheumatoid factor macroscopic particle aggregation or agglutination ensues.

which detect IgM antiglobulins reactive with denatured human or rabbit IgG. The detection of RF activity residing in other immunoglobulin classes or reactive only with native homologous IgG, remains a useful research procedure.

All the conventional assay systems employ human or rabbit IgG antigen attached to a macroscopically visible carrier particle (Vaughan, 1966). Reaction between an added RF—present in the biological sample being tested—and the IgG antigen results in flocculation, then aggregation or agglutination of the carrier particle (Figure 4.11). This flocculation can be seen with the naked eye and/or a hand lens. By employing serial dilutions of the sample being tested (e.g. undiluted serum, the serum diluted in saline 1:1, 1:2, 1:4, 1:8, etc.) the weakest dilution containing enough antiglobulin to precipitate the antigen-coated carrier particle can be detected, and gives the 'RF titre.' The greatest dilution of sample associated with visible flocculation (i.e. the highest recordable titre) depends to some extent on the assay system used. Therefore, interpretation of the RF titre in a particular patient requires some knowledge of the specificity and sensitivity of the assay used.

The simplest and most widely used assay utilises latex or bentonite particles as the inert carrier—latex or bentonite fixation tests (Singer and Plotz, 1956). These are obtainable coated with heat-denatured (aggregated) human IgG extracted from pooled normal human sera. The IgG-coated particles can be used at a high concentration on a glass slide ('slide-latex test'), in the wells of a microtitre plate ('microtitre test'), or in a test tube ('tube-latex test'). When the coated particles are suspended in buffer they are finely dispersed and, if left undisturbed, precipitate as a clean 'button'. The addition of normal serum at any dilution followed by incubation at 37°C should not alter this. However, if the added serum contains RF, the particles are aggregated. This aggregation can usually be identified as flocculation within an hour although the clear end-point of aggregation (and thus the titre) may not be ascertained until 12 hours.

Some assay systems utilise a biological carrier rather than inert particles. The tanned sheep red cell is one such example (Zutshi et al, 1969). Tanning of red cells results in a surface onto which protein antigens will attach. When coated with Cohn's fraction II (salt-extracted human IgG) they serve as a useful indicator of RF activity. The tanned sheep cell test can conveniently be run in test tubes or on microtitre plates, the presence of RF resulting in visible red cell agglutination.

In the RF assays described above the IgG antigen is passively coated onto the carrier particle and, in the case of the latex test, the antigen is highly denatured. Other assays are available where the IgG antigen is itself an antibody directed against the surface of the carrier particle—in this case a sheep or human red cell. The red cell coated by specific IgG antibody is then used as the indicator system for detecting antiglobulin. Under such circumstances the IgG on the cell surface is relatively undenatured ('native') antigen. In fact, some degree of IgG denaturation would appear inevitable following its reaction with specific cell surface sites. This principle is exemplified in the sensitised sheep cell agglutination test which uses fresh sheep red blood cells as the carrier for rabbit IgG in a test tube or microtitre plate system. The washed cells are coated with antigen by the addition of rabbit IgG anti-sheep red cell antiserum (Haemolysin). The diluted IgG antiserum sensitises, but does not agglutinate the red cells. Once coated, the sheep cells provide a very sensitive marker for RF reactive with heterologous IgG. Normal individuals may have naturally occurring antibody reactive with sheep red cell coat antigens (heterophile antibodies). Therefore, in any test using sensitised sheep red cells as the carrier particle, it is essential to include as a control unsensitised cells—if necessary with all dilutions of the serum being tested. The difference between the highest dilution of serum agglutinating the sensitised cells and that agglutinating unsensitised cells (i.e. the heterophile titre) provides the end-result differential RF titre.

The 'Ripley agglutination test' is another useful assay which utilises a biological carrier particle. The test is named after Mr Ripley, a patient of Dr Marion V. Waller (Richmond, Va., USA), whose serum contains specific, high titre, incomplete IgG antibodies to the Rhesus antigen (CD antigen). Human type-O positive erythrocytes can be coated with the anti-CD IgG antibody without agglutinating them. This provides a system for detecting RF reactive with homologous, relatively 'native' (undenatured) IgG antigen. This test is best performed in small tubes where an immediate settling of agglutinated cells indicates the presence of RF.

Certain precautions must be observed in conducting and interpreting any RF assay. The biological sample being tested should be heat-inactivated at 56°C for 30 minutes to destroy complement and various other inhibitors. Failure to do this results in a disproportionately high number of false-positive latex fixation tests as well as promoting undue lysis of sheep cells. When testing synovial fluid it is helpful to pre-digest the sample with hyaluronidase. This reduces viscosity thereby lessening the likelihood of false-positive results. Conversely, the presence of synovial fluid hyaluronic acid may inhibit the detection of RF using the latex agglutination test. All assay systems should be standardised with a known negative control serum and a pool of high-titre positive sera kept stored at −20°C.

A serum may contain large amounts of RF yet give negative assay results when tested undiluted, reactivity with IgG antigen only being evident when the sample is tested at low concentrations. It follows that, unless the test system includes low concentrations of serum, antiglobulin activity may be missed. This is called the prozone phenomenon and is probably due to gross antibody excess. Similarly, gross IgG excess within the sample being tested may inhibit RF reactivity with the carrier particle IgG, resulting in inappropriately low titres. Various other mechanisms, including tightly bound RF–IgG complexes within the serum, may similarly lead to false-negative results.

All antiglobulin assays have varying degrees of sensitivities and specificities. In general, tests employing human IgG antigen (latex or bentonite fixation, tanned sheep cell test, Ripley agglutination test) are more sensitive, but rather less specific for rheumatoid arthritis. Tests employing heterologous IgG antigen (senitised sheep cell test) are somewhat less sensitive but rather more specific, with fewer false-positive results in normal subjects (Ziff, 1957). In all of the assays there is a wide margin of error and variability related mainly to reading the precise end-point of agglutination. Thus, alteration of RF titre cannot be considered significant unless there is a change by at least several dilutions. Moreover, low titre positive results can be obtained with normal sera. For this reason, each laboratory has a cut-off titre for their assays above which dilution titres are considered significant.

Rheumatoid factor may be detected in normal individuals as well as in those suffering from various chronic diseases. The highly sensitive, less specific, latex agglutination test is positive in up to 5 per cent of normal subjects over 60 years of age. However, high titre latex or sheep cell tests are unusual in normal subjects.

Patients with chronic infectious diseases (e.g. tuberculosis, leprosy, syphilis, leishmaniasis) frequently have high titre RF, which is often reactive only with human IgG. An interesting example of this association is seen in patients with subacute bacterial endocarditis. In that disease the antiglobulin could conceivably neutralise IgG opsonins. This might result in defective polymorph killing of bacteria in vivo thereby perpetuating chronic infection. Another remarkable association of RF and chronic infection is seen in malarious zones where the presence of IgM antiglobulins with specificity for human IgG is associated with IgM antimalarial antibodies.

IgM rheumatoid factor can be detected at some time in the serum of 70 to 80 per cent of all patients with RA; and, once present, it usually remains for the duration of the disease. Using specialised techniques IgG antiglobulins may be detected in many apparently seronegative patients. Further, the synovial fluid of seropositive patients nearly always contains detectable RF, although a prozone phenomenon appears to be common in tests utilising human IgG antigen and appears to be related to the presence of hyaluronic acid. Although the titre of serum RF usually exceeds that in synovial fluid, the converse may occur (Bland and Clark, 1963). Indeed, synovial fluid RF may be detected early in the disease course of patients with seronegative RA. The localisation of RF at the main site of the disease—the synovial cavity—is not surprising since, even in rheumatoid patients with negative tests on serum and synovial fluid, antiglobulin may be eluted from the excised synovial membrane. Lastly, the detection of high titre RF in a pleural or pericardial effusion is suggestive of mesenchymal rheumatoid disease.

The presence and amount of circulating rheumatoid factor correlates to some extent with disease activity and prognosis (Mongan et al, 1969). This correlation is only approximate; some seronegative patients may have widespread and disabling arthritis, and some high titre seropositive patients may manifest mild or quiescent disease. Nonetheless, the extra-articular manifestations of RA such as nodules, vasculitis, neuropathy, pleurisy and pericarditis, are almost invariably associated with marked seropositivity. Indeed, it is almost axiomatic that patients with rheumatoid nodules are seropositive. Accordingly, disease remissions and exacerbations may be reflected in RF titre. Thus, although not a highly sensitive index of disease activity, the RF titre is helpful in monitoring the therapeutic response to gold, penicillamine, steroids and immunosuppressive agents.

Pepsin agglutinators

Some antiglobulins react specifically with human type-O positive red cells sensitised by pepsin-treated anti-CD antibody (i.e. enzyme-fragmented IgG). This curious phenomenon might reflect a biological role for RF—the reaction with antibody fragments thereby facilitating their clearance by the reticulo-endothelial system. Pepsin agglutinators are not particularly characteristic of rheumatoid arthritis, but their presence in serum is described in patients with various connective tissue and chronic infectious diseases.

Other immune aberrations in rheumatoid arthritis

About 10 per cent of patients with classical RA have positive serum and/or synovial fluid LE cells and ANA tests (Condemi et al, 1965). Usually these patients have longstanding severe RA, many extra-articular manifestations of their disease and high titres of antiglobulins. The ANA found in rheumatoid disease appears to differ in some respects from that found in SLE, e.g. it is a relatively poor fixer of complement in vitro. Only occasionally is ANA detected in patients with early, non-erosive RA and under such circumstances consists mainly of IgM antibody. Frequently the synovial fluid may be positive for ANA and the serum negative. Indeed, depending on the sensitivity of the assay and the substrate used, up to 50 per cent of rheumatoid synovial fluids contain leucocyte-specific ANA. However, unless other cardinal features of SLE develop, the diagnosis and management of RA should not be influenced by the presence of ANA. Although only limited data are thus far available, DNA-binding appears to be normal in patients with RA, even when the ANA and LE cell tests are positive.

The role of complement in RA is unclear. Recent observations, including immunofluorescent detection of synovial membrane complement deposits, strongly suggest that increased complement consumption occurs specifically at the site of the inflammatory lesion. This is manifest as a marked reduction of synovial fluid total haemolytic (C H_{50}) and third component of complement (C3) levels, in sharp contrast to the overall increase of other plasma proteins within the inflammatory synovial exudate (Ruddy and Austen, 1970). Moreover, increased amounts of synovial fluid complement degradation products frequently accompany the lowered complement levels (Ward and Zvaifler, 1971). In contrast to synovial fluid, serum complement levels are normal or only slightly diminished in RA. The lower levels are found in patients with severe seropositive disease and vasculitis. Generally, serum complement levels tend to be lower in seropositive than in seronegative patients, although still within the normal range in most. Thus, a profound selective lowering of synovial fluid complement in the presence of a normal or mildly diminished serum level is a diagnostic feature of seropositive RA. Patients with milder seronegative disease may have normal or only slightly lowered synovial fluid complement levels. In that situation the investigation is less helpful in differential diagnosis. Lastly, the sharply reduced synovial complement levels accompanying crystal-induced or infective arthritis should be readily distinguished from RA by the identification of the offending crystal or microorganism.

Cryoglobulins are also sometimes present in rheumatoid synovial fluid. Their detection and characterisation is the same as for serum cryoproteins (see page 107). They are usually of the mixed type (IgG:IgM) and their components may selectively possess high titre RF and ANA activity.

Felty's syndrome

Although only about one per cent of patients with RA develop Felty's syndrome, the accompanying serological changes deserve comment (Louie and Pearson, 1971). These patients frequently have elevated serum immunoglobulin levels and, almost always, high titre RF. Antinuclear antibody (of IgG, IgA and IgM class) is usual, producing predominantly nuclear-rim immunofluorescent staining. There is some indication that the ANA in Felty's syndrome is leucocyte-specific and perhaps contributes to the leucopenia. However, there is no direct correlation between ANA titre and the degree of leucopenia; nor does the ANA fix complement in vitro (in contrast to the ANA typifying SLE). Lastly, serum complement levels are usually normal.

Sjögren's syndrome

Sjögren's syndrome may present as an idiopathic sicca complex (keratoconjunctivitis and xerostomia) or as part of a clearly defined connective tissue disease (Shearn, 1971). In either event, serological abnormalities are frequent usually in the form of hypergammaglobulinaemia, RF and ANA. In addition, serum antibodies reactive with salivary duct epithelium are demonstrable at some time in about 50 per cent of patients with this syndrome. This characteristic IgG or IgM organ-specific autoantibody is detected by indirect immunofluorescence using human salivary duct as the tissue substrate. Only about 20 per cent of patients with lone sicca complex have detectable antibody to salivary duct epithelium. In contrast, most patients with Sjögren's syndrome accompanying RA have the autoantibody. However, the antibody may not be a specific marker of salivary gland disease since it is present in patients with RA without overt Sjögren's syndrome. This observation might be explained by the fact that certain patients with RA have latent salivary gland involvement. Finally, antimitochondrial antibodies have been reported in about 8 per cent of patients with Sjögren's syndrome (see Systemic Sclerosis).

Juvenile rheumatoid arthritis

All of the immunological abnormalities accompanying adult-onset RA may be found in children with juvenile rheumatoid arthritis (JRA, Still's disease). The main difference is quantitative (Bluestone et al, 1970). Children with JRA have a much lower incidence of humoral aberrations than do adults with comparable disease. Mild elevations of serum immunoglobulin levels are found in about 25 per cent of patients with JRA and correlate with the presence of hip involvement and lymphadenopathy. Of interest is the detection of selective IgA deficiency in about 2 per cent of children with this disease. Whether the incidence of this selective immune deficiency occurs with greater frequency in association with JRA than by chance alone is not yet clear.

Only 15 to 20 per cent of patients with JRA with disease onset before five years of age have conventional serum RF. The incidence of antiglobulins is higher in children with later onset of disease but is still only about 15 to 30 per cent. Indeed, even patients with JRA and rheumatoid nodules are sometimes seronegative by all conventional tests. However, IgG antiglobulins have been demonstrated using specialised techniques in many patients with JRA (Torrigiani et al, 1969). As in adults there is a broad correlation between severity of JRA and seropositivity, particularly with respect to hip involvement and functional status. Antinuclear antibody is detected in only about 5 per cent of patients and, in contrast to the adult disease, does not appear to indicate widespread extra-articular manifestations. Marked selective lowering of synovial fluid complement is as prevalent in seropositive JRA as in adult RA.

Rheumatoid Variants

Certain diseases display many of the clinical and pathological features of rheumatoid synovitis yet clearly are different, and can be distinguished from, classical RA. Ankylosing spondylitis, although predominantly a disease of joints and connective tissue, is distinguishable on epidemiological and clinical grounds. Psoriasis and chronic inflammatory bowel disease (ulcerative colitis, regional enteritis, Whipple's disease) may be associated with a recurrent or chronic polyarthritis. Reiter's syndrome sometimes fails to resolve completely and may evolve as a chronic destructive polyarthritis. All of these diseases can conveniently be referred to as 'rheumatoid variants' without necessarily implying a common aetiology. Appropriate laboratory investigation may usefully supplement the clinical differentiation of these forms of polyarthritis.

Occasionally early or atypical clinical presentation may suggest RA. It is therefore important to note that the rheumatoid variants are almost always seronegative using conventional antiglobulin assays. Even using more sensitive research procedures the detection of serum or synovial fluid antiglobulins in these miscellaneous diseases is unusual. However, elevated levels of serum IgG antiglobulins have been reported in patients with ankylosing spondylitis and psoriatic arthropathy. The method used for demonstrating these antiglobulins and the results obtained await verification (Tapanes, Rawson and Hollander, 1972). Of course, psoriasis and RA are both common diseases and may coexist. In such patients, however, the clinical joint disease is more typical of classical RA including the presence of subcutaneous nodules and high titre RF. Other serum immune aberrations such as antibodies to cell nuclear constituents (ANA, LE cells, increased DNA-binding), false-positive biological tests for syphilis and depressed complement levels, appear to be unusual in the rheumatoid variants. Relatively little data is available on the synovial fluid complement levels in these diseases; most reports indicate levels close to or only slightly less than the simultaneous serum value (Townes and Sowa, 1970). This contrasts strikingly to the low synovial fluid complement levels found in RA and SLE. Conversely, serum complement levels appear to be somewhat increased in patients with Reiter's syndrome, and elevated synovial fluid levels are found both in patients with Reiter's syndrome and ankylosing spondylitis.

Recent observations from several independent sources have revealed a remarkably high association between the histocompatibility cell surface antigen (HL-A) W27 and ankylosing spondylitis (Schlosstein et al, 1973; Brewerton et al, 1973a). This haplotype is found in about 8 per cent of normal Caucasian populations but is present in over 90 per cent of patients with ankylosing spondylitis. The transplantation antigens are detected by a microdroplet lymphocyte cytotoxicity test using specific antisera from patients with multiple transfusions or pregnancies (Mittal et al, 1968). Most transplantation (i.e., tissue-typing) centres can thereby identify about 26 specificities, most individual haplotypes consisting of two pairs of antigens, each pair governed by a distinct chromosomal locus. This remarkable association has now been extended to Reiter's syndrome (with or without spondylitis) where the incidence of W27 is about 95 per cent (Brewerton et al, 1973b; Morris et al, 1974). The explanation for the strikingly increased incidence of W27 in patients with ankylosing spondylitis and Reiter's syndrome is unknown. However, the observation is proving of real clinical value. Thus, the presence of a W27 haplotype in a young man with low back pain, an elevated sedimentation rate but normal sacroiliac radiographs might strongly suggest a diagnosis of ankylosing spondylitis (especially in the presence of a positive family history). Likewise, the presence of W27 in a young man with a culture-negative urethral discharge and arthritis might help differentiate between acute gonococcal arthritis and Reiter's syndrome. Histocompatibility testing can be rapidly performed by most tissue-typing centres and requires heparinised blood which can, if necessary, withstand storage or mailing for several days.

Sarcoidosis (Gumpel, Johns and Shulman, 1967) may feature acute or chronic polyarthritis which superficially mimics RA. About 40 per cent of these patients are seropositive, although high titres of RF are unusual. Standard diagnostic procedures for sarcoidosis, including biopsy and histological studies, clarify the situation.

With the mass immunisation schedules for rubella prophylaxis, transient rubella synovitis is increasingly seen in teenagers and young adults (Lerman et al, 1971), as well as occurring in its naturally acquired form in young children. The viral arthopathy is usually associated with elevated titres of serum anti-rubella antibodies demonstrable by orthodox techniques (haemagglutination or complement fixation). Rarely do the serological stigmata of the connective tissue diseases appear.

Rheumatic Fever

During the last decade the problem of acute rheumatic fever has lessened considerably, although the disease is still endemic in certain regions in the world. Moreover, reactivation of the rheumatic process in adults with chronic rheumatic heart disease is an important and difficult diagnostic problem.

Acute rheumatic fever occurs as a sequel to infection by group A streptococcus (Stollerman et al, 1956). Experimental studies suggest a major role for immune-mediated mechanisms operative within the rheumatic lesions of the heart and other tissues (Kaplan and Rakita, 1971). Gamma globulin can be demonstrated bound to the tissue lesions and cross-antigenicity between streptococcal cell-wall polysaccharide antigen and heart muscle components appears to be important in this process. In particular, antistreptococcal wall antibodies cross-react with mammalian heart and valve glycoprotein in vitro and may well play a pathogenic role in vivo (Kaplan, 1963). Indeed, such antibodies can be detected by indirect immunofluorescence in the sera of some patients with acute rheumatism or chronic rheumatic valvulitis, manifest as sarcolemmal staining. Furthermore, patients with streptococcal infection do not develop acute rheumatism unless they generate an immune response to the organism. Hence, the magnitude of antistreptococcal antibody titres in a population correlates directly with the initial and recurrent rheumatic fever attack rate.

One of the major advances in the recognition of group A streptococcal infection has been a better understanding of the immune response to the organism, notably an appreciation of the antigenic extracellular bacterial products whose detection facilitates diagnosis (Feinstein, 1966). Previously, streptococcal throat infections could only be diagnosed by direct culture; this clearly suffered from several disadvantages. Firstly, the culture might be taken too late to give a positive result and, secondly, a positive culture does not necessarily prove systemic infection (Kaplan et al, 1971). Hence the importance of indirect tests to diagnose recent streptococcal infections. If used carefully, these indirect immunological tests provide a certain means of detecting recent infection (usually via the throat or skin) and constitute the most useful investigation in a patient suspected of having acute rheumatic fever. In addition, serial antibody studies provide a means of judging the effectiveness of antibiotic prophylaxis in patients where reinfection may well be asymptomatic.

Antistreptococcal antibodies

Antibody response to the polysaccharide cell-wall antigens of group A organisms certainly occurs, is type specific and may persist for many months after infection. Unfortunately, the detection of these important antibodies is difficult and awaits better standardised methods. The immune reaction to the extracellular proteins of the organism, although not group or type specific or as long-lasting, is easy to assay and provides a handy yardstick of antibody response. Proof of antistreptococcal antibody response usually requires sequential serum samples showing a change of titre. A single titre, whether high or low, may be unhelpful; serial samples must be compared in order to detect any titre change. This is important to remember since the diagnosis of acute rheumatic fever might depend heavily on proof of recent streptococcal infection, either as a very high antibody titre which later falls or as a proven rise in antibody titre. Thus, it is easier to exclude a diagnosis of acute rheumatism if all titres in sequential serum samples remain low.

There is a fairly broad spectrum of streptococcal extracellular antigens, the response to any one or combination of which might signify recent infection. The commonest antibody response is to the streptococcal toxin streptolysin O—so called because it is oxygen labile (Stollerman, 1967). The detection of antistreptolysin O antibody (ASO) is performed using dilutions of the patient's serum and adding a standard amount of streptolysin O antigen (Rantz and Randall, 1945). Following incubation red blood cells are added. In the absence of the antibody the available streptolysin haemolyses the red cells. However, if serum antibody to the streptolysin is present the bacterial haemolysin is neutralised and no haemolysis ensues. The antibody titre is then expressed as the reciprocal of the greatest serum dilution which completely neutralises the streptococcal haemolysin. A four fold rise in titre is fairly specific evidence of recent streptococcal infection, correlating closely with cervical adenitis, the exception being false-positive titres following *Clostridium welchii* immunisation. Todd originally used a standard antiserum which neutralised an arbitrary dose of haemolysin and, by convention, titres are expressed in Todd units. Normal school-going children rarely have levels greater than 200 Todd units.

About 20 per cent of streptococcal infections only evoke an antibody response to extracellular antigens other than streptolysin O. Thus, it is important to detect antibody titres to streptococcal hyaluronidase and deoxyribonuclease B (DNAse B) (Ayoub and Wannamaker, 1962). Only by screening sequential serum samples for a variety of antistreptococcal antibodies can one be sure of detecting a restricted immune response. Antistreptococcal hyaluronidase is detected by adding hyaluronidase to the patient's serum and then testing for the enzyme activity on its substrate (hyaluronic acid). The antibody titre is expressed as the highest dilution which completely inactivates the enzyme. Deoxyribonuclease B is one of four extracellular desoxyribonucleases produced by group A streptococci. Antibodies to this enzyme antigen are particularly evoked by streptococcal skin infection and are measured by assaying residual enzyme activity following incubation with the patient's serum. Levels greater than 250 units are detected in only about 20 per cent of the normal adult population.

In considering single-value antistreptococcal antibody titres it is apparent that the upper limit of normal varies with age. Both for ASO and antiDNAse B titres there is a peak 'background' titre during school age which presumably reflects greater endemic exposure to the organism and may somewhat mask a significant titre rise. However, a change in titre is still apparent (up or down) following recent systemic infection if sequential serum samples are tested, with maximal titres at about 21 days following infection. Antistreptococcal antibodies are always present in acute rheumatic fever if the disease is detected early enough, before the titres fall. This is true for both the initial attack and recurrences. Specifically, rheumatic fever polyarthritis is nearly always associated with high antibody titres which are most helpful in differential diagnosis. Thus, if raised antistreptococcal antibody titres are absent, rheumatic fever can virtually be excluded as a cause of a patient's polyarthritis. This is perhaps the most useful clinical application of measuring streptococcal antibodies in the differential diagnosis of acute polyarthritis. Conversely, in patients with lone carditis or chorea, titres may have long since declined and low titres are not so helpful. Once primed to streptococcal antigens—especially streptolysin O—a very brisk response is observed on reinfection, even in asymptomatic individuals. Therefore significant boosts in titre accompany even mild reinfection, the exception being in protected populations such as patients on prophylactic antibiotics.

Other immune aberrations

A few non-specific immunological abnormalities are recognised in acute rheumatism. Increased serum immunoglobulin levels have been described, in particular elevated IgA values. Normal or elevated total complement and C3 levels may accompany the acute stages of rheumatic fever, returning to normal with clinical remission. In some patients an inverse relationship between depressed complement levels and elevated ASO titres has been noted. More recently, the presence of lymphocytotoxins has been described in patients with the disease although antinuclear antibodies are rarely detected.

C-reactive protein (CRP)

This abnormal plasma protein is so named because of its coincidental precipitating reactivity with the C-polysaccharide of pneumococcal cell membrane (Sonnenwirth, 1963). CRP is released into the blood stream 6 to 24 hours after acute inflammation of any tissue, whether or not pneumococcal-induced. Hence its release follows bacterial infections, acute gouty arthritis, SLE, myocardial infarctions, surgical procedures, burn injuries and even some types of immunisations. It does not follow viral infections but is present in pregnancy and in patients with congestive cardiac failure. The detection of C-reactive protein in rheumatic fever is used both as a diagnostic test and as an indicator of disease activity. It is nearly always present in early, untreated rheumatic fever. However, it may not be truly indicative of disease activity since its presence may be perpetuated in clinically inactive cases, and its absence may coincide with continuing chronic rheumatic inflammation. Moreover, the CRP may disappear before the sedimentation rate falls following effective treatment. Clearly the presence of CRP lacks specificity; in particular it is present in about 75 per cent of patients with rheumatoid arthritis.

C-reactive protein is usually detected by means of a microprecipitation technique using specific rabbit antiserum. In this test the patient's serum is mixed with the antiserum in a capillary tube and any resulting macroscopic precipitation measured on a 0 to 4 scale. It is a very sensitive and rapid qualitative assay, a positive result sometimes being apparent within two hours. In contrast to the erythrocyte sedimentation rate, CRP can be detected in sterile stored serum. A latex particle agglutination test for CRP is also available, although this is probably not as sensitive as the capillary tube test.

References

Alarcon-Segovia, D. (1969) Drug-induced lupus syndromes. *Mayo Clinic Proceedings*, **44**, 664–681.

Alpert, E., Isselbacher, K. J. & Schur, P. H. (1971) The pathogenesis of arthritis associated with viral hepatitis. Complement-component studies. *New England Journal of Medicine*, **285**, 185–189.

Araujo, F. G., Barnett, E. V., Gentry, L. O. & Remington, J. S. (1971) False-positive anti-toxoplasma fluorescent-antibody tests in patients with antinuclear antibodies. *Applied Microbiology*, **22**, 270–275.

Ayoub, E. M. & Wannamaker, L. W. (1962) Evaluation of the streptococcal desoxyribonuclease B and diphosphopyridine nucleotidase antibody tests in acute rheumatic fever and acute glomerulonephritis. *Pediatrics*, **29**, 527–538.

Barnett, E. V., Bluestone, R., Kantor, G., Cracchiolo, A. & Goldberg, L. S. (1970) Cryoglobulinaemia and disease. *Annals of Internal Medicine*, **73**, 95–107.

Bland, J. H. & Clark, L. (1963) Rheumatoid factor in serum and synovial fluid. *Annals of Internal Medicine*, **58**, 829–836.

Bluestone, R., Katz, R., Marchessano, J., Calabro, J. & Goldberg, L. S. (1970) Juvenile arthritis: A serologic survey of 200 consecutive patients. *Journal of Pediatrics*, **77**, 98–102.

Boyle, J. & Buchanan, W. W. (eds) (1971) *Clinical Rheumatology*. Oxford: Blackwell Scientific.

Brewerton, D. A., Caffrey, M., Hart, F. D., James, D. C. O., Nicholls, A. & Sturrock, R. D. (1973a) Ankylosing spondylitis and HL-A 27. *Lancet*, **i**, 904–907.

Brewerton, D. A., Caffrey, M., Nicholls, A., Walters, D., Oates, J. K. & James, D. C. O. (1973b) Reiter's disease and HL-A 27. *Lancet*, **ii**, 996–998.

Burnham, T. K. & Fine, G. (1971) The immunofluorescent 'band' test for lupus erythematosus. III. Employing clinically normal skin. *Archives of Dermatology*, **103,** 24–32.

Christian, C. L. (1969) Immune-complex disease. *New England Journal of Medicine*, **280,** 878–884.

Cochrane, C. G. & Dixon, F. J. (1969) Cell and tissue damage through antigen–antibody complexes. *California Medicine*, **111,** 99–112.

Condemi, J. J., Barnett, E. V., Atwater, E. C., Jacox, R. F., Mongan, E. S. & Vaughan, J. H. (1965) The significance of antinuclear factors in rheumatoid arthritis. *Arthritis and Rheumatism*, **8,** 1080–1093.

Cooper, N. R., Polley, M. J. & Müller-Eberhard, H. J. (1971) Biology of complement. In *Immunological Diseases*, 2nd Edition, ed. Samter, M., Vol. 1, Sec. III, Ch. 16. Boston: Little, Brown.

Currie, S., Saunders, M., Knowles, M. & Brown, A. E. (1971) Immunological aspects of polymyositis. The in vitro activity of lymphocytes on incubation with muscle antigen and with muscle cultures. *Quarterly Journal of Medicine*, **40,** 63–84.

Dixon, F. J., Feldman, J. D. & Vazquez, J. J. (1961) Experimental glomerulonephritis. The pathogenesis of a laboratory model resembling the spectrum of human glomerulonephritis. *Journal of Experimental Medicine*, **113,** 899–919.

Dubois, E. L. (ed) (1966) *Lupus Erythematosus.* A Review of the current status of discoid and systemic lupus erythematosus and their variants. New York: McGraw-Hill.

Dubois, E. L., Chandor, S., Friou, G. J. & Bischel, M. (1971) Progressive systemic sclerosis (PSS) and localised scleroderma (morphea) with positive LE cell test and unusual systemic manifestations compatible with systemic lupus erythematosus (SLE): Presentation of 14 cases including one set of identical twins, one with scleroderma and the other with SLE. Review of the literature. *Medicine*, **50,** 199–222.

Feinstein, A. R. (1966) The natural histories of acute rheumatic fever. *Bulletin on the Rheumatic Diseases*, **17,** 423–428.

Friou, G. J. (1967) The LE cell factor and antinuclear antibodies. In *Laboratory Diagnostic Procedures in the Rheumatic Diseases*, ed. Cohen, A. S. pp. 114–167. Boston: Little, Brown.

Gumpel, J. M., Johns, C. J. & Shulman, L. E. (1967) The joint disease of sarcoidosis. *Annals of Rheumatic disease*, **26,** 194–205.

Hargraves, M. M. (1969) Discovery of the LE cell and its morphology. *Mayo Clinic Proceedings*, **44,** 579–599.

Hollander, J. L. & Rawson, A. J. (1968) Gamma globulin, rheumatoid factors and rheumatoid arthritis. *Bulletin on the Rheumatic Diseases*, **18,** 502–505.

Kabat, E. A. & Mayer, M. M. (1971) *Experimental Immunochemistry*. Springfield: Thomas.

Kaplan, M. H. (1963) Immunological relation of streptococcal and tissue antigens. I. Properties of an antigen in certain strains of group A streptococci exhibiting an immunological crossreaction with human heart tissue. *Journal of Immunology*, **90,** 595–606.

Kaplan, M. H. & Rakita, L. (1971) Myocardial disease. In *Immunological Diseases*, 2nd Edition, ed. Samter, M., Vol. II, Section III, Ch. 83. Boston: Little, Brown.

Kaplan, E. L., Top, F. H., Jr, Dudding, B. A. & Wannamaker, L. W. (1971) Diagnosis of streptococcal pharyngitis: Differentiation of active infection from the carrier state in the symptomatic child. *Journal of Infectious Diseases*, **123,** 490–501.

Koffler, D. & Kunkel, H. G. (1968) Mechanisms of renal injury in systemic lupus erythematosus. *American Journal of Medicine*, **45,** 165–169.

Koffler, D., Schur, P. H. & Kunkel, H. G. (1967) Immunological studies concerning the nephritis of systemic lupus erythematosus. *Journal of Experimental Medicine*, **126,** 607–624.

Kraus, S. J., Haserick, J. R., Logan, L. C. & Bullard, J. C. (1971) Atypical fluorescence in the fluorescent treponemal-antibody-absorption (FTA-ABS) test related to deoxyribonucleic acid (DNA) antibodies. *Journal of Immunology*, **106,** 1665–1669.

Lachmann, P. J. & Coombs, R. R. A. (1965) Complement, conglutinin and immunoconglutinin. In *Ciba Symposium: Complement*, ed. Wolstenholme, G. E. W. & Knight, J., pp. 242–280. London: Churchill.

Lerman, S. J., Nannkervis, G. A., Heggie, A. D. & Gold, E. (1971) Immunologic response, virus excretion, and joint reactions with Rubella vaccine. A study of adolescent girls and young women given live attenuated virus vaccine (HPV-77:DE-5). *Annals of Internal Medicine*, **74,** 67–73.

Louie, J. & Pearson, C. M. (1971) Felty's syndrome. *Seminars in Haematology*, **3,** 216–220.

Mackay, I. R. (1968) Lupoid hepatitis and primary biliary cirrhosis: Autoimmune diseases of the liver? *Bulletin on the Rheumatic Diseases*, **18,** 487–494.

Meltzer, M. & Franklin, E. C. (1966) Cryoglobulinemia: A study of 29 patients. *American Journal of Medicine*, **40,** 828–856.

Miescher, R. A., Rothfield, N. & Miescher, A. (1966) Immunologic phenomena in patients with systemic lupus erythematosus. In *Lupus Erythematosus*, ed. Dubois, E. L., pp. 93–103. New York: McGraw-Hill.

Mittal, K. K., Mickey, M. R., Singal, D. P. & Terasaki, P. I. (1968) Serotyping for homotransplantation. XVIII. Refinement of microdroplet lymphocyte cytotoxicity test. *Transplantation*, **6,** 913–927.

Mongan, E. S., Cass, R. M., Jacox, R. F. & Vaughan, J. H. (1969) A study of the relation of seronegative and seropositive rheumatoid arthritis to each other and to necrotizing vasculitis. *American Journal of Medicine*, **47,** 23–35.

Moore, J. E. & Lutz, W. B. (1955) The natural history of systemic lupus erythematosus: An approach to its study through chronic biologic false positive reactors. *Journal of Clinic Diseases*, **1,** 297–316.

Morris, R., Metzger, A. L., Bluestone, R. & Terasaki, P. I. (1974) HL-A W27—A clue to the diagnosis and pathogenesis of Reiter's syndrome. *New England Journal of Medicine*, **290,** 554–556.

Norton, W. L. (1970) Aleutian mink and New Zealand mice: models of viral-induced connective tissue disease. In *Rheumatology: An Annual Review*—The Immunochemistry and Biochemistry of Connective Tissue and Its Disease States, ed. Rotstein, J., pp. 194–223. Basel: Karger.

Oldstone, M. B. A. & Dixon, F. J. (1969) Pathogenesis of chronic disease associated with persistent lymphocytic choriomeningitis viral infection. I. Relationship of antibody production to disease in neonatally infected mice. *Journal of Experimental Medicine*, **129,** 483–499.

Oldstone, M. B. A. & Dixon, F. J. (1970) Pathogenesis of chronic disease associated with persistent lymphocytic choriomeningitis viral infection. II. Relationship of the anti-lymphocytic choriomeningitis immune response to tissue injury in chronic lymphocytic choriomeningitis disease. *Journal of Experimental Medicine*, **131,** 1–19.

Petz, L. D., Sharp, G. C., Cooper, N. R. & Irvin, W. S. (1971) Serum and cerebral spinal fluid complement and serum autoantibodies in systemic lupus erythematosus. *Medicine*, **50,** 259–275.

Pincus, T., Schur, P. H., Rose, J. A., Decker, J. L. & Talal, N. (1969) Measurement of serum DNA-binding activity in systemic lupus erythematosus. *New England Journal of Medicine*, **281,** 701–705.

Rantz, L. A. & Randall, E. A. (1945) Modification of the technic for the antistreptolysin titer. *Proceedings of the Society of Experimental Biology and Medicine*, **59,** 22–25.

Rheumatoid Factors and Their Biological Significance (1969) *Annals of the New York Academy of Sciences*, **168,** 1–207.

Ritzmann, S. E. & Levin, W. C. (1961) Cryopathies: A review, classification, diagnostic and therapeutic considerations. *Archives of Internal Medicine*, **107,** 186–204.

Ruddy, S. & Austen, K. F. (1970) The complement system in rheumatoid synovitis. I. An analysis of complement component activities in rheumatoid synovial fluids. *Arthritis and Rheumatism*, **13,** 713–723.

Schlosstein, L., Terasaki, P. I., Bluestone, R. & Pearson, C. M. (1973) High association of an HL-A antigen, W27, with ankylosing spondylitis. *New England Journal of Medicine*, **288,** 704–706.

Sharp, G. C. (1971) Autoantibodies and complement in SLE: A reexamination. *Hospital Practice*, November, 109–120.

Shearn, M. A. (1971) *Sjögren's Syndrome*, Vol. II, Philadelphia: Saunders.

Singer, J. M. & Plotz, C. M. (1956) The latex fixation test. I. Application to the serologic diagnosis of rheumatoid arthritis. *American Journal of Medicine*, **21,** 888–892.

Sonnenwirth, A. C. (1963) Miscellaneous serologic tests. In *Gradwohl's Clinical Laboratory Methods and Diagnoses*, Vol. 1. A textbook on laboratory procedures and their interpretation, ed. Frankel, S. & Reitman, S., pp. 838–848. St. Louis: Mosby.

Stollerman, G. H. (1967) Streptococcal antibodies in the diagnosis of rheumatic fever. In *Laboratory Diagnostic Procedures in the Rheumatic Diseases*, ed. Cohen, A. S., pp. 168–215. Boston: Little, Brown.

Stollerman, G. H., Lewis, A. J., Schultz, I. & Taranta, A. (1956) Relationship of immune response to group A streptococci to the course of acute, chronic and recurrent rheumatic fever. *American Journal of Medicine*, **20,** 163–169.

Tapanes, F. J., Rawson, A. J. & Hollander, J. L. (1972) Serum anti-immunoglobulins in psoriatic arthritis as compared with rheumatoid arthritis. *Arthritis and Rheumatism*, **15,** 144–152.

Terasaki, P. I., Mottironi, V. D. & Barnett, E. V. (1970) Cytotoxins in disease. Autocytotoxins in lupus. *New England Journal of Medicine*, **283,** 724–728.

Torrigiani, G., Ansell, B. M., Chown, E. E. A. & Roitt, I. M. (1969) Raised IgG antiglobulin factors in Still's disease. *Annals of Rheumatic Diseases*, **28,** 424–427.

Townes, A. S. & Sowa, J. M. (1970) Complement in synovial fluid. *The Johns Hopkins Medical Journal*, **127,** 23–37.

Vaughan, J. H. (1966) The rheumatoid factors. In *Arthritis and Allied Conditions*, ed. Hollander, J. L., pp. 85–98. Philadelphia: Lea & Febiger.

Ward, P. A. & Zvaifler, N. J. (1971) Complement-derived leukotatic factors in inflammatory synovial fluids of humans. *Journal of Clinical Investigation*, **50,** 606–616.

Ziff, M. (1957) The agglutination reaction in rheumatoid arthritis. *Journal of Chronic Diseases*, **5,** 644–667.

Zutshi, D. W., Reading, C. A., Epstein, W. V., Ansell, B. M. & Holborow, E. J. (1969) FII haemagglutination test for serum antigammaglobulin factors in arthritides seropositive and sero-negative by other tests. *Annals of Rheumatic Diseases*, **28,** 289–298.

5. Immunology of Endocrine Disease

C. G. BEARDWELL

Immunological phenomena and techniques are of great practical interest to the endocrinologist from several points of view. They appear clearly to be concerned in the pathogenesis of a number of common endocrine disorders; they may complicate the therapy of endocrine disease and they are of ever-increasing importance in diagnosis. The three major fields of concern may be summarised as follows:

1. Those endocrine disorders in which abnormalities of glandular function are associated with evidence of immunological reactions, cellular and humoral, apparently directed specifically against antigenic determinants present in the affected glands.
2. Interference with hormone therapy, resulting from the development of antibodies in the recipient to the hormone administered.
3. The technique of radioimmunoassay, in which specific hormone antibodies are used for the measurement of hormone concentration in the body fluids and tissues of man and other animals.

ENDOCRINE DISORDERS ASSOCIATED WITH THE PRESENCE OF ORGAN-SPECIFIC ANTIBODIES

This group of diseases includes most types of thyroid disease, some forms of adrenal, ovarian, testicular and parathyroid failure and may include a number of other forms of endocrine disorder.

In many of these disorders, circulating antibodies which appear to be directed specifically against glandular antigenic determinants can be easily detected. This, together with a considerable amount of other evidence, suggests that autoallergic factors may be concerned in initiating and/or perpetuating the disease process. It thus seems appropriate to consider, in general terms, ways in which such antibodies could be produced.

Possible Mechanisms of Autoantibody Production

In spite of a great deal of clinical and experimental work the exact mechanisms by which the majority of autoimmune diseases arise in man are still largely unknown. A number of hypotheses have been put forward, some of which will be considered below. Before doing this, however, it may be helpful to list a number of facts concerning autoimmune diseases for which any acceptable hypothesis should account. These are as follows:

1. Autoimmune disorders may arise in man apparently spontaneously, in association with stimuli such as infection, tissue damage or drug therapy or together with congenital or acquired disorders of the immune mechanism.
2. Genetic factors are clearly involved in many disorders and, in some cases, autoantibodies develop more commonly with increasing age.
3. Autoantibodies tend to occur in certain combinations of specificity, and in many disorders autoantibodies of several different immunoglobulin classes may be found.
4. Evidence of autoimmune reactivity involving both cellular and humoral compartments is common in autoimmune disease.
5. B lymphocytes with the capacity to react with normal tissue components may be found in normal subjects.
6. Autoantibodies to a variety of autoantigens can be readily produced in normal animals using appropriate experimental conditions.
7. Many naturally occurring autoimmune disorders appear to be chronic, self-perpetuating processes.

Burnet (1972) has suggested that autoantibody production commonly results from a primary abnormality of the immune mechanism. He proposes that during the process of lymphocyte differentiation cells are produced which have the ability to synthesise antibody capable of reacting with autoantigens. Normally those cells are eliminated or functionally inhibited. On occasion, however, especially in genetically predisposed individuals, changes due to somatic mutations (or possibly to other factors) may allow an immunocyte line to develop which has an undue resistance to elimination by antigenic contact and reacts specifically with an accessible body component. Such a cell may then initiate a 'forbidden clone' of directly or indirectly pathogenic cells and result in the development of autoimmune disease.

Several objections to this theory have been put forward. Points 5 and 6 above seem incompatible with the suggestion that elimination of autoantibody-producing cells normally occurs, while point 3 is difficult to account for on a basis of somatic mutation unless this occurs with inordinate frequency (Vaughan, 1971).

Burnet (1959) also put forward the suggestion that certain body components were secluded from the immune system. Because of lack of antigenic contact immune tolerance did not develop and autoantibody formation would occur if the secluded antigen later came into contact with immunocompetent cells. Although certain secluded antigens may exist, e.g. lens protein, which will rapidly provoke an immune reaction if released into the circulation, it seems unlikely that this explanation accounts for the failure of autoantibody formation except in certain special cases. Thyroglobulin, for example, appears always to be found in the serum of normal subjects in low concentration so that such a hypothesis cannot be used to explain the development of antibodies to this antigen.

Recent studies on the interaction of the T- and B-immunocyte systems have led to the formulation of a number of hypotheses which seem to link together the apparent production of autoantibodies as a result of a primary abnormality of the immune mechanism, as proposed by Burnet, and their production as a result of tissue damage or experimental administration of antigens. These have been summarised by Allison, Denman and Barnes (1971) and by Allison (1973).

Interaction of the T- and B-immunocyte systems

It is known that humoral antibodies are produced by B cells, and that their production is initiated by contact of an immunoglobulin receptor on the cell surface with an antigen of appropriate chemical constitution under appropriate conditions. In many cases it appears that the cooperation of specifically reactive T cells is needed for an adequate B-cell response. It is not necessary that the T-cell stimulus should be the same as that to which the B cell reacts, although it seems probable that the antigenic determinants should be on the same molecule, or at least very closely spatially related. Certain adjuvants, e.g. Freund's complete adjuvant, appear to act as non-specific T-cell stimulants, although the exact mechanism of their action remains uncertain.

Immunological tolerance, defined as a state of specific unresponsiveness to an antigen, can be induced, in some cases, by giving either repeated low doses of the antigen, or very large doses. In the former case, low dose tolerance, there is evidence that specific unresponsiveness of T lymphocytes is induced, while B lymphocytes remain able to produce antibody under suitable conditions, e.g. when antigens with structural similarities to those used to induce tolerance, i.e. cross-reacting antigens, are given or when antigen is injected with adjuvant. High dose tolerance appears to result from unresponsiveness, or absence of both T and B immunocytes. Low dose tolerance may be analogous to the situation prevailing in normal man where many autoantigens are normally present in low concentration in the circulation. If this is so, B lymphocytes capable of reacting with such antigens should normally be present and such lymphocytes capable of reacting with thyroglobulin have recently been detected in normal subjects (Bankhurst, Torrigiani and Allison, 1973). For plasma components normally found in high concentration, e.g. serum albumin, autoantibody formation may be prevented by mechanisms analogous to those seen in high dose tolerance and, indeed, no B lymphocytes capable of reacting wich such antigens have yet been detected.

If these statements are correct, autoantibody formation against antigens normally protected by low dose tolerance might occur if there is either some abnormality in the control of B lymphocytes by T lymphocytes, or if the need for the 'helper' effect of T lymphocytes can be bypassed.

Control of B lymphocytes by T lymphocytes

As already mentioned, there is now evidence that, in some cases, antibody production by B lymphocytes requires the 'helper' effect of T lymphocytes stimulated by either the same or a different antigen associated with that against which antibody is directed. This mechanism has been invoked to explain autoantibody formation associated with virus infections, the administration of drugs or other chemicals, and adjuvants.

Virus infections. Following viral infection viral antigen may be found on the surface of infected cells and cell antigens on the surface of virus particles. This would seem to provide appropriate conditions for stimulation of T cells bearing an antivirus receptor which could then stimulate B cells with an anti-self-antigen receptor to produce autoantibody. There is considerable experimental evidence that such a mechanism exists and the occurrence of autoallergic manifestations after viral or mycoplasma infections in man lends further support.

Haptens and drugs. Animals can be sensitised to certain haptens, e.g. dinitrophenol. If this is then coupled to host cells or to protein antigens administration of the complex may lead to the formation of autoantibodies directed against the cellular or protein antigen. Thyroglobulin antibodies have been produced experimentally by such a mechanism. It has been suggested that this type of reaction could account for the Coombs' positive haemolytic anaemia occasionally seen in patients treated with methyldopa.

Adjuvants. It has already been mentioned that autoantibodies can readily be produced experimentally if antigens are administered in Freund's complete adjuvant, possibly as a result of non-specific T-cell stimulation. The essential ingredient of this adjuvant appears to be killed mycobacteria and it seems possible that some of their effectiveness may result from an ability to form complexes with antigens. Although there is little evidence that bacterial infection in man has adjuvant effects it must, at present, remain a possibility.

Suppression of antibody formation by T lymphocytes

As well as having a 'helper' effect in antibody formation it appears that T lymphocytes can, in some situations, exert a suppressing effect on antibody formation. It has been shown that T cells from mice made unresponsive to sheep red cells can block the formation of antibody to this antigen. Antilymphocyte serum (which is mainly active against T cells) results in an increase in antibody formation against pneumococcus type III polysaccharide in mice, a reaction for which a T-cell helper effect is not required. Autoantibody formation might therefore result from a failure of normal T-cell suppression of B lymphocytes capable of producing autoantibodies. Considerable evidence for such a mechanism has come from experiments using NZB mice, a strain remarkably liable to develop spontaneous autoimmune disease. It has been shown that T cells from young animals can delay, or prevent, autoantibody formation in old animals. Transfer of spleen cells from old to young animals (mainly B lymphocytes) results in transiently positive Coombs tests in many of the recipients; treatment with antilymphocyte serum increases and perpetuates the formation of autoantibody. Further evidence for a failure of T-cell control of antibody formation in these animals is provided by the findings that T and B cells seem to be unusually resistant to the production of unresponsiveness to various antigens and that T-cell function, as judged by the capacity to mount graft versus host reactions, seems to decline rapidly with age.

There is, at present, little or no direct evidence in man that failure of T-cell control results in autoantibody formation. However, by analogy with the experimental situation such a mechanism would seem to account satisfactorily for the genetic factor in autoimmune disease in man, the increased incidence of autoantibodies with ageing, the continued production of antibodies in the absence of a continued antigenic exposure, the association of certain types of autoantibody and the varied immunoglobulin classes of the antibodies produced. Such a mechanism would seem more likely to be responsible for the chronic autoimmune disorders than the T-cell 'helper' mechanism which would seem to be self-limiting in the absence of continued antigenic exposure—as indeed are most virus- or drug-induced autoimmune disorders.

Mechanisms by which direct B-lymphocyte stimulation, without the intervention of T cells, could occur remain at present speculative. However, a number of ways, other than those already mentioned in which autoantibody formation might be stimulated, have been suggested. Tissue damage, resulting from infection or other causes, might result in minor modifications of tissue antigens resulting in the release of substances detected by the immune system as cross-reacting antigens capable of breaking immune tolerance. Such a mechanism might account for the production of antibodies to liver antigens following carbon tetrachloride poisoning or the occasional finding of antinuclear antibodies following pulmonary infarction.

An alternative form of the sequestered antigen concept may also account for autoantibody formation in some cases. This suggests that tissue damage or other stimulus might result in the exposure of antigenic determinants which are normally concealed within a molecule. Tolerance to such antigens would never have been established and an immune reaction would develop. Rheumatoid factor, which appears to be an antibody to aggregated IgG or to IgG which has taken part in an antigen–antibody reaction, could be an example.

The hypotheses presented above by no means include all those that have been suggested. They do, however, seem to provide a basis for experiments in man and other animals to test their validity. It seems likely that more definite evidence to confirm or refute them will soon appear.

Pathogenetic mechanisms in autoimmune disease

There seems no reason to think that autoantibodies differ in their reaction with antigens from any other type of antibody. Cytotoxic autoantibodies certainly occur and Arthus-like (immune complex) reactions may play a part in the production of autoimmune disease.

In many disorders, as will be discussed below, tissue damage appears to correlate much better with evidence of delayed hypersensitivity (cell mediated) to tissue antigens than with circulating antibody concentrations. However, the rôle of antibody fixed to tissue antigens or of cellular and humoral immune interactions has not yet been well defined. The immuno-pathogenic mechanisms differ in the different autoimmune diseases and will be further considered in the appropriate section of this chapter.

Thyroid

In man, evidence of autoimmune reaction to components of the thyroid gland is provided by the detection of circulating antibodies, apparently directed specifically against thyroid antigens. These may be found in high concentration and are sometimes accompanied by hyperglobulinaemia. They are commonly associated with histological changes in the gland suggesting an immunological reaction against thyroid tissue. Evidence of delayed hypersensitivity reactions to thyroidal components may also be found.

In this review it is not proposed to give a comprehensive coverage of the whole subject but to concentrate on those aspects which are of particular interest to the clinician. More detailed reviews have recently been provided by Bastenie and Ermans (1971), by Shulman (1971), by Doniach and Roitt (1968), and by Volpé et al (1974).

Evidence for the involvement of autoimmunity in thyroid disease

Antibodies reacting with several different thyroid antigens have now been described. These are given as follows.

Antibodies to thyroglobulin. Thyroglobulin antibodies were the first type of thyroid antibody to be found in man. Several methods have been described for their detection. Those most commonly used are described as follows.

The precipitin test. This is usually carried out in agar gel. The patient's serum is placed in one well and either a simple saline extract of human thyroid or thyroglobulin purified by salt fractionation in another. If antibody is present in the patient's serum a precipitin line forms between the two wells. The test is relatively insensitive and will detect only high concentrations of antibody.

Latex agglutination test. Latex particles coated with thyroglobulin will, under appropriate conditions, agglutinate in the presence of thyroglobulin antibody. This test is only slightly, if at all, more sensitive than the precipitin test. It can, however, be carried out rapidly and may be used as a screening test. False positive results may be obtained with sera containing rheumatoid factor unless the serum is used at a dilution of 1 in 20 or greater.

A similar technique, in which thyroglobulin is adsorbed to Bentonite particles, has also been described.

Tanned red cell test. This test is similar in principle to the latex test but, instead of latex particles, formolised red cells are coated with thyroglobulin. This results in a considerable increase in sensitivity so that this test is approximately 1000 times more sensitive than the precipitin reaction.

Immunofluorescence. Antithyroglobulin antibodies can be readily demonstrated by the indirect immunofluorescent technique. Alcohol-fixed sections of thyroid are used. In these, microsomal antigen (see below) is destroyed but antigens present in the colloid are unaffected. The sensitivity of this method is intermediate between that of the precipitin and tanned red cell tests.

A number of other methods have also been described including a more sensitive immunodiffusion technique for precipitins and a competitive protein binding method, apparently more sensitive than the tanned red cell technique. These are not, however, at present widely used.

There is evidence that more than one type of thyroglobulin antibody may exist in man. Antithyroglobulin activity has been found associated with the IgG, IgM and IgA classes of immunoglobulins. IgG is usually the predominant class but the proportions of the three classes differ in different sera. As well as this heterogeneity of immunoglobulin class, it also seems likely that there is more than one antigenic site on the thyroglobulin molecule against which antibodies are directed. Although, in general, sera giving positive precipitin tests show high titres of antibody by the tanned red cell test (greater than 1 in 25 000), this is not invariably so and precipitation is occasionally seen with sera giving a titre of as little as 1 in 1000. Furthermore, different types of precipitin reaction are sometimes seen with different sera. Largely on this basis, Roitt, Torrigiani and Doniach (1968) have suggested that thyroglobulin contains two pairs of autoantigenic determinants with two corresponding antibodies, the proportions of which differ in different patients.

Antibodies to the microsomal antigen. This antigen is found within the cells forming the thyroid follicles. After homogenisation of the cells and ultracentrifugation it is found with the microsomal fraction and appears to be an insoluble lipoprotein intimately attached to vesicle membranes. It is present in relatively low concentration in the normal gland but is several times more concentrated in the thyrotoxic gland. Preparations of such glands are usually used for detection of antibodies. The methods most commonly used are as follows.

Complement fixation test. This is carried out with a preparation of microsomes from a thyrotoxic gland. Although convenient to carry out it is a less sensitive technique than immunofluorescence.

Immunofluorescence. The indirect immunofluorescent method is used and is carried out with sections of unfixed thyroid gland (free of colloid).

Other methods which have been used include a haemadsorption test and a competitive protein binding assay.

As with the thyroglobulin antibodies, it seems likely that more than one type of antimicrosomal antibody exists. Studies with tissue cultures of thyroid cells have shown that certain sera from patients with thyroid disease contain a cytotoxic factor which requires complement for its activity and appears to be specific for thyroid cells. It seems likely that this factor is identical with the antimicrosomal antibody detected by immunofluorescence but not with that detected by the complement fixation test, since there is only a poor correlation between the concentrations of immunofluorescent/cytotoxic antibody and that of complement-fixing antibody.

Occasionally, sera giving positive tests for thyroid microsomal antibody will also react with microsomes from other tissues, such as brain or liver. This indicates that the antibody is not thyroid specific, and its presence does not have the same significance as does that of the more usual antibody. Such a non-organ specific antibody may be found in patients with primary biliary cirrhosis or chronic active hepatitis. Occasionally it is also seen in systemic lupus erythematosus or rheumatoid arthritis. The tissue specificity of the microsomal antibody can be checked by including a rat kidney homogenate in the complement fixation test and human kidney sections in the fluorescent test.

Antibodies to the second colloid antigen. If indirect immunofluorescent tests are carried out with certain sera using alcohol-fixed thyroid sections a uniform, specific staining of the acinar colloid is seen, quite different from the floccular or 'cracked' staining of the colloid produced by antibodies to thyroglobulin. The antigen against which this antibody is directed has not yet been fully characterised but it appears to be a non-iodine containing protein, quite distinct from thyroglobulin.

The frequency with which these three types of antibody may be found in normal subjects and in those with various thyroid diseases is shown in Table 5.1.

Table 5.1. Percentage of patients with various diseases giving positive results in thyroid antibody tests

Diagnosis	Thyroglobulin antibodies		Microsomal antibodies.	Second colloid antigen	Fluorescent tests only[a]
	Precipitin	Tanned red cell	Complement fixation		
Hashimoto's disease	55	85	82	74	4
Primary hypothyroidism	17	64	52	26	13·5
Graves' disease	4	59	41	28	26
Non-toxic goitre	0	25	13	12	21
Thyroid carcinoma	0–24	19	18	30	7
Pernicious anaemia	0	29	31	–	–
Addison's disease (idiopathic)	0	39	22[b]	–	–
Diabetes mellitus (insulin dependent)	0	8	18	–	–
Hyperglobulinaemic states[c]	0	0–22	0·5–36	–	–
Normal subjects	0	11[d]	9[d]	3	–

The figures given are the mean percentages derived from a large number of reports.

[a]Includes antibodies to thyroglobulin, microsomal antigen and second colloid antigen not detected by other methods.

[b]Detected by immunofluorescence (Irvine et al, 1970).

[c]Includes connective tissue disorders; hepatic diseases and paraproteinaemias (Skanse and Nilsson, 1962).

[d]Percentage varies with age and sex.

The long-acting thyroid stimulator (LATS). In 1956 Adams and Purves reported the detection of a thyroid-stimulating substance in the serum of the thyrotoxic patients which differed from thyroid-stimulating hormone in the time of onset and the duration of its action. This substance is known as the long-acting thyroid stimulator.

The assay method usually used is that described by McKenzie (1958).

Mice are rendered iodine deficient by feeding them a diet low in iodine. They are then given a single injection of radioactive iodine and treated with thyroxine to suppress endogenous thyroid-stimulating hormone (TSH) release. Under these conditions, uptake of radioactive iodine by the mouse thyroid is high, and release from the gland is inhibited. After a suitable time period to allow excretion of radioiodine not taken up by the thyroid, a control blood sample is taken and its radioactivity measured. Standard or test solutions are then injected and further blood samples taken at appropriate times for measurement of radioactivity. Thyroid-stimulating activity is shown by an increased release of radioactive iodine from the gland into the blood, and results are usually expressed as the ratio of radioactivity at the peak of the response to that in the control blood sample. Following TSH injection peak blood radioactivity is usually seen after 2 to 3 hours, while LATS has a more gradual effect with peak blood radioactivity being seen 12 to 16 hours after injection.

There is now a considerable body of evidence supporting the concept that LATS is an antibody. Using a variety of chemical methods, it has been shown that LATS activity is always associated with the IgG fraction of the serum proteins. Techniques designed for the study of IgG structure have shown that the thyroid-stimulating activity of LATS is due to the presence of certain chemical groupings in the Fd fragment of the heavy chain of the LATS–IgG molecule. The antigen–binding sites of known antibodies are also located, at least in part, in the Fd fragment. LATS is thus an IgG molecule, identical in structure to other antibodies and quite unrelated to TSH. Antisera to human IgG or to the κ and λ chains of the immunoglobulins can neutralise the LATS activity of serum while having no effect on TSH activity. Conversely, antibodies to TSH inhibit its biological activity while having no effect on that of LATS. Like other immunoglobulins LATS appears to be produced by lymphoid cells. A LATS effect can be obtained with proteins from a culture medium in which phytohaemagglutinin-stimulated leucocytes from thyrotoxic patients have been grown.

In spite of a great deal of work the antigen to which LATS appears to be an antibody remains unknown. If serum containing LATS is incubated with whole thyroid homogenate, the LATS activity can apparently be absorbed out. Early experiments with thyroid subcellular particles suggested that the microsomal fraction was the most effective, but more recently it has been suggested that the LATS-absorbing material may be found in soluble form in the supernatant after all subcellular particles have been removed by centrifugation. Some of the results of these experiments are open to doubt for technical reasons and no clear picture of either the site or nature of the antigen has yet emerged.

LATS activity is found mainly in the serum of patients who have, or have had, thyrotoxicosis. It has, however, also been found occasionally in patients with other conditions. In spite of the fact that it can be found in a high proportion of patients with thyrotoxicosis and its undoubted thyroid-stimulating activity, it is by no means universally accepted that it plays the main aetiological rôle in the development of thyrotoxicosis. This will be discussed further below.

A second gamma globulin occurring in the serum of thyrotoxic patients has been described more recently and named the LATS protector (Adams and Kennedy, 1967, 1971). It was observed that the LATS activity of thyrotoxic sera was inhibited to a very variable extent by human thyroid extracts and that the degree of inhibition did not correlate with the concentration of LATS in the serum. This suggested that certain sera might contain a substance which protected LATS from neutralisation. Further studies showed that a substance could indeed be found in sera from patients with Graves' disease which could prevent neutralisation of LATS activity by human but not by mouse thyroid extracts. Fractionation of the serum proteins showed that this protective activity was a property of the gamma globulin fraction. It could be detected in either the serum or globulin concentrates of all patients with Graves' disease studied, but not in serum from patients with toxic adenoma, hypothyroidism or normal thyroid function. It has been suggested that this material might be a thyroid stimulator capable of reacting only with the human thyroid, and thus not detectable by the conventional McKenzie bioassay. Evidence in favour of this view has been produced by Shishiba et al (1972). They showed that LATS protector produced a dose-related increase in intracellular colloid droplet formation (an index of thyroid stimulation) in human thyroid tissue comparable to that produced by LATS. Normal human IgG, concentrated fourfold, produced no such effect.

Onaya et al (1973), using a similar assay system, showed that 47 of 56 sera from thyrotoxic patients would induce colloid droplet formation in slices of human thyroid while control sera from normal subjects had no such effect. In only 5 of these 47 sera could LATS be demonstrated by the McKenzie bioassay. They also showed that LATS-negative sera, while able to induce colloid droplet formation in human thyroid, would not do so in mouse or guinea-pig thyroid. It is not clear whether the thyroid stimulating substance so demonstrated is LATS protector or another substance.

It seems reasonable to conclude that serum from thyrotoxic patients may contain two or more thyroid stimulating agents, only one of which, LATS, can be detected by the McKenzie assay technique.

Histological and other features of thyroid disease

Macroscopic and microscopic changes occurring in the thyroid and other tissues in certain thyroid disorders, especially Hashimoto's disease and Graves' disease, support the concept that autoimmune reactions are involved in their pathogenesis.

In Hashimoto's disease the gland commonly shows generalised infiltration with lymphocytes, plasma cells and macrophages. Lymphoid follicles with germinal centres are common. The thyroid follicles themselves show variable changes. In some cases the cells are hyperplastic and the colloid content somewhat reduced, while in others variable degrees of follicular disorganisation are seen with almost complete loss of colloid, and enlarged follicular cells with numerous eosinophilic granules (Ashkanazy cells or oncocytes) or masses of swollen cells with clear eosinophilic cytoplasm, sometimes vacuolated. Chronic inflammatory cells may sometimes be seen within these degenerate follicles and variable degrees of fibrosis may be seen within the gland.

The histological picture has been likened to that seen in an allogeneic graft undergoing rejection.

Similar, though less widespread, changes may be seen in thyroid glands from patients with almost any other thyroid disease, when localised or focal lymphocytic thyroiditis is said to be present. In patients with primary hypothyroidism, the gland is usually atrophic and densely fibrosed, but even at this stage, lymphocytic and plasma cell infiltration can still be seen. Patients at an earlier stage of the disease may show a greater degree of inflammatory infiltration ranging almost up to the picture seen in Hashimoto's disease.

In Graves' disease there are several pathological features, both intra- and extra-thyroidal, which suggest involvement of the immunological system. Lymphadenopathy may occur, lymphocytosis is common, splenomegaly may be found, and, in autopsy studies, thymic enlargement is seen in about half the cases examined. Recently, immunofluorescent studies have shown the presence of IgG, IgM and IgE and complement in the connective tissue stroma and the follicular basement membrane of a high proportion of thyroids from patients with Graves' disease (Werner et al, 1972). Fibrinogen was not detected, suggesting that the presence of immunoglobulin and complement could not be attributed simply to leakage from capillaries, and study of control glands, either from normal subjects or from patients with toxic or non-toxic multinodular goitre, showed no evidence of the presence of immunoglobulin or complement.

Delayed hypersensitivity reactions

Evidence of cell-mediated immunity to thyroid antigens has been sought mainly in patients with Hashimoto's disease and Graves' disease. Techniques used have included skin tests using thyroid antigens and in vitro methods such as studies of lymphoblast transformation with lymphocytes from patients with thyroiditis exposed to thyroid antigens, leucocyte migration studies and rosette formation tests.

Although cutaneous reactions to thyroglobulin have been reported in patients with Hashimoto's disease, it seems likely that these represent Arthus reactions rather than being a manifestation of delayed hypersensitivity.

The results of in vitro tests have been somewhat variable. Positive leucocyte migration inhibition tests have been reported in patients with lymphocytic thyroiditis and in those with Graves' disease. In the latter both thyroid extracts and extracts of retrobulbar tissue have been shown to produce inhibition, especially when leucocytes from patients with exophthalmos are used.

On balance, although the evidence in man is not yet complete, it seems very likely that cell-mediated immune reactions to thyroid antigens occur in thyroiditis and Graves' disease as well as humoral immune reactions.

Experimental thyroiditis

Some of the most powerful support for the concept that human thyroiditis has an autoimmune basis comes from animal studies involving immunisation with thyroid antigens. These studies stem largely from the work of Rose and

Witebsky, who have recently reviewed the entire subject (Rose and Witebsky, 1971).

In 1956 they showed that rabbits immunised with a crude saline extract of rabbit thyroid developed antibodies to the thyroid extract which could be detected by complement fixation, precipitation, tanned red cell haemagglutination and passive cutaneous anaphylaxis. The antibodies were specific for thyroid extract and showed no cross reaction with other rabbit organs. They were also shown to be true autoantibodies, in the sense that they would react with extracts of the animal's own thyroid and could be produced by injection of such extracts made following thyroidectomy.

The antibodies were shown to be directed against thyroglobulin and could be produced by the use of partially purified thyroglobulin as antigen. Skin reactions of delayed hypersensitivity type to thyroid extract or thyroglobulin could also be demonstrated.

In many of the rabbits obvious histological abnormalities were seen in the thyroid. Areas of dense cellular infiltration were seen around the follicles, consisting mainly of lymphoid cells and eosinophils, areas of follicular damage and fibrosis were present and in some cases there were large accummulations of lymphocytes with lymphoid follicles.

Subsequent experiments have confirmed these observations and have defined, to some extent, the conditions necessary for the production of experimental thyroiditis and the pathogenetic mechanisms involved. Although this work has suggested ways in which spontaneous thyroiditis might arise in man, the experimental disease shows certain differences from the human disease and, so far, it has not proved possible to induce experimental thyroiditis without using thyroglobulin either in chemically modified form or emulsified in various adjuvants. Although chemical modification of thyroglobulin may occur in vivo and initiate the disease in man there is, as yet, no direct evidence that this occurs.

Thyroiditis may persist for as long as two years in guinea pigs following a single injection of antigen, but in most animals repeated injections must be given if the antibody response and the thyroiditis are to persist. In rabbits initially immunised with chemically modified thyroglobulin, antibody titres can be increased if injections of native thyroglobulin are given or if thyroglobulin release from the animal's own thyroid occurs as a result of autotransplantation of part of the gland or treatment with radioactive iodine. Usually, however, experimental thyroiditis does not seem to be a self-perpetuating process.

In most animals immunisation with thyroid extract results in the production of thyroglobulin antibodies. These differ from those found in man in that they are able to fix complement. Usually other antibodies have not been detected. There is, however, one important exception—the rhesus monkey. If this animal is immunised with autologous thyroid extract in Freund's complete adjuvant, thyroglobulin antibodies, thyroid microsomal antibody and a cytotoxic antibody active against both monkey and human thyroid cells can be found. The antibodies resemble those seen in man in that complement is not fixed by the thyroglobulin antibody but is by the microsomal antibody and is needed for the cytotoxic effect.

There has been much speculation as to whether thyroiditis in the immunised animal results from cellular damage due to circulating antibodies or from cellular immune responses.

Many workers have attempted to correlate the severity of thyroiditis with the titre of circulating antibody but, in general, no close correlation has been found. It has also proved possible, by varying the immunisation procedure, to dissociate antibody production and thyroiditis. Thus, immunisation with alum-precipitated thyroid extract produces a good antibody response but no thyroiditis, while the same antigen given in Freund's complete adjuvant produces antibodies, thyroiditis and evidence of a delayed hypersensitivity response. Other techniques have also been used to suppress antibody formation or the delayed hypersensitivity response selectively. Only depression of the latter appears to prevent the development of thyroiditis.

Attempts to transfer thyroiditis passively to non-immunised animals using serum from immunised animals have generally been unsuccessful. However, this has now been achieved in the rabbit (Nakamura and Weigle, 1969) using serum taken from thyroidectomised donor animals soon after immunisation. It seems possible that thyroidectomy may be necessary to prevent uptake of the toxic factor from serum and thus to allow a higher concentration to be transferred.

In general, it has proved easier to correlate the frequency of development and severity of thyroiditis with evidence of delayed hypersensitivity to antigen rather than with the serum antibody response. It has also proved possible to transfer thyroiditis to histocompatible recipient animals using spleen cells or lymphoid cells from immunised donors.

In spite of much work it is still not possible to say definitely whether cellular or humoral factors are more important in the development of experimental thyroiditis. Both may be involved, e.g. cellular attack may be necessary to allow antibody to reach antigenic sites in the gland where it can exert a cytotoxic effect, or interaction of antibody and lymphoid cells may be necessary to 'sensitise' the cells and to confer the appropriate target specificity upon them. However, many other factors may be involved including genetic ones.

Relationship of experimental thyroiditis to human disease

Although experimental thyroiditis has much in common with spontaneous thyroiditis occurring in man and has provided a basis for many theories and experiments on the nature of the human disease, it is, perhaps, reasonable to be cautious in extrapolating from animals to man. Experimental thyroiditis appears, usually, to be a self-limiting disorder and the relationship, if any, between the methods used to bring about its production and the mechanisms resulting in the spontaneous development of thyroiditis in man remain almost entirely speculative. Perhaps the closest human analogy to experimental thyroiditis is provided by de Quervain's (subacute) thyroiditis. Here damage to the gland, probably by viral infection, results quite commonly in the development of thyroid antibodies. However, these usually disappear spontaneously as the disease subsides. The development of chronic, self-perpetuating thyroiditis would seem to need the presence of factors other than simple thyroid damage with antigen release.

Genetic factors in human thyroid disease

Familial aggregations of thyroid disease have been reported on many occasions. Although some of these studies have been criticised on epidemiological grounds there seems to be little doubt that relatives of patients with Hashimoto's disease, primary myxoedema or thyrotoxicosis show a higher incidence of clinically apparent thyroid disease and of positive tests for thyroid antibodies than do the relatives of controls. Thyroid abnormalities found in such families include not only these disorders but also colloid goitre and thyroid adenoma. Overall, evidence of thyroid disorder appears to be four or five times more common in the relatives of patients with chronic thyroiditis, myxoedema or thyrotoxicosis than it does in the relations of controls.

There is general agreement that other organ-specific disorders thought to be of autoimmune aetiology, e.g. idiopathic adrenal atrophy, pernicious anaemia and primary hypoparathyroidism are also associated with autoimmune thyroid disease. Thus, approximately 30 per cent of patients with thyroiditis have gastric parietal cell antibodies, while between 40 and 50 per cent of patients with idiopathic adrenal atrophy have either clinical or serological evidence of thyroiditis.

An association between thyroiditis and the non-organ specific autoimmune disorders, such as rheumatoid arthritis or systemic lupus erythematosus, has also been suggested, but the validity of such an association remains doubtful.

Further evidence that genetic factors may be involved in the development of autoimmune thyroid disease comes from studies carried out on the families of subjects with chromosomal anomalies. Patients with Down's syndrome show an unusually high frequency of thyroid antibodies as also do their parents and it has been suggested that a similar situation prevails in Turner's syndrome. The exact relationship between thyroiditis and these chromosomal anomalies remains uncertain.

Clinical aspects of autoimmune thyroiditis

On the basis of the evidence discussed above, it is now generally held that the association of a typical histological picture with circulating antithyroid antibodies indicates the presence of autoimmune thyroiditis. This may occur either as a diffuse process throughout the gland, or as scattered foci of lymphocytic infiltration.

When present in diffuse form progressive destruction and fibrosis of the gland may occur without glandular enlargement. This process leads to primary hypothyroidism. In other cases, the destructive process is balanced by hyperplasia and proliferation of thyroid cells, at least for a time. As a result, the gland enlarges and the patient remains euthyroid (Hashimoto's disease). Later on, destruction may proceed to a point where the number of thyroid cells remaining is inadequate to maintain normal function and hypothyroidism develops.

In these disorders the situation seems relatively clear cut. However, from the point of view of the clinician interested in using thyroid antibody tests or even thyroid biopsy as an aid to diagnosis, the situation is greatly complicated by the fact that histological and serological evidence of thyroiditis may be found in patients with any type of thyroid disease, including carcinoma, multinodular goitre and thyrotoxicosis, while thyroid antibodies may also be detected in patients with no other evidence of thyroid disorder. To complicate the situation further, certain patients, who have been shown histologically to have diffuse autoimmune thyroiditis, may have no thyroid antibodies detectable by the methods usually available.

Thus, thyroid antibody tests and even thyroid biopsies can never be used alone to make a diagnosis, but must always be considered in conjunction with the clinical picture and tests of thyroid function.

Hashimoto's disease

This disorder is characterised by enlargement of the thyroid gland, histological evidence of diffuse thyroiditis and, usually, high titres of thyroid antibodies in the serum.

Estimates of the incidence of the disease vary somewhat depending upon the diagnostic criteria used. It appears to be approximately nine times as common in women as in men, and the incidence in both sexes increases with age. In women it occurs most commonly between the ages of 30 and 60, the mean age of most series being about 45, while in men the mean age is nearer 60. However, the disease is occasionally seen in children and in the very old.

Population studies have suggested an overall incidence in women aged 30 to 60 of about 74 cases per 100 000 population, while the overall incidence at necropsy has been estimated as 0·8 per cent. The disease is certainly more commonly diagnosed now than formerly but whether this indicates a true increase in incidence or a change in diagnostic criteria is not entirely certain.

The usual presentation is that of progressive enlargement of the thyroid in a middle-aged woman. Occasionally, the gland enlarges rapidly, the goitre becoming obvious in a period of only a few weeks, but more commonly enlargement is more gradual, occurring over a period of one or two years. A few patients complain of pain in or around the gland, usually in the early stages, and enlargement of the regional lymph nodes has been described though this appears to be very unusual. Dyspnoea is not uncommon and dysphagia is seen in 10 to 20 per cent of patients.

On examination, the thyroid is usually diffusely enlarged, rather firm with a very well-defined outline and a finely granular surface.

A number of variant forms of the disease have been described:

The fibrous variant. Dense fibrosis develops in part of the gland, producing an asymmetrical goitre, the fibrous part of which is firmer than the remainder. The cellular infiltrate contains a higher proportion of plasma cells than usual.

The hyperplastic variant of adolescence (oxyphil). Young subjects may rapidly develop a diffuse, symmetrical goitre which is less firm than that usually seen in adults. The cellular infiltrate consists mainly of small lymphocytes with a few plasma cells.

Hashimoto's disease with exophthalmos. Occasional patients with otherwise typical Hashimoto's disease have eye signs identical with those more commonly seen in thyrotoxicosis.

Thyroid function. The majority of patients with Hashimoto's disease are either euthyroid or mildly hypothyroid when first seen. Those who are euthyroid may show no obvious progression of the disease for many years, but a proportion, variously estimated as lying between 10 and 50 per cent, will insidiously develop hypothyroidism.

In the advanced case which has progressed to definite clinical hypothyroidism, thyroid function tests usually present no difficulty in interpretation. However, in the earlier stages they may be somewhat misleading. There is often a defect in the organification of iodine, the intrathyroidal iodine pool is smaller than normal and abnormal iodinated compounds may be secreted. These defects lead to an increase in the ^{131}I uptake, especially within 6 hours of administration, when it may be well into the thyrotoxic range, though at 24 hours the uptake may have fallen into the normal range or even below. The perchlorate discharge test may also be positive and the $PB^{131}I$ is commonly higher than normal. The protein bound iodine level (PBI) may also be elevated, as a result of the secretion of abnormal iodinated compounds. More specific tests for thyroxine usually show that the concentration is either normal or low. Thus, the combination of a raised ^{131}I uptake, a high PBI and an elevated $PB^{131}I$ may suggest the diagnosis of thyrotoxicosis in a patient who is, in fact, euthyroid or even mildly hypothyroid. However, the elevated ^{131}I uptake can be suppressed with tri-iodothyronine, unlike that in the thyrotoxic patient, and the serum TSH level will be either normal or mildly elevated, whereas in the thyrotoxic case it is nearly always undetectable.

Some patients present with symptoms suggestive of thyrotoxicosis and in these thyroid function tests must be carefully chosen to allow thyroid status to be correctly assessed. In most of these patients the clinical impression of thyroid overactivity cannot be confirmed but a few have been described in whom there seems no doubt that thyrotoxicosis was indeed present. Such patients may show remission of the hyperthyroid state after a few months and may progress through a euthyroid phase to hypothyroidism. The exact relationship between thyrotoxicosis and Hashimoto's disease remains unclear. The occurrence of exophthalmos in a few patients with Hashimoto's disease has already been mentioned and LATS has also been detected in some subjects. Conversely, thyrotoxic patients commonly show evidence of autoimmune thyroiditis (see below). At present it seems most profitable to consider thyrotoxicosis and Hashimoto's disease as two separate disorders, which may, not uncommonly, co-exist.

Antibody studies (see Table 5.1). Thyroid antibodies can be detected in virtually every patient with Hashimoto's disease. Doniach and Roitt (1968), using precipitin, tanned red cell, complement fixation and immunofluorescent tests, found 99·7 per cent of patients to give positive results when all tests were considered together. Thus failure to detect thyroid antibodies by any of these tests makes the diagnosis of Hashimoto's disease very unlikely. Immunofluorescent tests are not always routinely available, but even if these are excluded, 94 per cent of patients still give positive results with the other tests.

Hyperglobulinaemia has been found in up to 60 per cent of patients with Hashimoto's disease, whereas it is extremely rare in other types of thyroid disease. The elevation may be of either $alpha_2$ or gamma globulin.

Although it has been claimed that the concentration of circulating antibodies correlates directly with the degree of inflammatory infiltration of the gland, the relationship is certainly not a very close one. The wide variation in the proportions of antibodies present makes it difficult to define any very clear-cut relationship. There is some evidence that the titre of antibodies tends to decrease in patients with long-standing disease who have advanced thyroid destruction.

Treatment. Many patients with Hashimoto's disease who are euthyroid and have small- to moderate-sized goitres need no treatment, but should simply be observed, after assessment of their thyroid function, to detect the development of pressure symptoms or of hypothyroidism.

Those who already have pressure symptoms or who are worried by the size of the gland should be treated with replacement doses of thyroxine (0·1 to 0·3 mg daily). In many patients, especially those with diffuse goitres of recent onset, this will cause a marked decrease in the size of the gland in a period of two to three months. Once having started such treatment it should probably be continued for life. Certainly, if it is stopped, the patients should be closely observed for further enlargement of the gland and to confirm that they remain euthyroid.

Patients who present hypothyroid will, of course, need replacement therapy for life.

The only indications for surgery now are: (a) suspicion of carcinoma; (b) serious pressure symptoms not responsive to thyroxine treatment; or (c) for cosmetic reasons in those unwilling to take, or who are unresponsive to, thyroxine. These indications are rare and if surgery is carried out thyroxine replacement should always be given.

Following treatment with thyroxine or surgery, or both, antibody titres may fall but do not always do so.

Primary hypothyroidism

The clinical and biochemical features of this disease are too well known to need discussion here. As mentioned above the disease is thought to represent the end result of progressive diffuse autoimmune thyroiditis leading to glandular destruction and fibrosis.

The disease is approximately five times as common in women as in men and the incidence increases progressively with age. Pathologically the thyroid is usually markedly atrophic and the histological picture ranges from changes similar to those seen in Hashimoto's disease to virtually complete fibrosis of the gland with almost total absence of follicular cells and only sparse lymphocytic infiltration. Thus, there appears to be no clear dividing line between Hashimoto's disease progressing to hypothyroidism and primary hypothyroidism.

Overall, thyroid antibodies can be found in over 90 per cent of patients with primary hypothyroidism. Although there is a tendency for titres to be lower than in Hashimoto's disease there is a very considerable overlap in the results obtained in the two conditions.

Asymptomatic atrophic thyroiditis

This term has been used by Bastenie and his collaborators (Bastenie and Ermans, 1972) to indicate the presence of lymphocytic thyroiditis in a patient who has neither thyroid enlargement nor clinical signs of thyroid disease. The diagnosis is made either by the detection of thyroid antibodies during life, or by necropsy studies. The latter have shown a surprisingly high incidence of the disorder, evidence of thyroiditis being found in about 20 per cent of post-mortem studies when patients with known thyroid disease are excluded. It occurs two to four times as commonly in women as in men, and in about ten per cent of affected subjects the thyroiditis is found to be extensive.

Studies of the incidence of thyroid antibodies in patients without clinical evidence of thyroid disease have given rather similar results. The incidence varies with sex and age but, overall, thyroglobulin antibodies can be detected by the tanned red cell test in about eleven per cent of patients, while microsomal antibodies can be found in nine per cent by the complement fixation test. When tests for both antibodies are considered together, 20 per cent of women admitted to hospital for non-thyroid disease give positive results, as do 10 per cent of men. The incidence of positive tests for thyroglobulin antibodies increases with age, at least up to the age of 80, in both sexes but at all ages positive tests are two to three times as common in women as in men. Thus in the 70 to 79-year-old age group 23 per cent of women and 9 per cent of men are positive, while in those aged 15 to 39 years positive results are seen in 9 per cent of women and 3 per cent of men.

When the titre of antithyroid antibodies found during life is considered together with the extent of thyroiditis found at necropsy, there appears to be a fairly good correlation. Thus, a tanned red cell titre of 1 in 125 or greater and/or positive tests for microsomal antibodies appear always to be associated with histological evidence of thyroiditis.

From the point of view of thyroid function these patients appear to form a mixed group. In some no abnormality can be detected and the thyroiditis appears to be non-progressive and of little significance. In others minor degrees of hypothyroidism exist and in the third group tests show abnormalities similar to those seen in euthyroid patients with Hashimoto's disease (see above).

Since this disorder is, by definition, asymptomatic the significance of its existence to the practising clinician remains uncertain. Apart from indicating that minor degrees of thyroid dysfunction are, perhaps, more common than previously realised it may also have significance for another reason. Bastenie and his co-workers have claimed that there is an association between thyroiditis, diabetes mellitus, hypertension, ischaemic heart disease and atheroma. They have produced evidence that it is the presence of thyroiditis itself, rather than of any impairment of thyroid function, which is associated with an increased incidence of the other disorders. Although their evidence for this association is compelling it has not yet been fully substantiated by other studies and the factors linking thyroiditis and the other disorders are far from clear.

Whether patients without symptoms in whom thyroid antibodies are detected should receive any treatment is also uncertain. Those with definite biochemical evidence of hypothyroidism should clearly receive replacement doses of thyroxine. In those who have normal thyroid function tests, but who show an elevated TSH level, a state which might be defined as compensated thyroid failure is presumably present. Since it seems likely that the thyroiditis in these patients will be progressive, replacement therapy with thyroxine should probably be given. In those in whom no abnormality can be detected other than the presence of thyroid antibodies the position is less clear. It is not known what proportion of such patients will eventually become hypothyroid and there is, as yet, no evidence that treatment will reduce the incidence of myocardial infarction. At present, the best course would seem to be to follow such patients carefully and to institute treatment if a rising TSH concentration or other tests of thyroid function suggest progressive impairment of thyroid hormone production.

The thyroiditis itself seems to be little affected by thyroxine treatment. In some patients a progressive fall in antibody titre is seen after therapy is started, but an equal number show no change.

Thyrotoxicosis

Hyperthyroidism resulting from the development of single or multiple autonomous adenomas is not thought to have an autoimmune basis and will not be further discussed.

In the most common type of hyperthyroidism (Graves' disease) clinical and biochemical evidence of thyroidal overactivity is associated with diffuse enlargement of the thyroid with, or without, exophthalmos and pre-tibial myxoedema. Evidence of autoimmune thyroiditis is common in this disorder, but the discovery of the long-acting thyroid stimulator provided the main stimulus to the idea that autoimmune factors play a role in the aetiology of the disease. Some of the evidence suggesting that LATS is an antibody has been discussed above.

Reasons for concluding that LATS plays a major rôle in the development and maintenance of thyrotoxicosis may be briefly summarised as follows:

1. LATS can be detected in the serum of up to 85 per cent of patients with Graves' disease, if procedures for the concentration of IgG are used.
2. LATS has been shown to have thyroid-stimulating activity in vivo in both man and experimental animals as well as in vitro.
3. Transient thyroidal overactivity may occur in neonates born to mothers with high serum LATS concentrations. This appears to result from trans-placental passage of LATS.
4. Serum TSH is usually undetectable in untreated patients with Graves' disease and thyroidal overactivity cannot be suppressed with exogenous thyroid hormone, indicating the presence of a thyroid-stimulating factor other than TSH.
5. A correlation has been claimed to exist between LATS concentration, radioactive iodine turnover and thyroid mass (Carneiro, Dorrington and Munro, 1966).
6. It has been claimed that LATS is found only in the serum of patients with untreated or treated thyrotoxicosis or in their relatives.

Although nobody would deny that LATS has thyroid-stimulating activity its rôle in the pathogenesis of Graves' disease has recently been challenged for several reasons:

1. Although assay techniques have been increasingly refined it has not, so far, proved possible to detect LATS in all patients.

2. A number of patients with thyrotoxicosis have now been described who show suppression of radioactive uptake when given tri-iodothyronine both before and during treatment with antithyroid drugs. There is no correlation whatever between the degree of suppression seen and the serum LATS concentration.
3. Several studies have failed to confirm the presence of any correlation between the degree of hyperthyroidism and serum LATS concentrations. Thus Chopra et al, (1970) in a study of 35 patients were unable to find any correlation between LATS concentration and any test of thyroid function or thyroid size.
4. LATS has been found in the serum of a number of euthyroid patients. These include subjects with Hashimoto's disease, euthyroid patients with exophthalmos, euthyroid relatives of patients with Graves' disease, including some relatives of hyperthyroid patients without detectable LATS and occasional normal subjects with no evidence of thyroid disease. A few patients have also been described who have been found to have high LATS concentrations while euthyroid and have later become thyrotoxic without any obvious change in LATS concentration.

In some of these patients it has been suggested that LATS is unable to produce hyperthyroidism because of the presence of concomitant thyroiditis, which diminishes thyroid reserve to such a degree that increased function is no longer possible. However, thyroid antibodies have been detected in only a small proportion of LATS positive euthyroid relatives of patients with Graves' disease. Other subjects have been found to show increased thyroid function after TSH stimulation and some patients show normal suppressibility of ^{131}I uptake after tri-iodothyronine in spite of the presence of high LATS concentrations.

In general, the incidence of positive LATS assays has been found to correlate more closely with the number of manifestations of Graves' disease present in a group of patients than with the severity of any one of them. Thus about 90 per cent of patients with hyperthyroidism, pre-tibial myxoedema and exophthalmos give positive results in assays on concentrated serum, as against about 50 per cent in patients with only one manifestation.

For these reasons it is difficult to accept the concept that hyperthyroidism in Graves' disease results simply from thyroidal stimulation by LATS. The finding of other thyroid stimulating substances in the serum of thyrotoxic patients, as discussed above, goes some way to answering these problems, however.

As already mentioned above, evidence of autoimmune thyroiditis is common in patients with Graves' disease. Thyroid antibodies can be detected in 80 to 90 per cent of patients. Usually titres are fairly low and in about 25 per cent only immunofluorescent tests are positive.

Autoimmune thyroiditis in other thyroid disorders

As shown in Table 5.1 thyroid antibodies can be detected in about 50 per cent of patients with multinodular goitre and thyroid carcinoma. Antibody titres are usually, though not invariably, low, and in multinodular goitre immunofluorescent tests only are positive in about half the patients in whom antibodies can be detected.

Histological evidence of thyroiditis can be found in a similar proportion of patients, usually in the form of scattered areas of lymphocytic infiltration.

Subacute thyroiditis (de Quervain's) is a disease thought possibly to be of viral origin. It occurs mainly in adults aged between 20 and 60 and is some 2 to 3 times as common in women as in men. Its onset is usually characterised by non-specific symptoms such as general malaise, mild dysphagia and diffuse pain in or around the neck. Fever is common. After a short prodromal phase, the temperature rises further and the thyroid becomes swollen and often acutely painful and tender. Sometimes the swelling is asymmetrical. Later, symptoms gradually subside and the gland returns to normal over a period of a few weeks, or sometimes a few months. Remissions and relapses are not uncommon.

Tests of thyroid function show release of large amounts of thyroxine in the early stages of the disease, together with other iodinated compounds. Symptoms suggesting hyperthyroidism may be seen at this stage. Radioiodine uptake, however, is low or absent. Following the early phase of release, the gland remains depleted of thyroxine for a variable period, so that a hypothyroid phase may ensue before glandular function returns gradually to normal.

Tests for thyroid antibodies give positive results in about 50 per cent of patients. Antibodies cannot be detected in the early stages of the disease and usually appear somewhere between 4 and 12 weeks after the onset. Antibodies to the second colloid antigen are most commonly detected; those to thyroglobulin or to the microsomal antigen also occur but are usually present in low titre. In most cases the antibodies disappear following recovery from the disease. Very occasionally, patients with apparently straightforward subacute thyroiditis have been reported in whom titres of thyroglobulin and microsomal antibodies show a progressive increase to reach high levels. In such subjects subacute thyroiditis has apparently been transformed into chronic, lymphocytic thyroiditis and the development of hypothyroidism has been reported. Such a sequence of events seems to be extremely rare and in those few patients who do become permanently hypothyroid the usual cause seems to be unusually severe damage to the gland by subacute thyroiditis with no definite evidence that autoimmune processes are involved.

Diagnostic value of thyroid antibody tests

In routine clinical practice, thyroid antibody tests have only limited value. The most common situations in which they may be useful are as follows.

The differential diagnosis of goitre. The most important problem is that of the patient who presents with a rapidly enlarging gland or with pressure symptoms. Failure to detect thyroid antibodies or hyperglobulinaemia makes a diagnosis of Hashimoto's disease virtually untenable. By contrast, a positive precipitin test is strongly in favour of such a diagnosis, although occasional positive results have been reported in patients with thyrotoxicosis, carcinoma and subacute thyroiditis. The finding of high titres in both the tanned red cell test (greater than 1 in 25 000) and the complement fixation test (greater than 1 in 64) has not been reported except in Hashimoto's disease and, occasionally, in thyrotoxicosis.

Rapidly developing Hashimoto's disease may occasionally be confused with subacute thyroiditis; however, titres of thyroid antibodies are usually high in Hashimoto's disease of this type. In subacute thyroiditis antibodies are usually absent in the first few weeks and thereafter, if present, are usually found only in low titre.

The finding of high concentrations of either thyroglobulin or microsomal antibodies alone, of low concentrations of either or both, or of positive immunofluorescent tests only, is of no value in differential diagnosis.

For these reasons antibody tests must always be considered in conjunction with clinical observations and carefully chosen tests of thyroid function. If there is any suspicion of malignancy thyroid biopsy should be carried out, especially since lymphoma may occasionally complicate lymphocytic thyroiditis.

In thyrotoxicosis. In the young patient one of the commonest problems is the differentiation of mild thyrotoxicosis from an anxiety state. In those patients in whom tests of thyroid function are equivocal the detection of thyroid antibodies would tend to support a diagnosis of thyrotoxicosis, especially if they are present in high titre and if the thyroid is only slightly enlarged. In the elderly woman this test becomes of little value, since the finding of thyroid antibodies is so common in patients with no evidence of thyroid disease. In patients with an obvious goitre the test is of no value.

There is some evidence that thyrotoxic patients with tanned red cell and, especially, complement fixation tests positive in high titre (TRC $>$ 1/640; CFT $>$ 1/64) show a higher incidence of hypothyroidism following partial thyroidectomy than do patients with low titre or no detectable antibodies. Such patients may also show a higher incidence of hypothyroidism following radioiodine therapy but the difference seems to be less marked. Antibody tests seem to be of no value in predicting whether or not remission will occur following a course of medical treatment. If remission does not occur the choice between surgery and radioiodine will usually be made on grounds such as age of the patient, size of the gland and the patient's preference. The major value of antibody tests would then seem to be in picking out a group of patients particularly at risk of developing hypothyroidism, thus alerting the clinician to the need for careful follow-up. However, since hypothyroidism commonly follows either procedure, in any case, it is to be hoped that all patients will be followed with care.

Differentiation of primary and secondary hypothyroidism. In those areas where it is available, the measurement of serum TSH has completely replaced all other methods for the differentiation of hypothyroidism resulting from primary thyroid disease from that of pituitary or hypothalmic origin. If this test is not available detection of thyroid antibodies would favour primary thyroid disease, especially in the young patient. However, there is no reason why autoimmune thyroiditis should not co-exist with pituitary disease, especially in the elderly.

In patients with mild hypothyroidism. These patients may present with such relatively non-specific complaints as weight gain, constipation, hair loss or dryness of the skin. In such subjects routine tests of thyroid function may fall within the normal range and it may not be possible to differentiate such patients from the much larger group of subjects with similar complaints but without thyroid disease. Positive tests for thyroid antibodies are found in up to 95 per cent of patients with mild hypothyroidism, so that completely negative antibody tests make it unlikely that the patient's symptoms result from thyroid disease or will respond to treatment with thyroxine. Conversely, detection of antibodies suggests either that more sophisticated tests of thyroid function should be carried out, or, if these are not readily available, that a trial of thyroxine therapy is justifiable.

In both these situations measurement of the serum TSH concentration seems a much more precise method of detecting primary thyroid abnormality.

Patients with an unexplained elevation of the ESR and hyperglobulinaemia. In occasional patients presenting with this picture the detection of thyroid antibodies might suggest thyroiditis as a reasonable explanation for the findings.

Adrenal and Parathyroid

Primary adrenocortical failure may result from destruction of the glands by infections such as tuberculosis or fungal disease, by carcinomatous metastases or by infarction. However, the majority of cases now result from the process known as idiopathic atrophy of the adrenal cortex. There is much evidence to suggest that autoimmune factors play a major part in the pathogenesis of this disease.

Adrenal antibodies

Circulating antibodies to adrenal tissue in patients with Addison's disease can be demonstrated either by indirect immunofluorescent methods or by a complement fixation test. The latter method is now rarely used. With the former, two major types of antibody have now been demonstrated.

1. That most commonly found reacts specifically with adrenal cortical cells, but not with those of the medulla or of other organs. The antigens involved have not been fully characterised but appear to be present in both the microsomal and mitochondrial fractions of adrenal homogenates. The amount of antigen present appears to be dependent upon glandular activity, being increased in hyperplastic glands. For this reason adrenals removed from patients with Cushing's syndrome due to bilateral adrenal hyperplasia provide the best material for the demonstration of antibodies, but glands removed for other reasons or obtained post mortem can also be used. Adrenals obtained from experimental animals can be used, but are least satisfactory. As a result of the wide variation in antigen content between different adrenal glands, it is essential to carry out control studies with known positive sera and with adrenals of known antigen content before deciding whether or not an unknown serum contains antibodies (Irvine and Barnes, 1972). Positive sera usually give a finely granular immunofluorescent staining of the cytoplasm of the cells of the whole thickness of the adrenal cortex.

2. Antibody to steroid-producing cells; this second type of antibody reacts

not only with adrenal cortical cells but also with steroid-producing cells of other organs, namely testis, ovary and placenta (Anderson et al, 1968). This type of antibody occurs in a smaller proportion of patients with idiopathic Addison's disease than does the first type.

Adrenal antibodies are rarely found except in patients with idiopathic Addison's disease or primary hypoparathyroidism. When Addison's disease results from tuberculosis, adrenal antibodies are almost invariably absent, and, as evidence accumulates, it seems increasingly likely that the occasional positive report in this condition results from misdiagnosis. The incidence of adrenal antibodies in various disease states and in control subjects is shown in Table 5.2.

Table 5.2. Percentage of patients with various diseases giving positive results in the immunofluorescent test for anti-adrenal antibody

Diagnosis	Percentage positive
Idiopathic Addison's	58
Tuberculous Addison's	0
First-degree relatives of patients with idiopathic Addison's	6
Primary hypoparathyroidism[a]	40
Hashimoto's disease	4
Normal subjects and patients with other adrenal or autoimmune disorders	Occasional single cases only

The results of tests for antibody to steroid-producing cells are not included. Figures are derived from the data of Irvine and Barnes (1972), Blizzard et al (1966) and Nerup et al (1966).

[a]Excluding patients with associated Addison's disease.

Histology

The histological picture of idiopathic adrenal atrophy is fully compatible with the suggested autoimmune basis. The normal cortical architecture is disrupted and the cortical cells replaced by lymphocytes and plasma cells. In the early stages, islands of lipid-depleted cortical cells remain, surrounded by the cellular infiltrate and variable amounts of fibrous tissue. Later, fibrosis increases, cortical cells almost or entirely disappear and the inflammatory infiltrate may become less prominent.

The adrenal medulla is entirely uninvolved, except for areas where small numbers of cortical cells extend into it. Thus, unlike the situation in tuberculosis where the entire gland is often destroyed, idiopathic atrophy leaves medullary function unimpaired.

Cellular immune reactions

Very little work has been reported suggesting the existence of cell-mediated reactions to adrenal tissue in man. Nerup and Bendixen (1969) studied 30 patients with idiopathic Addison's disease using the leucocyte migration inhibition test with pooled fetal adrenal extracts as antigen. They reported that in 14 patients (46 per cent) there was an abnormally low migration index. No such reaction was noted in patients with tuberculous Addison's disease. Blast transformation experiments with leucocytes from the patients with idiopathic disease grown in cell culture and exposed to adrenal antigen were negative. Of the 30 patients, 22 were shown to have circulating adrenal antibodies, and considering both these and the evidence of cellular immunity they claimed that 27 of the 30 patients showed evidence of humoral and/or cellular hypersensitivity to adrenal antigens.

Experimental adrenalitis

Allergic adrenalitis has been produced in a variety of experimental animals by the injection of whole adrenal homogenates emulsified in Freund's complete adjuvant. Guinea pigs, rabbits and rats have been mainly used.

In guinea pigs immunised with isologous or homologous adrenal extracts the adrenalitis produced is characterised by lesions in both cortex and medulla. Adrenal cells show degenerative changes of all grades up to complete destruction and infiltration with histiocytes, macrophages, lymphocytes, plasma cells and eosinophils is seen. Circulating antibodies, specific for guinea-pig adrenal homogenates, can be detected by complement fixation, tanned red cell haemagglutination and double diffusion in agar gel. These antibodies do not react with extracts of other guinea-pig organs, nor with adrenal extracts from other species. They will, however, react with extracts of the immunised animals' own adrenal gland and thus are true autoantibodies. The adrenal antigen against which they are directed has not been well characterised but appears to be thermolabile and may be a protein (Colover and Glynn, 1958; Milgrom and Witebsky, 1962). There appears to be no clear-cut relationship between the occurrence of antibodies and the development of adrenalitis.

The rabbit immunised with homologous adrenal extract appears to behave somewhat differently. Antibodies can be demonstrated in the same way as in guinea-pigs, but will react not only with homologous adrenal extracts but also with extracts of adrenal from other mammalian species. Further, Barnett, Dumonde and Glynn (1963) found that the antibodies could also be shown to react by immunofluorescent methods with antigens in the cytoplasm of ovarian and testicular cells (Leydig cells and spermatozoa). They also found that the rabbit adrenal antigen was heat labile and that the antibody responsible for both complement fixation and immunofluorescence could be absorbed by the ultracentrifuged sediment of adrenal or ovarian extract. In spite of this evidence of antibody production, histological evidence of adrenalitis in the rabbit is rarely seen unless heterologous antigen is used.

In certain strains of rat, allergic adrenalitis can readily be induced by single injections of rat adrenal emulsified in Freund's complete adjuvant given into the foot pad together with pertussis vaccine given at a neighbouring site (Levine and Wenk, 1968; Werdelin and Witebsky, 1970). The adrenalitis so produced involves the cortex only and can be transferred to non-immunised animals by the injection of suspensions of large numbers of cells obtained from the regional lymph nodes of animals with actively induced disease.

The experiments show striking similarities between experimental adrenalitis and spontaneous idiopathic adrenal atrophy in man. Although species differences exist in terms of the types of antibody produced, the extent of adrenal damage and the ease with which this can be produced, it is clear that autoimmune processes can lead to adrenal cortical destruction. As with experimental thyroiditis, the relative roles of humoral and cellular immune processes are still uncertain, as are the mechanisms leading to activation of the adrenal-damaging immune mechanism in man.

Genetic factors in adrenal disease

The occurrence of idiopathic Addison's disease in more than one member of the same family and in identical twins has been described on several occasions. Members of affected families also show a higher incidence, than would be expected by chance, of idiopathic hypoparathyroidism, mucocutaneous moniliasis, pernicious anaemia, thyroid disease, premature ovarian failure and diabetes mellitus, either alone or in various combinations with, or without, Addison's disease. First-degree relatives of patients with Addison's disease also show an increased incidence of adrenal antibodies as compared to controls.

So strong does the genetic element appear to be in family studies of patients with idiopathic adrenal atrophy that it has been suggested that the disease may be inherited as an autosomal recessive characteristic.

In conclusion, the case for considering that idiopathic adrenal atrophy in man is a disease resulting from autoimmune adrenal damage in a genetically predisposed individual is a strong one. The situation appears somewhat simpler than that seen in thyroid disease, in that there is little or no evidence that autoimmune adrenalitis plays either a primary or secondary role in any other adrenal disorder. In particular, although it has been suggested that certain cases of Cushing's syndrome might be due to adrenal stimulation by an antibody analogous to LATS, no proof for such a hypothesis has yet appeared.

Clinical aspects of Addison's disease

Addison's disease is a comparatively rare disorder. Studies in both this country and the United States suggest that the incidence is roughly 40 cases for each million of the population. Approximately one-third of these result from tuberculosis and the remaining two-thirds from idiopathic adrenal atrophy. In this country, other causes are extremely rare.

Although tuberculosis was formerly a more common cause, in the last 10 to 15 years the percentage of cases due to this disease has fallen markedly. In a series of cases diagnosed in the ten years up to 1938, 79 per cent were of tuberculous origin, but in another series diagnosed between 1962 and 1972, this percentage had fallen to 21 per cent (Irvine and Barnes, 1972).

Patients with idiopathic atrophy most commonly present between the ages of 20 and 50, but cases may also be seen in childhood and in old age. Below the age of 20 the disease is more common in boys, between 20 and 30 the sex incidence is equal, while after this age, women predominate.

Symptoms and signs of the disease develop insidiously and in many patients the diagnosis is made only when they present in adrenal crisis. The early symptoms are vague and non-specific. Weakness, tiredness and anorexia with resultant weight loss are usual. Later vague abdominal discomfort with occasional episodes of nausea, vomiting, diarrhoea or constipation may occur. Symptoms of postural hypotension may be seen in the later stages and hypoglycaemia after prolonged fasting may develop. Increasing pigmentation is seen in nearly all patients but rarely forms a cause for complaint, being usually attributed to a healthy sun tan. Vitiligo is seen in about 20 per cent of patients. Amenorrhoea may occur and some loss of pubic and axillary hair is not uncommon. Adrenal crisis may develop gradually, commonly being preceded by nausea and vomiting, often attributed to gastritis, or may be precipitated by acute infection, accident or surgery. Consciousness is usually impaired to a variable extent, the blood pressure is low and other signs of salt depletion are present. Serum sodium and chloride are low, potassium usually elevated and the blood urea almost invariably raised. The blood glucose may also be low.

Since the clinical features seen in the early stages are not at all uncommon in a variety of disease states, diagnosis depends upon the demonstration of low normal or low levels of plasma cortisol and 17 oxogenic steroids together with failure of the adrenal to respond to exogenous ACTH. Tests for adrenal antibodies have no place in diagnosis at this stage, but once the diagnosis has been made their finding gives assurance that adrenal failure results from idiopathic atrophy and is not due to tuberculosis or other cause. Since antibodies are found in only just over 50 per cent of patients with idiopathic atrophy, failure to detect them does not, of course, necessarily indicate another aetiology. In patients with adrenal tuberculosis, adrenal calcification, visible radiologically, is usual as is evidence of active or quiescent tuberculosis elsewhere.

Once the diagnosis is established treatment consists essentially of replacement of the sodium deficit and the lifelong administration of adequate replacement doses of a glucocorticoid, usually cortisone acetate or cortisol, together with a mineralocorticoid, such as fludrocortisone, although the latter is not always necessary. The glucocorticoid dose must, of course, be increased to cover any stressful situations, such as febrile illnesses or operations.

Although many patients will remain in perfect health on this regime without any need for modification, lifelong follow-up would seem wise in view of the frequent and unpredictable occurrence of associated disorders.

Disorders associated with Addison's disease

As has already been mentioned a number of other disorders may occur in members of the family of patients with Addison's disease and also in patients who themselves have this disease. Many of these associated disorders are also thought to have an autoimmune basis. That the association is with idiopathic adrenal atrophy, and not simply with abnormal adrenocortical function, is shown by their failure to occur in patients with tuberculous adrenal destruction. These patients, in fact, form an ideal control group for patients with idiopathic atrophy.

Two large series of patients have been studied with particular emphasis on the incidence of associated disorder. 118 patients were studied by Blizzard, Chee and Davis (1967) and 174 by Irvine and Barnes (1972). In the discussion that follows data from these two series has been combined where this seems appropriate.

Of the total 292 patients, 134 had a second disorder. Of 46 patients with tuberculous adrenal disease, another disorder was found in only 2.

Thyroid disease. The association of thyroid disease and non-tuberculous adrenal failure has been recognised for many years. Thyrotoxicosis, Hashimoto's disease and primary hypothyroidism may all be seen with unusual frequency. Subclinical thyroiditis is also more common than in normal controls or tuberculous patients, as shown by post-mortem histological studies and measurement of thyroid antibodies. In the combined series mentioned above, 57 of 292 patients had clinically apparent thyroid disease while thyroid antibodies could be detected in about 30 per cent of the patients in whom they were sought. No cases of clinically apparent disease were seen in a control group of patients with tuberculous Addison's disease, and although thyroid antibodies were detected in some of these patients, the frequency was the same as that seen in a group of normal control subjects.

Pernicious anaemia. Clinically apparent pernicious anaemia was found in 17 of the 292 patients. Antibodies to gastric parietal cells and to intrinsic factor were also more common than in control groups, being found in about 22 per cent of the patients. In subjects in whom such antibodies were detected, but who did not have clinically apparent pernicious anaemia, impairment of gastric acid secretion was common. No cases of pernicious anaemia were found in 46 patients with tuberculous Addison's disease.

Diabetes mellitus. This was present in 28 of the 292 patients, and in the majority was of the insulin-dependent type. Other authors have also commented upon the increased incidence of diabetes in these patients. Once again, there appears to be no association with tuberculous Addison's disease.

Gonadal failure. A number of authors have commented upon the association of idiopathic Addison's disease with an early menopause. Blizzard et al (1967) found four patients out of 57, while Irvine and Barnes (1972) found amenorrhoea in 27 out of 102 patients, primary in 5 and secondary in 22. Antibody to steroid-producing cells was found in all of the former and in 15 of the latter. No such antibodies could be found in patients with amenorrhoea or oligomenorrhoea not associated with Addison's disease or in patients with gonadal dysgenesis. In most patients amenorrhoea developed at about the time at which Addison's disease was diagnosed, suggesting the possibility that similar autoimmune processes were involved in both adrenal and ovarian failure. Ovarian histology in these patients has shown changes ranging from lymphocytic infiltration around developing ovarian follicles to complete replacement of the ovary by fibrous tissue.

Testicular failure may also occur in association with Addison's disease. Turkington and Lebowitz (1967) reported 3 cases in a series of 6 men selected because of the association of Addison's disease and another disorder. Irvine and Barnes (1972) found steroid cell antibodies in 2 of 52 male patients with idiopathic adrenal atrophy but no evidence of hypogonadism could be detected. Testicular histology does not seem to have been studied in detail in these patients and although it seems probable that autoimmune factors are involved, further studies are needed to clarify the situation.

Idiopathic hypoparathyroidism. This is an exceedingly rare disease which shows a strong association with Addison's disease. In the two large series previously referred to 30 of the 292 patients with Addison's disease also had idiopathic hypoparathyroidism. In the majority of these the diagnosis of Addison's disease was made in childhood.

The parathyroid glands in such patients show atrophy and lymphocytic infiltration and Blizzard, Chee and Davis (1966), using indirect immunofluorescent techniques, reported the detection of antibodies reacting with human parathyroid tissue in 38 per cent of 74 patients with idiopathic hypoparathyroidism. They also found these antibodies in 26 per cent of patients with Addison's disease, 12 per cent of patients with Hashimoto's disease and 6 per cent of 245 controls. They also reported that the antibodies were not directed against parathyroid hormone and did not cross react with sections of gastric mucosa, thyroid, adrenal, liver or kidney. Other authors have been unable to confirm this high incidence of parathyroid antibodies.

Patients who present with idiopathic hypoparathyroidism also show an increased incidence of gastric, thyroid and adrenal antibodies.

The disorder commonly presents with symptoms of hypocalcaemia, predominantly tetany, but abnormalities of the skin, hair and nails are common. These may include chronic mucocutaneous moniliasis. Cataracts, aplasia or hypoplasia of the teeth and basal ganglion calcification are also often seen. The serum calcium is low, sometimes being reduced to as little as 4 mg/100 ml while the inorganic phosphate is elevated. Treatment consists of giving a high calcium–low phosphate diet together with sufficient vitamin D to maintain the serum calcium in the normal range. In view of the high frequency of other autoimmune disorders in this condition, evidence of their presence should be sought at the time of first presentation and the possibility that they may develop later should always be kept in mind.

Other disorders. Irvine (1971) has also described the occurrence of a variety of neurological disorders in patients with idiopathic adrenal atrophy. These include Schilder's disease, spastic paraplegia, idiopathic epilepsy, suspected multiple sclerosis and mental retardation with deafness.

Vitiligo occurs in about 9 per cent of patients and may also be seen in association with evidence of thyroid and gastric-autoimmune disease.

The occurrence of mucocutaneous candidiasis in idiopathic hypoparathyroidism has already been mentioned, but it may also occur in patients with idiopathic adrenal atrophy alone.

Alopecia has also been reported, as have a number of other disorders (Irvine and Barnes, 1972).

Testis

The association of testicular atrophy with Addison's disease has been mentioned above. Apart from this association, autoimmune reactions to spermatozoal antigens have been suggested as a possible cause of infertility in both men and women.

Experimental studies have shown that allergic orchitis can be produced in male animals immunised with autologous or homologous testicular homogenate in Freund's complete adjuvant. Guinea pigs appear to be particularly susceptible and, in this species, testicular damage may be seen between two and eight weeks following immunisation. Inflammation and oedema are seen between the tubules and infiltration with plasma cells and lymphocytes occurs. Degenerative changes are seen in sperm cells at all stages of maturation together with widespread sloughing of the germinal epithelium. The Sertoli cells appear less affected and the Leydig cells remain normal. Azoospermia may persist for several months, but, eventually, sperm production returns to normal. A similar picture can be produced if spermatozoa themselves are used as the antigen rather than testicular homogenate.

Circulating antibodies, apparently directed specifically against an antigen located in the acrosome of spermatozoa and spermatids, can be demonstrated in such animals. Exposure of motile spermatozoa to these antibodies commonly results in immobilisation and agglutination. Evidence of cell-mediated immunity can also be found and its presence appears to correlate more closely with the occurrence and severity of allergic orchitis than does that of circulating antibodies.

Anti-spermatozoal antibodies can also be readily induced in female animals, using the same techniques of immunisation. More interestingly however, as far as problems of human fertility are concerned, these antibodies may also develop following administration of antigen plus adjuvant by the intravaginal route. Once produced, the titre may increase following deposition of sperm in the vagina without adjuvant. As well as being present in the blood, antibodies can also be found in vaginal and uterine secretions, and, in some animals, impairment of fertility has been noted.

Experimental and clinical studies in man

Mancini et al (1965) have shown that autoimmune orchitis can be induced experimentally in man and resembles that seen in the guinea pig. No definite naturally occurring counterpart has, however, yet been identified.

Studies designed to test the hypothesis that circulating antibodies to spermatozoal antigens may be associated with infertility in men have yielded generally rather disappointing results. Methods used for the detection of antibodies include observations of microscopic or macroscopic agglutination of spermatozoa exposed to patient's serum and haemagglutination reactions using various antigens derived from sperm or semen. Studies of large numbers of infertile men by these techniques have shown antibodies to be present in only a small proportion and in many patients antibodies were associated with inflammatory or obstructive disease of the testis and ducts. Surgical relief of the obstruction in some patients has led to restoration of fertility even though antibody titres remain unaffected.

Anti-spermatozoal antibodies have been detected in a small proportion of infertile women, though in some series these were also detected in the similar proportions of fertile women. There have been a few reports of decrease in antibody titres when seminal contact is prevented by the use of a condom, with the occurrence of pregnancy when unrestricted intercourse was resumed (Franklin and Dukes, 1964).

From the evidence at present available it seems unlikely that autoimmune factors play any major part in the development of infertility in either men or women. It may be that studies of cell-mediated immunity will be more relevant than those of circulating antibodies but comparatively little work has yet been done in this field.

Diabetes Mellitus

In spite of an enormous amount of work the aetiology of diabetes mellitus remains essentially unknown. Some features of the disease, especially of the juvenile onset type, have led to the suspicion that autoimmune factors may be involved. These include the following features.

The association of diabetes with other disorders of presumed autoimmune aetiology

An increased incidence of diabetes, especially when insulin-dependent, has been reported in patients with pernicious anaemia, Hashimoto's disease, myxoedema and idiopathic Addison's disease. Certain autoantibodies also seem to occur with greater frequency in insulin-dependent diabetics than they do in those who are not insulin-dependent or in normal controls. Irvine et al (1970) studied 521 men and 533 women with diabetes of both types and found an increased incidence, compared to that in controls, of thyroid microsomal and gastric parietal cell antibodies in insulin-dependent diabetics of all ages. The difference was particularly striking in patients under 40, where 22 per cent and 20 per cent of female patients gave positive tests for thyroid microsomal and gastric parietal cell antibodies respectively. The comparable figures for female controls were 6 per cent and 5 per cent. Male patients also showed an increased incidence of similar proportions but the total percentage positive in both groups was about four times less. In patients over 40 the incidence of these two antibodies was also increased in insulin-dependent-patients compared both to controls and to younger diabetics. The incidence of thyroglobulin antibodies was not significantly increased except in men over 40. Non-insulin dependent diabetics differed only to a minor extent from controls, although gastric parietal cell antibodies were more common in the elderly diabetic and thyroid microsomal antibodies in young male patients. As this would suggest, gastric parietal cell and thyroid microsomal antibodies were significantly more common in insulin-dependent patients than in the non-insulin-dependent.

Whittingham et al (1971) reached very similar conclusions though in insulin-dependent patients over 60 they found a lower incidence of thyroid and gastric antibodies than in controls, and they suggested that diabetics with autoantibodies died earlier than those without. They also found an increased incidence of antinuclear factor in young diabetics whose disease had been present for more than 20 years. Non-insulin-dependent diabetics in this study showed no increase in the incidence of autoantibodies.

Evidence of insulitis

In young diabetics inflammatory infiltrates may be seen around and within the pancreatic islets. That such lesions might occur had been known for many years, but they were thought to be rare. Le Compte (1958) suggested that they might be less uncommon than previously thought. This was confirmed by Gepts (1965) who found such lesions in pancreatic tissue obtained post-mortem from 15 out of 22 young diabetics whose disease had been present for 180 days or less. The infiltrates, composed of lymphocytes, reticular cells and a few polymorphs were found in and around islets showing degenerative changes. They were not seen around normal islets or in tissue from juvenile diabetics with disease of longer duration.

Such lesions are not seen in experimental diabetes produced by alloxan or injection of pituitary extracts but have been produced in rabbits and cows following immunisation with heterologous or homologous insulin (Toreson, Lee and Grodsky, 1968; Renold et al, 1966). In the rabbit such lesions appear soon after immunisation, before circulating anti-insulin antibodies can be detected, and may persist for up to 62 weeks. In some animals they are associated with evidence of damage to the β cells of the islets and in these diabetes may develop. It is suggested that cell mediated immunity may be the dominant aetiological mechanism.

Evidence of humoral or cellular immune reactions to pancreatic antigens

Studies designed to show direct evidence of humoral or cellular autoimmune reactions against pancreatic antigens in untreated diabetes have produced conflicting results.

As mentioned in another section (p. 162), insulin antibodies can be detected in almost all insulin-treated patients. Some early studies in which complement fixation tests were used for insulin-antibody detection suggested that such antibodies might also be present in a high proportion of untreated patients. However, these results have not been confirmed by other techniques and most authors would now accept that evidence of insulin-antibody formation in untreated patients occurs very rarely, if at all. Følling and Norman (1972) have recently described a patient with mildly impaired glucose tolerance and reactive hypoglycaemia whose serum appeared to contain an IgG globulin capable of binding both porcine and human insulin. This material was studied by a variety of methods and appeared to have all the characteristics to be expected of an insulin antibody. There was no evidence that the patient had ever been treated with insulin. Studies of the patient's relatives and of control subjects showed no evidence of insulin binding. There was some evidence that the antibody was monoclonal in type. It seems clear, however, from other studies that such a finding is an extremely rare event and its relevance to the problem of the aetiology of more usual types of diabetes is uncertain.

Several authors have suggested that some of the complications of diabetes might result from immunological reactions. Attention has been focussed particularly on vascular and renal lesions. It has been reported that fluorescein-labelled insulin binds to basement membranes and glomerular nodules from kidneys of diabetic patients. Several workers have also reported the finding of immunoglobulins and complement components in kidney, retina and skin of diabetics. Many of these studies can be criticised on technical grounds and the involvement of insulin antibodies seems unlikely since, as already stated, these can rarely if ever be detected in diabetics not treated with insulin, although renal and vascular lesions are not uncommon in such subjects. That other types of immunological reaction may be involved, cannot, however, be definitely excluded.

Little work has been done on cellular immune reactions to pancreatic components in diabetes. Nerup et al (1971) carried out leucocyte migration tests with white cells from 22 insulin-dependent diabetics and 18 normal controls. As antigen they used the 104 000 g precipitate from a homogenate made from porcine pancreas removed from animals whose pancreatic ducts had been ligated 8 weeks previously. Liver and kidney homogenates and porcine and bovine insulin were used as controls. In half the diabetics the migration index was significantly reduced on exposure to pancreatic antigen. Other antigens had no effect and a similar reduction in migration was seen in only one control. They showed that this effect occurred in diabetics not treated with insulin and in whom no insulin antibodies could be detected, as well as in insulin-treated patients.

Intradermal tests in four diabetics also showed a delayed-type reaction to pancreatic antigen, but not to porcine insulin present in the same concentration as in the pancreatic preparation. Controls gave negative responses.

Conclusion

The strong association of juvenile-onset diabetes with disorders of suspected autoimmune aetiology, the reports of inflammatory islet-cell lesions and the evidence of delayed hypersensitivity to pancreatic components make it tempting to assume that autoimmune factors play a causative role in diabetes. However, the evidence remains inconclusive at present.

IMMUNOLOGICAL REACTIONS TO EXOGENOUS HORMONES

An increasing number of polypeptide hormones are being used for the treatment of disease in man. Since all these are readily destroyed by proteolytic enzymes in the gut they are usually given by injection or, occasionally, in the form of nasal sprays or as snuff. Immunological reactions to such hormones can commonly be demonstrated in the recipients and are of importance in that they may interfere with therapy.

In general two types of reaction are seen, described as follows.

Local or generalised cutaneous or vascular reactions

Erythema and inflammation or localised urticaria may be seen at the injection site. Generalised urticaria and angioneurotic oedema are also seen and acute anaphylactic reactions may occur.

Circulating antibodies

These may develop and bind the hormone in plasma or extracellular fluid, reducing the ease with which it gains access to tissue receptors where it exerts its biological effect and results in alterations of hormonal metabolism.

The frequency and severity with which such reactions develop depend upon a number of factors; these may include the following.

The genetic constitution of the patient

Local reactions are more likely to occur in individuals with an atopic constitution. Genetic factors are probably also concerned in the development of other types of immunological reaction but are of relatively minor importance compared with other considerations.

The chemical nature of the hormone given

Polypeptide hormones used for therapeutic purposes may be divided into three groups.

Those that are chemically identical with the natural human hormone. These may be either extracted from material of human origin, e.g. human anterior pituitary tissue obtained post mortem, or chemically synthesised.

In view of the obvious difficulties in obtaining human tissue, hormones derived from such a source are only used where the analogous hormones from other species are not biologically active in man. Human growth hormone is an example. Even though a hormone is extracted from human tissue it cannot necessarily be assumed that the end product is chemically identical with the natural hormone. Minor chemical modifications may occur during the extraction procedure, and there is increasing evidence that many polypeptide hormones occur in the natural state in several chemical forms, either as precursor molecules of high molecular weight or as partially metabolised forms which may, or may not, have biological activity.

Chemical synthesis of polypeptide hormones is, at present, only possible on a large scale for those of low molecular weight, e.g. arginine vasopressin, oxytocin, and certain of the hypothalamic releasing hormones. Even when synthetic material is used it is unwise to assume that only a single molecular species of hormone is present. 'Error peptides' are produced during synthesis and chemical changes, including polymerisation, may occur during storage.

Hormones obtained from species other than man. Polypeptide hormones obtained from different species show varying degrees of chemical identity. Most types of mammalian and even non-mammalian insulin are biologically active in man even though there are a number of differences in the amino-acid constitution of the basic insulin molecule. The same is true of ACTH, TSH and glucagon.

Biologically active hormone fragments of synthetic or natural origin. For many hormones the entire 'natural' molecule is not needed for biological activity. The human ACTH molecule contains 39 amino acids, but only the N-terminal 24 are needed for full biological activity. The molecule containing these amino acids has been synthesised and is available for therapeutic use (tetracosactrin). Chemical modifications of other hormones can also be made without impairing biological activity to more than a minor extent. Thus the 8 C-terminal amino acids of the B chain of the insulin molecule can be removed (desoctapeptide insulin) and other minor chemical modifications can also be made.

From the immunological point of view, such modifications may be of value in that the chemical differences in the hormones derived from various species sometimes are found only in that part of the molecule not needed for full biological activity. In the ACTH molecule, for example, amino acids 1–24 are the same in all species, but there are differences in amino acids 25–39. Removal of these thus eliminates species differences from the molecule while leaving biological activity unimpaired. This type of modification may, therefore, reduce the antigenicity of the molecule.

The degree of purity of the hormone preparation

Hormones derived from natural sources may be contaminated by a variety of non-human proteins and peptides. These may, themselves, be antigenic and may be responsible for some of the local reactions seen to hormone preparations. As extraction procedures and synthetic techniques improve this is becoming a diminishing problem.

The pharmaceutical formulation of the hormone preparation

Polypeptide hormones usually have short biological half-lives in the circulation and are rapidly destroyed by proteolytic enzymes in the tissues. It is often desirable, therefore, to increase the duration of action by using depot preparations of hormones, designed to ensure delayed release from, and destruction in, the tissues. This may be achieved by chemically modifying the molecule, by the addition of foreign proteins such as protamine, by preparing the hormone in macrocrystalline or aggregated form or by suspension of the hormone in oil. Many of these manoeuvres are reminiscent of the use of adjuvants and other procedures used by the immunologist to increase the immunogenicity of an antigen preparation.

The duration of treatment

Once started, treatment with polypeptide hormones must often be continued for many years, thus ensuring a prolonged stimulus to the immunological system. Intermittent courses of treatment are sometimes given, and these appear to be particularly favourable to the development of severe allergic reactions.

A number of other considerations may also apply in the case of specific hormones, and reactions to these will be considered individually.

Insulin

Evidence of the formation of antibodies in patients receiving insulin for any length of time is almost universal.

Local reactions

These usually occur within a few days of starting treatment. A sensation of stinging or itching may be felt at the injection site and erythema, swelling and tenderness may occur and persist for 24 to 48 hours. These reactions usually cease spontaneously after 2 to 4 weeks, or occasionally after a longer interval.

In a few patients more severe reactions, such as generalised urticaria or angioneurotic oedema may be seen. Anaphylactic shock has been reported but seems to be extremely rare. These reactions may occur in patients receiving insulin for the first time, but appear to be more common in those who have received previous insulin therapy which was discontinued.

There is now a large body of evidence that these reactions are due to the presence of reaginic antibody directed against insulin itself. Most commercial insulin is a mixture of beef and pork insulins. Patients showing local reactions do not usually show any allergy to beef or pork proteins other than insulin, but do show reactions to insulin prepared from other species. Prausnitz–Küstner reactions can often be demonstrated in normal subjects, following administration of serum from a sensitive patient. The antibody responsible for these local reactions is heat labile, being destroyed by heating to 57°C for 2 hours and may persist for three weeks or longer at the sensitised site in the skin of a normal subject. Passive transfer of sensitivity can no longer be shown if the serum is treated with rabbit anti-reaginic antibody or if heat-inactivated serum from a patient with circulating anti-insulin antibodies is added to the serum used in transfer experiments, presumably because of the 'blocking' effect of circulating antibodies. Electrophoretically the skin-sensitising antibody migrates with the beta globulins rather than the gamma globulin and cannot be removed from serum by absorption with an antiserum to IgA. In vitro tests, e.g. tests for histamine release from the peripheral blood leucocytes of sensitive patients after incubation with insulin, have usually been unsuccessful in demonstrating the presence of hypersensitivity.

The antibody thus appears to be a reagin and the local reactions are probably mainly type I of Gell and Coombs (1968). Since, however, other types of antibody are commonly also present in insulin-treated patients, it is difficult to exclude the possibility that some local reactions may be of type II (cytotoxic) or III (Arthus type). The immunoglobulin class of the reaginic antibody has not yet been definitely established.

Patients showing local reactions to beef–pork insulin show sensitivity on direct intradermal testing to a wide variety of insulins from various species including human insulin, either synthetic or extracted from the plasma of a sensitive patient. Attempts to show cutaneous hypersensitivity in patients whose endogenous insulin concentration has been increased by giving tolbutamide, have been unsuccessful.

These results seem to leave no doubt that the antibody is directed against insulin rather than a contaminating protein. However, it is less certain whether it is the insulin molecule itself that is antigenic or slightly altered forms of insulin present in most commercial preparations. Once-crystallised beef insulin, for example, has been shown to contain not only insulin but also proinsulin, insulin dimer, insulin ethyl ester and mono-desamido insulin as well as a number of other unidentified components.

Circulating insulin antibodies

It has been known for more than thirty years that circulating anti-insulin antibodies may be found in insulin-treated patients, that these could reduce the biological activity of insulin and that these antibodies were quite distinct from the skin-sensitising antibody. However, the development of such antibodies was thought to be a rare event until Berson et al (1956) showed that they could be demonstrated in most, if not all, patients treated with insulin for more than a few weeks. These antibodies bind administered insulin in the plasma in the form of soluble antigen–antibody complexes. This results in a considerable prolongation of the plasma half-life of administered insulin and limits its ability to diffuse into the extracellular space where it exerts its biological effect. In most patients the antibody concentration is relatively low and is sufficient to bind only five to ten units of insulin per litre of plasma; however, in certain subjects, especially those showing insulin resistance (defined as an insulin requirement greater than 200 units daily in the absence of ketosis, infection, etc), sufficient antibody may be present to bind up to 1000 units per litre. Although antibody-bound insulin is in dynamic equilibrium with free insulin in the circulation, the affinity of the antibodies may be so high that only a small proportion of the total plasma insulin is in free form unless massive doses are given, and it seems likely that it is only the free fraction which exerts biological activity. The antigen–antibody complexes are presumably removed from the circulation by phagocytosis and the insulin then rapidly destroyed by insulinase. Since new antibody is continually being formed the patient continues to need large doses of insulin to produce a biologically effective concentration of free hormone. It has been estimated that if the insulin-binding capacity is 60 units per litre, over 100 units of insulin will be wasted each day by the destruction of antigen–antibody complexes.

Insulin-binding antibodies can be readily demonstrated in plasma by mixing it with radioactively labelled insulin and carrying out chromatoelectrophoresis. In the absence of antibody, labelled insulin remains adsorbed at the site of application of the mixture to the paper strip, while if antibody is present it travels with the globulin (Berson et al, 1956). In order to exclude the possibility of non-specific binding, suitable controls must be set up. A number of other techniques, such as radioimmunoelectrophoresis, have also been used.

Insulin antibodies in most patients appear to be heterogeneous. The most common is of IgG class. IgA antibodies can be found together with IgG in about 25 per cent of patients, but IgM antibodies are rare. The affinity of the antibodies for insulin also appears to vary considerably.

Like the skin-sensitising antibody, circulating antibodies will react with most types of insulin, including human. Studies in patients with high titres suggest that beef insulin is more strongly bound than porcine, while sheep and fish insulins are relatively weakly bound. In both man and animals, very highly purified insulin preparations (single peak or monocomponent insulin), which contain 1 per cent or less of substances other than insulin itself, produce little or no antibody response, while the less pure, more widely used, preparations are much more immunogenic, presumably because of their content of chemically altered forms of insulin.

Clinical significance and treatment of immunological reactions to insulin

Local reactions usually subside spontaneously within a few weeks or months and rarely provide a serious problem. This tendency makes it difficult to assess the value of the various forms of treatment that have been proposed. Often a change from subcutaneous to intramuscular injection for a few days or weeks is enough to overcome the problem, but in patients with more severe reactions it may be necessary to change the type of insulin used. Substitution of pork insulin for the usual beef–pork mixtures is sometimes successful and good results have been claimed with the very highly purified preparations referred to above. However, not all workers using these preparations have found a reduction in the frequency of occurrence of local reactions. The use of sheep insulin or of desalaninated pork insulin, in which the C-terminal alanine of the beta chain has been removed, has also been recommended.

Rapid desensitisation, starting with doses of insulin as small as 0·001 unit has also been carried out in a few patients with more severe reactions, and appears to have been successful in some.

In those patients in whom the local reaction is transient, allergy to insulin can often be shown to persist indefinitely by intradermal testing or by Prausnitz–Küstner reactions. Similarly, in those patients in whom local reactions disappear after a change of insulin type, evidence of formation of antibodies to the new form of insulin can often be found even though no local reactions occur.

From data derived from studies in both man and animals it seems clear that circulating antibodies to insulin can decrease its biological effectiveness and high titres are commonly found in patients showing insulin resistance. The choice of treatment in such patients lies between changing the type of insulin used, as for local reactions, or the use of glucocorticoids. The choice will usually be determined by the availability of the different forms of insulin and the urgency of the situation.

Since antibodies to exogenous insulin usually also react with the patients' own endogenous insulin, the development of high titres may occasionally be implicated in the development of severe hyperglycaemia and ketosis in patients with maturity-onset diabetes treated with exogenous insulin. Thus, Karam, Grodsky and Forsham (1969) report the case of an obese diabetic woman who developed severe insulin resistance and ketosis when treated with insulin, together with extremely high titres of anti-insulin antibodies. When insulin treatment was stopped, the patient's clinical state improved and the titre of antibodies fell. They suggest that the antibodies bound both exogenous and endogenous insulin and led to a state of relative insulin deficiency.

The possibility that circulating insulin-antibody complexes might be involved in the development of certain diabetic complications, such as vasculitis or nephropathy, has been put forward. However, the evidence in favour of this view is unconvincing and such complications certainly occur in patients who have never received insulin and in whom no antibodies can be demonstrated.

Adrenocorticotropic hormone (ACTH)

In patients treated with ACTH, immunological reactions very similar to those occurring in insulin-treated patients may be seen.

Local reactions

Localised oedema at the injection site, urticaria, fever and anaphylactic reactions have all been described in patients receiving porcine ACTH by intramuscular, subcutaneous or intravenous injection. Passive cutaneous anaphylaxis has been demonstrated using serum from such patients with various preparations of ACTH. Direct intradermal testing with highly purified porcine ACTH preparations suggests that the antibody responsible for those reactions is directed against the ACTH molecule itself, rather than against impurities in the preparation, in most cases. Some patients also react against highly purified human ACTH, suggesting that the antigenic site in the molecule includes not only the species-specific portion (amino acids 25–39) but also amino acids 1–24 which are common to all types of ACTH.

Circulating antibodies

A high proportion of patients treated with ACTH preparations for more than a few weeks develop circulating antibodies. These can be demonstrated by chromatoelectrophoresis using radioactively labelled ACTH, and by a variety of other techniques.

Landon, Friedman and Greenwood (1967) found ACTH antibodies in 13 of 19 children treated with porcine ACTH gel for 5 to 200 weeks. There was no relation between the length of treatment or total dose and the presence or absence of antibodies. The reaction was not affected by heating the plasma to 56°C for 60 minutes and on electrophoresis the bound ACTH was found to run in the inter β–γ zone. In patients with the highest antibody titres the binding capacity was estimated to range from 16 to 48 ng/ml of plasma. Antibodies from 4 subjects were tested for their ability to bind bovine ACTH and tetracosactrin (synthetic α 1–24) as well as porcine ACTH. Cross reaction with both these substances was shown, but reaction was weakest with tetracosactrin and variable with bovine ACTH.

No obvious abnormality in the adrenal response to either endogenous or exogenous ACTH was found in patients with antibodies.

Fleischer et al (1967) obtained very similar results in a group of patients treated with porcine zinc ACTH. They were able to show, however, that patients in whom antibodies were present had higher endogenous ACTH levels than normal subjects although plasma cortisol levels were similar. Acidification of the plasma from such patients increased the biological activity in a bioassay for ACTH, presumably by disrupting ACTH-antibody complexes. Incubation of known amounts of either porcine or human ACTH with antibody-containing plasma before bioassay reduced the biological activity considerably while incubation with plasma from normal subjects had no such effect. The biological half-life of ACTH was also considerably prolonged in patients with antibodies. These results suggest that antibody-binding of ACTH does reduce biological activity, but the amount of antibody present rarely, if ever, seems to be sufficient to disturb seriously the adrenal response to exogenous or endogenous ACTH.

Glass and Daly (1971) suggested that there may be more than one antibody-combining site on the ACTH molecule. They detected antibodies in patients treated with gelatin-linked porcine ACTH and also in 12 of 38 treated with tetracosactrin. By using various peptide fragments of the complete ACTH molecule they showed that antibodies were present which reacted with antigenic determinants at the species-specific C-terminal end of the molecule but that reaction could also be shown against the N-terminal portion which shows no species differences.

As might be expected, there is no definite correlation between the titre of circulating antibodies and the occurrence of local reactions.

Clinical significance of ACTH antibodies

Local reactions are rarely a problem in clinical practice, but in the occasional case where they cause trouble it would seem reasonable either to change the ACTH preparation or to use oral glucocorticoids instead.

Circulating antibodies rarely seem to cause ACTH resistance comparable to insulin resistance, but if this should occur it might be treated in the same way as local reactions.

Growth Hormone

Growth hormone, extracted from human pituitaries, is used in the treatment of short stature in children, resulting from growth-hormone deficiency. Formation of antibodies to the injected material appears to be relatively common and can occur in normal subjects as well as in those with growth-hormone deficiency, resulting from hypothalamic or pituitary disease.

Using radioiodine labelled human growth hormone, antibodies can be detected in normal subjects within 30–60 days of starting injections (Roth et al, 1964). The binding capacity of the antibodies was of the order of 300–500 μg/l. When injections were stopped the antibody concentrations fell rapidly, indicating that endogenous growth hormone was unable to sustain the immune response.

In children treated with growth hormone the true incidence with which antibodies occur is not yet known, although several studies are in progress. From previous reports on small series of patients it appears that between 25 and 50 per cent of all patients develop antibodies, although this is likely to be a minimal estimate since in early reports the rather insensitive haemagglutination technique was sometimes used. In most cases the antibodies are present only in low concentration, but significant binding of ^{131}I-labelled growth hormone has been reported in a few patients with plasma dilutions of up to 1 in 10 000, and binding capacities of up to 100 mg/litre have been estimated. In normal subjects endogenous serum growth hormone concentrations rarely exceed 10 μg/litre so it might be expected that patients with high antibody concentrations would show resistance to the biological effect of exogenous growth hormone. That this does occur is suggested by several reports describing children who showed an initially good metabolic response with acceleration of growth but later failed to respond and were found to have developed high titres of antibodies. In most patients, however, antibody concentrations seem to be insufficient to interfere with biological effectiveness of the hormone. It has also been shown that incubation of human growth hormone with antibody-containing serum neutralises its biological effect on cartilage growth in the hypophysectomised rat.

The antibodies seem to be relatively specific and appear to cross react with endogenous human growth hormone. Parker, Mariz and Daughaday (1964) studied the antibody from one patient and stated that it did not cross react with monkey growth hormone or with the chemically closely related hormone, human chorionic somatomammotrophin. Frasier and Smith (1966) again studying one patient, stated that the antibody was specific for primate growth hormone. They also showed that it was an IgG antibody and were unable to detect any binding to IgM or IgA. Prader et al (1964), using a haemagglutination technique, showed that the reaction could be inhibited by absorption of the patient's serum with human growth hormone or with serum from an acromegalic subject.

Vasopressin

Various preparations of vasopressin have been used for the long-term treatment of diabetes insipidus resulting from endogenous vasopressin deficiency. These may consist of relatively crude preparations of bovine or porcine posterior pituitary given as snuff or by intramuscular or subcutaneous injection or of preparations of synthetic vasopressin given either as a nasal spray or by injection.

Human vasopressin is a nonapeptide with arginine in position number 8. The same molecule is found in all other mammalian species, except in the pig family, where the natural vasopressin differs only by substitution of lysine for arginine (lysine vasopressin). This type is therefore to be found in preparations derived from porcine posterior pituitary, and is also present, together with arginine vasopressin, in many commercial preparations containing a mixture of bovine and porcine material. Commercially available synthetic vasopressin is also of this type.

The crude preparations also contain a wide variety of other proteins and peptides and not uncommonly cause immunological reactions. Pepys et al (1966) studied these reactions in patients treated with posterior pituitary snuff. Allergic reactions occurred in 5 out of 9 patients. Asthma, rhinitis, itching of the eyes and face, miliary infiltration of the lungs and faintness were seen.

Skin tests and nasal tests showed reactions to the crude pituitary preparations in several patients and some were also apparently positive with synthetic lysine vasopressin. In one patient porcine and bovine serum also produced strong reactions.

Serological and immunofluorescent tests suggested that most of the immunological reactions were directed against antigens present in bovine and porcine serum and pituitary but were not directed specifically against vasopressin.

Circulating antibodies directed specifically against vasopressin were, however, detected in a patient by Roth et al (1966). Using vasopressin labelled with ^{131}I, they showed, by equilibrium dialysis, that antibody was present in the plasma of one patient treated with pituitary snuff for two months, but were unable to detect antibodies in eight other patients treated with snuff or pitressin tannate in oil. The antibody cross reacted with arginine vasopressin to some extent, but only minimally with oxytocin. The positive patient had shown no local allergic reactions, whereas these had been seen in some of the other patients.

The frequency with which such antibodies occur is still unknown as also is whether they play any part in the resistance to vasopressin sometimes found to develop in previously sensitive patients.

Other Hormones

Other polypeptide hormones used on a long-term basis include calcitonin and luteinising and follicle-stimulating hormones. Immunological reactions to all three have been reported but have not so far been shown to cause serious interference with therapy. From the evidence available it seems probable that antibody formation will always be a problem in patients treated with peptide hormones, even though refinement in preparation may reduce its occurrence.

RADIOIMMUNOASSAY

The technique of radioimmunoassay was first developed by Berson, Yalow and their collaborators as an extension of their studies on the development of antibodies to exogenous insulin in insulin-treated diabetics (Berson et al, 1956).

Essentially, they found that, if insulin labelled with ^{131}I was mixed with the serum of the patient and the mixture was then subjected to chromato-electrophoresis on paper strips under appropriate conditions, the labelled insulin remained at the point of application if no antibodies were present, but travelled with the gamma globulins if antibody was contained in the serum. They then showed that if unlabelled insulin was added to the mixture the proportion of labelled insulin travelling with gamma globulin decreased as the amount of unlabelled insulin added increased. A curve could then be drawn relating the amount of unlabelled insulin present in the serum sample to the percentage of labelled insulin travelling with gamma globulin. If serum containing an unknown amount of insulin was then added to the system and the percentage of antibody-bound labelled insulin measured after chromo-electrophoresis the amount of unlabelled insulin present could be determined by reference to the standard curve.

On the basis of these findings a series of assays have been developed and have since been applied to the measurement of most human hormones, as well as to an ever-increasing variety of non-hormonal substances.

In general, any substance can be measured by radioimmunoassay provided that five requirements can be met. These are described as follows.

Availability of a suitable antiserum

It was soon found that immunisation of animals with insulin in Freund's complete adjuvant resulted in the production of antibodies of much higher titre and with a much greater affinity for antigen than could be found in diabetic patients. Using such antisera much more sensitive assays could be developed and it is now possible to measure hormone concentrations as low as 10^{-12}M, or even lower, without undue difficulty.

Ideally the antiserum used should react only with the substance that it is desired to measure and show no reaction either with chemically related substances or with fragments of the original antigen produced during metabolic breakdown. These requirements can usually be met, although it may be necessary to raise many antisera before a really suitable one is found. Many antisera show a remarkable degree of specificity; those raised against the nonapeptide arginine vasopressin, for example, usually show virtually no reaction with the chemically very closely related hormone oxytocin, which differs from vasopressin in only two amino-acid residues. Many of them will also clearly distinguish arginine from lysine vasopressin, where the difference is confined to one amino acid.

Reaction of antisera with hormone fragments produced during metabolic breakdown has not proved a major problem in most assays, provided that antisera are carefully chosen to minimise such reactivity. From this point of view it is desirable that the antigenic determinant with which the antibody reacts should include, or at least be near, the biologically active site of the molecule. Otherwise alterations to the hormone might occur in vivo which would render it biologically inactive while not affecting its immunoreactivity. Under these circumstances hormone concentrations determined by immunoassay might be quite different from the biologically active concentrations.

In order to obtain a sensitive assay the antibody used must have a high affinity constant which, it has been shown theoretically, should be of the same order of magnitude as the minimum concentration of hormone it is desired to measure (Berson and Yalow, 1964). For practical reasons it is also desirable that the titre of the antibody should be high, so that once a suitable antiserum is found it can be used for many thousands of assays. In some cases antisera can be used in the assay at final dilutions of greater than 1 in 10^6 and 1 or 2 ml will last for many years.

Numerous techniques have been used to produce antibodies in many species of animals. No one method has been conclusively proved better than any other although some, such as direct injection into spleen or lymph nodes or multiple intradermal injections, seem to enable good antisera to be produced with the minimal amount of antigen—an important consideration since some antigens are extremely scarce. Freund's complete adjuvant is usually used. Most polypeptide hormones can be injected directly, after emulsification in adjuvant, and appear to be good antigens. This applies even to peptides as small as arginine vasopressin (mol. wt. 1084) and antibodies can often be raised even with autologous hormones. The hormone preparation used for immunisation need not necessarily be pure and indeed, relatively crude preparations often seem to produce the best antibodies, though very many sera may need to be raised before one of suitable specificity is found.

Smaller molecules, such as steroids or thyroid hormones and some of the smaller polypeptides, are usually combined with larger molecules, such as bovine albumin, and can then be used for immunisation. Again, highly specific antibodies can be produced, e.g. antibodies raised against a tri-iodothyronine–albumin complex will react with tri-iodothyronine (and bovine serum albumin), but will often show very little reaction with thyroxine. In the case of steroids, antibody specificity can be determined to some extent by linking the carrier molecule to the steroid molecule at various different sites so that functional groupings on the steroid can be exposed or concealed as desired.

Availability of a suitably labelled form of the hormone

The introduction by Greenwood, Hunter and Glover in 1964 of a rapid, simple and effective method for labelling polypeptides with radioactive iodine allowed a tremendous expansion in the use of radioimmunoassay. Their technique uses chloramine T, a mild oxidising agent, to convert radioactive iodide to iodine, and possibly other highly reactive compounds, which then react with tyrosine residues in the peptide molecule to produce iodotyrosyl derivatives. After a suitable time the reaction is halted, usually by the addition of sodium metabisulphite, and the labelled hormone is then separated from damaged hormone and the other components of the reaction mixture by any one of several techniques depending on which hormone is concerned.

With this method labelled hormones of high specific radioactivity can easily be produced. By using appropriate conditions this can be done while damaging the hormone little, if at all. This is important since, in the ideal assay, labelled and unlabelled hormone should react identically with the antiserum. In order to allow this it is essential that a pure preparation of the hormone, identical with the native form, should be available.

This method is by far the most widely used technique and can be employed with either ^{131}I or ^{125}I. For certain hormones, e.g. those that do not possess tyrosine residues or some that are very easily damaged, other techniques are available.

In the case of steroids ^{3}H or ^{14}C labelled compounds are usually used.

Availability of a suitable preparation of hormone for use as standard

Where a pure preparation of the hormone, identical with the native form, is available this will normally be used as the standard. For steroids, thyroid hormones and those polypeptides which have identical structure in several different species or which can be synthesised, this presents no problem. However, where polypeptide hormones show large species differences, e.g. growth hormone, prolactin, it may be difficult to obtain adequate supplies of pure, human material. In such cases it is sometimes possible to use either impure material, in the form of a crude gland extract or serial dilutions of a serum or plasma known to contain large amounts of the material to be measured. These can then be used as arbitrary standards provided that sufficient material of homogeneous constitution is available for many assays. Alternatively, if the antiserum fails to distinguish between the hormone to be measured and the analogous hormone from another species, a preparation of the latter can be used to establish a heterologous assay system.

Availability of the hormone to be measured in a form suitable for assay

Radioimmunoassays are most widely used to measure hormones in plasma or serum. In many systems this can be done directly by introducing a small volume of plasma into the assay system and comparing its effect with that of standard hormone either in buffer or in an equal volume of hormone free plasma. For some systems, however, extraction of the hormone from plasma is necessary before assay. This may be because:

1. The assay system is insufficiently sensitive to detect normal plasma concentrations of hormone and extraction and concentration is therefore necessary.

2. The antiserum used cross reacts with other hormones in plasma, so that the hormone to be measured must first be separated from these. This applies particularly to steroids.
3. Plasma contains non-hormonal substances which interfere with the binding of labelled and unlabelled hormone by antiserum or with the procedure used to separate antibody bound and free hormone. A variety of substances, acting through different mechanisms, may produce such interference. Proteolytic enzymes capable of attacking labelled or unlabelled hormone or antiserum may be responsible in some cases, but often the nature of the interfering substance is obscure. This situation is seen most strikingly in the case of assays for vasopressin.

With some steroids and the thyroid hormones the situation is rather different. Here plasma normally contains specific binding proteins which, unless inactivated, will compete with antiserum for labelled and unlabelled hormone. Thus, before assay either endogenous hormone must be displaced from binding protein and further hormone binding prevented by a suitable blocking agent, or the hormone must be displaced and extracted, usually with an organic solvent which denatures the binding protein.

Availability of a suitable technique for separating antibody-bound and free hormone

The technique of chromatoelectrophoresis has now been largely superseded by simpler and more rapid methods. These fall into three main groups.

Precipitation of antibody. Antibody together with bound hormone (labelled and unlabelled) is rendered insoluble and then separated from unbound hormone by centrifugation. The supernatant, containing unbound hormone, is removed and the amount of labelled hormone attached to antibody determined by counting the radioactivity in the precipitate. Antibody is precipitated either by immunological means, using an appropriate concentration of anti-gamma globulin antibody (the double antibody technique) or by use of other substances in which gamma globulin is insoluble such as ethanol, dioxan or ammonium sulphate.

Adsorption and precipitation of hormone not bound to antibody. Under appropriate conditions, a number of adsorbents, e.g. charcoal, talc, can be used to adsorb free hormone, while leaving bound hormone in solution.

Solid-state methods. Antibody can be linked to insoluble particles, or adsorbed to the walls of the assay tube, without affecting its ability to combine with antigen. Assays can then be carried out by adding the other reagents to a suspension of adsorbed antibody or to the antibody-coated tube. After reaction has occurred antibody + bound hormone is separated either by centrifugation or, in the case of antibody-coated tubes, by decanting the other reagents.

As should be clear from the above discussion, that the general principles of radioimmunoassay remain the same whatever the substance being measured. The practical details of assay systems, however, vary quite widely depending upon such factors as the nature of the substance being measured, the characteristics of the antiserum being used, the availability of reagents and apparatus and the personal preference of the user. Fuller reviews of the theoretical and practical aspects of immunoassays may be found elsewhere (Kirkham and Hunter, 1971; Odell and Daughaday, 1971; Sonksen, 1974).

Uses of Radioimmunoassay

The major use of radioimmunoassay is to measure concentrations of hormones in body fluids such as plasma or urine, or in tissue extracts. For certain hormones, e.g. growth hormone, for which no adequate bioassay is available, it is only the introduction of radioimmunoassay which has allowed measurement of the hormone in physiological amounts. For many other hormones, however, other methods of assay, either biological or chemical,

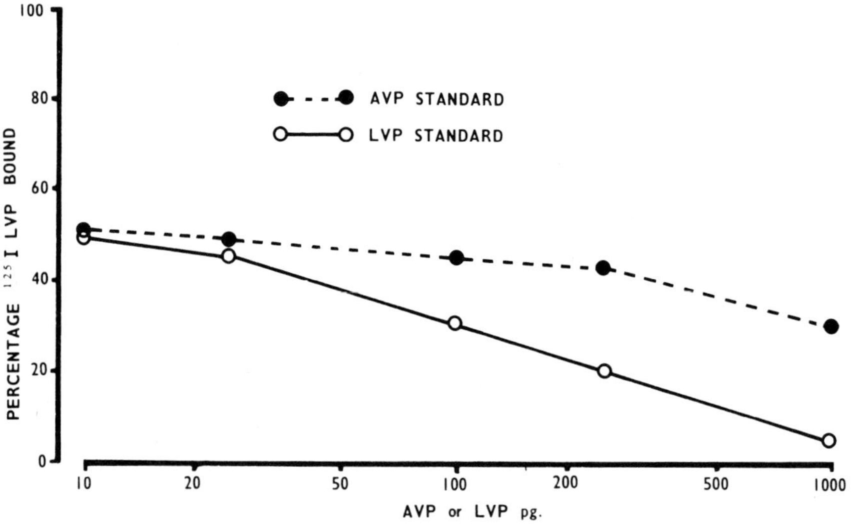

Figure 5.1. Displacement curves obtained with arginine and lysine vasopressin standards using an antiserum raised against lysine vasopressin and ^{125}I labelled lysine vasopressin as tracer. The curves are clearly not parallel indicating that the affinity of the antiserum for the two forms of vasopressin differs.

are also available and the choice of which assay technique to use depends upon a number of factors. In general the advantages of radioimmunoassay compared to bioassay are that: the assay technique is simpler; more samples can be dealt with in a shorter time; in some cases immunoassay is more sensitive and, often, more specific. However, as mentioned above, unless the antibody is directed specifically against the biologically active site of the hormone, the concentration of immunoreactive material may not be the same as the concentration of biologically active substance. Conversely of course, bioassay may detect a number of substances having the same biological activity while immunoassay will detect only those which have identical antigenic determinants. Thus, although radioimmunoassay is rapidly superseding bioassay in many situations it must always be remembered that the two techniques are complementary, rather than being alternatives.

For those hormones which can be measured by chemical techniques radioimmunoassay seems likely to supersede these only where they are extremely difficult and time-consuming, e.g. steroids such as aldosterone, or where interference by contaminants is a major problem.

Since variations in hormonal structure may result in modifications of the antigenic determinants, radioimmunoassay can sometimes be used to detect structural differences between hormones which may have similar biological activity. If such structural differences result in a change of affinity for antibody, assay of serial dilutions of the various hormonal forms will result in curves that do not run parallel with each other. An example of two such curves is shown in Figure 5.1. Such methods have been used to detect immunological differences between analogous hormones from various species and also to detect chemically different forms of the same hormone in a single species. It is now becoming increasingly clear that hormones such as insulin, parathormone, glucagon and others exist in different chemical forms in man. In some cases, the first clue that this might be so was provided by observations of differences in immunological reactivity of hormone preparations from different human sources.

Immunoassays Currently in Use

As can be seen from Table 5.3 immunoassays are now available for most human hormones and are finding an ever-increasing application in the diagnosis of endocrine disease, as well as in other fields of medicine. The available assays differ, to some extent, from each other in technical details and in their ease of execution but these will not be discussed here. A fairly typical immunoassay schedule is, however, shown in Table 5.4.

Table 5.3. List of hormones for which radioimmunoassay techniques have now been developed

Peptide hormones	
1. Pituitary	Growth hormone; Luteinising hormone; follicle-stimulating hormone; thyroid-stimulating hormone; prolactin; adrenocorticotrophic hormone; neurophysin; vasopressin; oxytocin; beta melanocyte-stimulating hormone
2. Thyroid and parathyroid	Parathormone; calcitonin
3. Pancreas	Insulin; glucagon
4. Gastro-intestinal	Gastrin; secretin; entero-glucagon; vasoactive intestinal peptide
5. Placenta	Placental lactogen; chorionic gonadotrophin
6. Miscellaneous	Erythropoietin; angiotensin I and II; renin; bradykinin
Steroids	Oestradiol; oestrone; oestriol; progesterone; testosterone; aldosterone; deoxycorticosterone, etc
Thyroid hormones	Thyroxine; tri-iodothyronine

There can be little doubt that, in practical terms, the greatest contribution made to endocrinology by immunology has been the development of radioimmunoassay.

Table 5.4. TSH radioimmunoassay

Tubes set up as follows:	
2 tubes with no antiserum	100 μl PBSA 200 μl TSH–free serum 100 μl PBSA–NIGP–EDTA
2 tubes with excess antiserum	100 μl PBSA 200 μl TSH–free serum 100 μl 1/2000 TSH antiserum[a]
4 tubes for OμU TSH point on standard curve	100 μl PBSA 200 μl TSH–free serum 100 μl TSH antiserum[a] diluted 1 in 80 000
2 tubes for each standard	100 μl TSH standard 200 μl TSH–free serum 100 μl TSH antiserum[a] diluted 1 in 80 000
4 tubes for each unknown serum	100 μl PBSA 200 μl serum 100 μl TSH antiserum[a] diluted 1 in 80 000

Mix, incubate at 4°C for 3 days.
Add 100 μl TSH–^{125}I (c.10 000 cpm) to each tube and also to 4 empty tubes (to check amount of radioactivity contained in 100 μl).
Mix, incubate further 2 days at 4°C.
Add to all tubes (except those containing TSH–^{125}I only) 100 μl of suitable dilution of rabbit anti-guinea pig gamma-globulin antiserum (2nd antibody).
Incubate overnight at 4°C.
Add 1·5 ml distilled water to each tube (except TSH–^{125}I only, tubes).
Centrifuge at 2500 rev/min at 4°C for 25 minutes.
Aspirate supernatant; count radioactivity in precipitate.

PBSA = phosphate buffered saline with 0·25 per cent bovine albumin.
NIGP = non-immune guinea pig serum.
EDTA = ethylene diamine tetra-acetic acid.

[a]Antiserum diluted in PBSA, NIGP, EDTA.

References

Introduction

Allison, A. C. (1973) Interactions of thymus-dependent and bone-marrow-derived lymphocytes in immunological tolerance. *Proceedings of the Royal Society of Medicine*, **66,** 463–465.

Allison, A. C., Denman, A. M. & Barnes, R. D. (1971) Cooperating and controlling functions of thymus-derived lymphocytes in relation to auto-immunity. *Lancet*, **ii,** 135–140.

Bankhurst, A. D., Torrigiani, G. & Allison, A. C. (1973) Lymphocytes binding human thyroglobulin in healthy people and its relevance to tolerance for autoantigens. *Lancet*, **i,** 226–230.

Burnet, F. M. (1959) *The Clonal Selection Theory of Acquired Immunity*. Cambridge: Cambridge University Press; Nashville, Tennessee: Vanderbilt University Press.

Burnet, F. M. (1972) *Auto-immunity and Auto-immune Disease*. Lancaster: Medical and Technical Publishing Co.

Vaughan, J. H. (1971) Autoallergic diseases; concepts and general considerations. In *Immunological Diseases*, ed. Samter, M. Vol. II, Ch. 59. Boston: Little, Brown.

Thyroid

Adams, D. D. & Kennedy, T. H. (1967) Occurrence in thyrotoxicosis of a gamma globulin which protects LATS from neutralisation by an extract of thyroid gland. *Journal of Clinical Endocrinology and Metabolism*, **27,** 173–177.

Adams, D. D. & Kennedy, T. H. (1971) Evidence to suggest that LATS Protector stimulates the human thyroid gland. *Journal of Clinical Endocrinology and Metabolism*, **33,** 47–51.

Adams, D. D. & Purves, H. D. (1956) Abnormal responses in the assay of thyrotropin. *Proceedings of the University of Otago Medical School*, **34,** 11.

Bastenie, P. A. & Ermans, A. M. (1971) *Thyroiditis and Thyroid Function.* Oxford: Pergamon.

Carneiro, L., Dorrington, K. J. & Munro, D. S. (1966) Relationship between LATS and thyroid function in thyrotoxicosis. *Lancet*, **ii,** 878–880.

Chopra, I. J., Solomon, D. H., Johnson, D. E. & Chopra, V. (1970) Thyroid gland in Graves' disease: victim or culprit? *Metabolism*, **19,** 760–772.

Doniach, D. & Roitt, I. M. (1968) Thyroid auto-allergic disease. In *Clinical Aspects of Immunology*, ed. Gell, P. G. H. & Coombs, R. R. A. Ch. 35. Oxford & Edinburgh: Blackwell Scientific Publications.

McKenzie, J. M. (1958) The bioassay of thyrotropin in serum. *Endocrinology*, **63,** 372–382.

Nakamura, R. M. & Weigle, W. O. (1969) Transfer of experimental autoimmune thyroiditis by serum from thyroidectomised donors. *Journal of Experimental Medicine*, **130,** 263–286.

Onaya, T., Kotani, M., Yamada, T. & Ochi, Y. (1973) New in vitro tests to detect the thyroid stimulator in sera from hyperthyroid patients by measuring colloid droplet formation and cyclic AMP in human thyroid slices. *Journal of Clinical Endocrinology and Metabolism*, **36,** 859.

Roitt, I. M., Torrigiani, G. & Doniach, D. (1968) Immunochemical studies on the thyroglobulin autoantibody system in human thyroiditis. *Immunology*, **15,** 681–696.

Rose, N. R. & Witebsky, E. (1971) Experimental thyroiditis. In *Immunological Diseases*, ed. Samter, M. Vol. II, Ch. 72. Boston: Little, Brown.

Shishiba, Y., Shimizu, T., Yoshimura, S. & Shizume, K. (1972) Direct evidence for human thyroidal stimulation by LATS protector. *Proceedings of the Fourth International Congress of Endocrinology, Excerpta Medica Congress Series*, **256,** 193.

Shulman, S. (1971) Thyroid antigens and autoimmunity. *Advances in Immunology*, **14,** 85–185.

Skanse, B. & Nilsson, S-B. (1962) Hypergammaglobulinaemia and thyroid antibodies. *Acta Medica Scandinavica*, **172,** 505–512.

Volpé, R., Farid, N. R., von Westarp, C. & Row, V. V. (1974) *Clinical Endocrinology*, **3,** 239.

Werner, S. C., Wegelius, O., Fierer, J. A. & Hsu, K. C. (1972) Immunoglobulins (E,M,G) and complement in thyroid of Graves' disease. *New England Journal of Medicine*, **287,** 421–425.

Adrenal and parathyroid

Anderson, J. R., Goudie, R. B., Gray, K. & Stuart-Smith, D. A. (1968) Immunological features of idiopathic Addison's disease: an antibody to cells producing steroid hormones. *Clinical and Experimental Immunology*, **3,** 107–117.

Barnett, E. V., Dumonde, D. C. & Glynn, L. E. (1963) Induction of autoimmunity to adrenal gland. *Immunology*, **6,** 382–402.

Blizzard, R. M., Chee, D. & Davis, W. (1966) The incidence of parathyroid and other antibodies in the sera of patients with idiopathic hypoparathyroidism. *Clinical and Experimental Immunology*, **1,** 119–128.

Blizzard, R. M., Chee, D. & Davis, W. (1967) The incidence of adrenal and other antibodies in the sera of patients with idiopathic adrenal insufficiency (Addison's disease). *Clinical and Experimental Immunology*, **2,** 19–30.

Colover, J. & Glynn, L. E. (1958) Experimental autoimmune adrenalitis. *Immunology*, **1,** 172–178.

Irvine, W. J. (1971) Adrenalitis, hypoparathyroidism and associated diseases. In *Immunological Diseases*, ed. Samter, M. Vol. II, Ch. 74. Boston: Little, Brown.

Irvine, W. J. & Barnes, E. W. (1972) Adrenocortical insufficiency. *Clinics in Endocrinology and Metabolism*, **1**, 549–594.

Levine, S. & Wenk, E. J. (1968) The production and passive transfer of allergic adrenalitis. *American Journal of Pathology*, **52**, 41–53.

Milgrom, F. & Witebsky, E. (1962) Immunological studies on adrenal gland. II. Immunisation with adrenals of the same species. *Immunology*, **5**, 67–78.

Nerup, J. & Bendixen, G. (1969) Anti-adrenal cellular hypersensitivity in Addison's disease. II. Correlation with clinical and serological findings. *Clinical and Experimental Immunology*, **5**, 341–353.

Turkington, R. W. & Lebowitz, H. E. (1967) Extra-adrenal endocrine deficiencies in Addison's disease. *American Journal of Medicine*, **43**, 499–507.

Werdelin, O. & Witebsky, E. (1970) Experimental allergic rat adrenalitis. A study on its elicitation and lymphokinetics. *Laboratory Investigation*, **23**, 136–143.

Testis

Mancini, R. E., Andrada, J. A., Saraceni, A., Bachmann, A. E., Lavieri, J. C. & Nemirowsky, M. (1965) Immunological and testicular response in man sensitised with human testicular homogenate. *Journal of Clinical Endocrinology and Metabolism*, **25**, 859–875.

Franklin, R. R. & Dukes, D. C. (1964) Further studies on sperm agglutinating antibodies and unexplained infertility. *Journal of the Americal Medical Association*, **190**, 682–683.

Diabetes mellitus

Følling, I. & Norman, N. (1972) Hyperglycaemia, hypoglycaemic attacks and production of anti-insulin antibodies without previous known immunisation. *Diabetes*, **21**, 814–826.

Gepts, W. (1965) Pathologic anatomy of the pancreas in juvenile diabetes mellitus. *Diabetes*, **14**, 619–633.

Irvine, W. J., Clarke, B. F., Scarth, L., Cullen, D. R. & Duncan, L. J. P. (1970) Thyroid and gastric autoimmunity in patients with diabetes mellitus. *Lancet*, **ii**, 163–168.

Le Compte, P. (1958) 'Insulitis' in early juvenile diabetes. *Archives of Pathology (Chicago)*, **66**, 450–457.

Nerup, J., Andersen, O. O., Bendixen, G., Egeberg, J. & Poulsen, J. E. (1971) Anti-pancreatic cellular hypersensitivity in diabetes mellitus. *Diabetes*, **20**, 424–427.

Renold, A. E., Steinke, J., Soeldner, J. S., Antoniades, H. N. & Smith, R. E. (1966) Immunological response to the prolonged administration of heterologous and homologous insulin in cattle. *Journal of Clinical Investigation*, **45**, 702–713.

Toreson, W. E., Lee, J. C. & Grodsky, G. M. (1968) The histopathology of immune diabetes in the rabbit. *American Journal of Pathology*, **52**, 1099–1115.

Whittingham, S., Matthews, J. D., Mackay, I. R., Stocks, A. E., Unger, B. & Martin, F. I. R. (1971) Diabetes mellitus, autoimmunity and ageing. *Lancet*, **i**, 763–766.

Immunological reactions to exogenous hormones

Berson, S. A., Yalow, R. S., Bauman, A., Rothschild, M. A. & Newerly, K. (1956) Insulin–I^{131} metabolism in human subjects: demonstration of insulin binding globulin in circulation of insulin treated subjects. *Journal of Clinical Investigation*, **35**, 170–190.

Fleischer, N., Abe, K., Liddle, G. W., Orth, D. N. & Nicholson, W. E. (1967) ACTH antibodies in patients receiving depot porcine ACTH to hasten recovery from pituitary-adrenal suppression. *Journal of Clinical Investigation*, **46**, 196–204.

Frasier, S. D. & Smith, F. G. (1966) Antibodies to human growth hormone. *American Journal of Diseases of Children*, **112**, 383–388.

Glass, D. & Daly, J. R. (1971) Development of antibodies during long term therapy with corticotrophin in rheumatoid arthritis. I. Porcine ACTH. II. Zinc tetracosactrin. *Annals of the Rheumatic Diseases*, **33**, 589–596.

Karam, J. H., Grodsky, G. M. & Forsham, P. H. (1969) Insulin resistant diabetes with autoantibodies induced by exogenous insulin. *Diabetes*, **18,** 445–464.

Landon, J., Friedman, M. & Greenwood, F. C. (1967) Antibodies to corticotrophin and their relation to adrenal function in children receiving corticotrophin therapy. *Lancet*, **i,** 652–655.

Parker, M. L., Mariz, I. K. & Daughaday, W. H. (1964) Response to human growth hormone in pituitary dwarfism. *Journal of Clinical Endocrinology and Metabolism*, **24,** 997–1004.

Pepys, J., Jenkins, P. A., Lachmann, P. J. & Mahon, W. E. (1966) An iatrogenic autoantibody: immunological responses to pituitary snuff in patients with diabetes insipidus. *Clinical and Experimental Immunology*, **1,** 377–389.

Prader, A., Wagner, H., Szeky, J., Illig, R., Tauber, J. L. & Maingay, D. (1964) Acquired resistance to human growth hormone caused by specific antibodies. *Lancet*, **ii,** 378–382.

Roth, J., Glick, S. M., Yalow, R. S. & Berson, S. A. (1964) Antibodies to human growth hormone (HGH) in human subjects treated with HGH. *Journal of Clinical Investigation*, **43,** 1056–1065.

Roth, J., Glick, S. M., Klein, L. A. & Petersen, M. J. (1966) Specific antibody to vasopressin in man. *Journal of Clinical Endocrinology and Metabolism*, **26,** 671–675.

Radioimmunoassay

Kirkham, K. E. & Hunter, W. M. (eds) (1971) *Radioimmunoassay Methods*. Edinburgh & London: Churchill Livingstone.

Odell, W. D. & Daughaday, W. H. (eds) (1971) *Principles of Competitive Protein-Binding Assays*. Philadelphia: J. B. Lippincott.

Sonksen, P. H. (ed) (1974) Radioimmunoassay and saturation analysis. *British Medical Bulletin*, **30,** 1.

6. Immunology of the Gastro-Intestinal Tract and Liver

JONATHAN BROSTOFF
GEOFFREY WALKER

The importance of immunological phenomena in human disease is increasingly recognised, although the exact part that these mechanisms play in the aetiology and pathogenesis of alimentary disorders in particular is not clear. We plan to discuss those immunological phenomena related to gastro-intestinal pathology which either help in the clinical diagnosis or management of the patient or throw light, however little, on to actual disease processes. The situation in which immunological tests are the most useful to the clinician is in the field of liver disease.

GASTRO-INTESTINAL TRACT

Aphthous Ulcers

Recurrent aphthous ulceration is one of the most common lesions affecting the oral mucosa, one in three to one in ten of the population suffering from this disorder at one time or another. The aetiology of the condition is still unknown, although many factors have been suggested. Among the causes that have been discounted are trauma, vitamin deficiency, infection and food allergy. The highest incidence of ulcers is found in children whose parents also suffer from the same complaint.

There are no useful immunological tests that need to be performed in this condition as the diagnosis is usually self evident. Of interest are the observations that lymphocytes from patients with aphthous ulcers are stimulated by extracts of oral mucosa and haemagglutinating antibodies against the same antigen are found in about 80 per cent of patients.

In the condition known as Behçet's syndrome, in addition to oral ulceration, there may be changes in many epithelial surfaces. In this context it is of interest that mucosae from many sites share common antigenic determinants, and this might explain the widespread involvement in this disease.

Sjögren's Syndrome

Sjögren's syndrome comprises the triad of keratoconjunctivitis sicca, xerostomia with or without salivary gland enlargement and, in over one half of patients, rheumatoid arthritis (RA) or some other form of collagenosis. When the latter feature is lacking it is usual to refer to the condition as 'Sicca syndrome'.

Patients with Sjögren's (or 'Sicca') syndrome show a wide variety of immunological phenomena, mainly in the form of organ specific and non-organ specific serum auto-antibodies and dysgammaglobulinaemia. Associated disorders are frequent in patients with this condition and include pulmonary complications and chronic bronchitis, pernicious anaemia, thyroid disease, renal glomerular and tubular defects, peripheral neuropathy, myasthenia gravis, focal myositis, pancreatic disease, diabetes mellitus, purpura and vitiligo. There is also, interestingly, an association with malignant lymphoreticular neoplasms and with certain types of chronic liver disease (see also the section on Liver). These patients are also susceptible to the development of drug allergy.

Serological tests

Serum immunoglobulins. Male and female patients with Sjögren's syndrome and RA, and female patients with the Sicca syndrome, show significantly higher serum IgG levels than matched controls. Both IgM and IgA are frequently elevated in cases associated with collagenosis whereas secretory IgA is raised independently of the presence of the collagen disorder.

Very occasionally macroglobulinaemia and cryomacroglobulinaemia occur in Sjögren's syndrome and rarely hypogammaglobulinaemia, if a malignant lymphoma develops.

Rheumatoid factors. RA-latex agglutination tests are positive in over 95 per cent of cases associated with clinical rheumatoid arthritis. In the absence of the latter feature they are positive in about 50 per cent of patients. Screening for IgG antiglobulin factors against rabbit and horse serum FII fractions frequently produces positive results in 'sero-negative' Sjögren's and 'Sicca' cases.

Antinuclear antibodies (ANA). These autoantibodies are present in about one third of 'Sicca' cases and in just over half of patients having an associated collagenosis. The staining pattern is usually homogenous but nucleolar, speckled and membraneous appearances may be seen. In about three per cent of cases, with or without rheumatoid disease, LE latex tests for antibody to nucleoprotein are positive and, of course, this figure is very much higher when the 'Sicca' syndrome is associated with systemic lupus erythematosus. LE cell preparations are, however, occasionally positive in the absence of the latter clinical sydrome.

Native DNA-binding capacity elevation may be detected when frank lupus erythematosus is present and occasionally in its absence. In about 25 per cent of patients with Sjögren's syndrome it is possible to demonstrate antibodies reactive with heat-denatured DNA.

Salivary duct antibodies. These antibodies may be shown on immunofluorescence in some 10 per cent of Sicca patients. The incidence rises to about 65 per cent when rheumatoid disease co-exists. These antibodies are distinct from mitochondrial antibodies which may also stain salivary duct epithelium. The true Sjögren antibody stains only the salivary ducts.

Mitochondrial antibodies (AMA). Between 5 and 10 per cent of patients with a Sicca or Sjögren's syndrome have mitochondrial antibodies (see Liver section) in their serum, and this figure is higher when clinical systemic lupus erythematosus is present. These AMA-positive patients almost invariably have a 'subclinical' hepatitis with features akin to either primary biliary disease or chronic active hepatitis. If AMA are present, the salivary duct antibodies cannot be seen.

Thyroid autoantibodies. Between 20 and 33 per cent of patients with a Sicca or Sjögren's syndrome have thyroglobulin autoantibodies as detected by passive haemagglutination tests. Microsomal thyroid antibodies occur in 20 to 50 per cent of cases. With both types of antibody the incidence appears to be higher in the absence of clinical rheumatoid disease or collagenosis.

Gastric parietal cell antibodies. These occur in just over a quarter of Sicca/Sjögren's patients and are an invariable accompaniment of pernicious anaemia occurring in this context (which is the case in about 3·5 per cent of patients).

Coombs tests. These are positive in 10 per cent of patients with Sjögren's syndrome but would appear to be very uncommon in those having only a Sicca component.

The incidence of various antibodies in this disorder is summarised in Table 6.1.

Significance of immunological changes

Serum levels of all three major immunoglobulins are elevated and these changes are most marked in the IgG component and least marked in the IgA fraction. This can probably be attributed to a generalised immunological hyper-reactivity. The measurements are of no great value, however, in clinical diagnosis. The presence of rheumatoid and antiglobulin factors is striking but the presence of such factors in a wide variety of arthritides suggest they simply indicate the presence in the body of a chronic inflammatory process. The rheumatoid factors in Sjögren's syndrome appear to be directed against different antigenic determinants on the IgG molecule than are rheumatoid factors in Sicca cases. Anti-Gm specificity is of much higher incidence in the former group of patients.

Patients with positive ANA tests who do not have clear-cut clinical lupus erythematosus (SLE) but who have serum antibodies to native DNA, should be followed closely as they may well develop SLE as time progresses. Raised serum DNA-binding capacity correlates closely with subsequent development of lupus nephritis.

The significance of the other autoantibodies described in Sjögren's and Sicca syndrome is unclear and their role in pathogenesis (if any) is totally obscure. There is a striking set of inter-relationships between the presence of AMA, Sjögren's or Sicca syndrome and the presence of sub-clinical liver

Table 6.1. Incidence of main antibody reactions in patients with Sicca or Sjögren's syndrome

	Gastric parietal cell	Mitochondrial	Thyroglobulin	Thyroid Microsomal	RA Latex test	ANF	Salivary duct	Coombs test
Sicca syndrome	25%	5–10% (both groups)	35%	45%	50%	35%	10%	Rare
Sjögren's syndrome (i.e. RA or collagenosis present)	25%		20%	20%	95%	50%	65%	10%

Based on data of Whaley et al, 1973.

disease or primary biliary cirrhosis (see also Liver section) and renal tubular acidosis. The mechanisms inter-linking these phenomena and the pathogenesis of the lesions involved is unknown at the present time.

When lymphoid neoplasms develop in Sjögren's syndrome, a steady fall of serum globulin and autoantibody levels occurs. These changes may precede the clinical onset of malignancy and the Ig changes are most striking in the IgM component. The reason for such progression to lymphoma is not known.

Oesophagus—Post-Cricoid Web

The only condition of the oesophagus where immunological phenomena have been studied with positive results is that of post-cricoid web (PCW).

The association of this disorder with iron deficiency anaemia is well established; why only a small proportion of patients with this common deficiency get post-cricoid webs is unclear. It is known, however, that such patients may suffer from a variety of associated conditions including thyroid disease, pernicious anaemia, ulcerative colitis and Sjögren's syndrome.

Serological tests

Thyroid cytoplasmic antibodies occur in about a quarter of patients with PCW and the incidence is more than double that in iron deficient 'control' subjects who do not have webs. Antibodies to thyroglobulin, ANA and gastric parietal cell antibodies are all more common in 'webbed' patients, but the difference in incidence from iron deficiency control subjects does not achieve statistical significance. The only difference between iron deficient and healthy controls is in the increased incidence of gastric parietal cell antibodies. Intrinsic factor antibodies do not occur in iron deficient or webbed patients in the absence of concurrent pernicious anaemia (see Stomach section). Sera from PCW patients do not contain antibodies directed against human or animal pharynx. Serum immunoglobulin studies reveal no differences between 'webbed' subjects and a control population.

Significance of immunological changes

Achlorhydria and gastric atrophy are common in iron deficiency but no more so in those patients who develop a post-cricoid web. However, pernicious anaemia is more common in patients with a web, as is the incidence of gastric parietal cell antibodies, when compared with normal controls. There is no significant difference in incidence between patients with webs and iron deficient controls. These findings would fit in with Witts' view that primary iron deficiency leads to atrophic gastritis and achlorhydria, which may then in some subjects be followed by the development of a web and/or pernicious anaemia.

The increased incidence of thyroid disease and thyroid autoantibodies in 'webbed' patients is significantly different from controls both with and without iron deficiency. An explanation for the clinical and immunological association between webs and thyroid disease might lie in a common genetic predisposition to both or in similar environmental factors. Preliminary studies have suggested the possibility of familial clustering of the PCW syndrome, while a family history of pharyngo-oesophageal malignancy appears to be more common than in healthy controls.

Pancreas

There are no established immunological tests in routine use in the investigation of patients with pancreatic disease. There is no good evidence that pancreatic disorders result from autoallergic reactions. Attempts to produce autoantibodies in experimental animals have not so far resulted in antibodies which react with the animals' own pancreas. There are recent reports of detection of an onco-fetal antigen in patients with carcinoma of the pancreas and, if this is confirmed, it offers some hope of an immunological diagnosis in this condition in the future.

Stomach

Atrophic gastritis

The clinical presentation of patients with atrophic gastritis is very varied; whilst they may be symptomless or present with the haematological or other manifestations of pernicious anaemia and total gastric atrophy, others display a symptomatology closely akin to peptic ulceration or gastric carcinoma. There are many causes of acute gastritis, such as exposure to alcohol, aspirin or other irritant substances, but often no direct cause is established. There is usually no direct relationship between acute and chronic gastritis in that the majority of acute lesions heal without sequelae.

Pernicious anaemia (PA)

The problem of whether classical Addisonian PA is merely an end stage of progressive atrophic gastritis is not resolved. It appears likely, however, that PA patients represent a distinct group of subjects, suggested by the fact that very few patients with chronic gastritis who are followed for lengthy periods are found to develop PA and by immunological studies which suggest that these two groups are different.

Serological tests

Antibodies against gastric parietal cells. These organ-specific autoantibodies may appear in the serum or gastric juice and react with an antigen of the gastric parietal cell which is present in the microsomal fraction.

The antibodies are usually of IgG and less often of IgA class, and interestingly there is no correlation between the classes of antibody in serum and gastric juice. It seems likely that antibodies in juice and serum are derived separately, and that those in serum may be produced outside the stomach in local lymph nodes.

Patients with chronic gastritis may develop antibodies to gastric parietal cells although the histopathology of the mucosa itself is similar whether antibodies are present or not. It is uncertain when in the evolution of the gastric disease the antibodies appear in serum, lymphoid cells or gastric juice, or if their appearance is the cause or the result of the disease. There is a positive correlation between the degree of gastritis and the appearance and titres of these antibodies. Gastric parietal cell antibodies may be demonstrated by the immunofluorescent technique in 80 to 100 per cent of pernicious anaemia patients. (Figure 6.2.)

In patients without pernicious anaemia but with gastric atrophy the incidence of parietal cell antibodies is lower, being about 50 per cent, but this is still much higher than in healthy controls where the incidence is approximately 11 per cent. The latter figure, however, varies with age, being less than 5 per cent

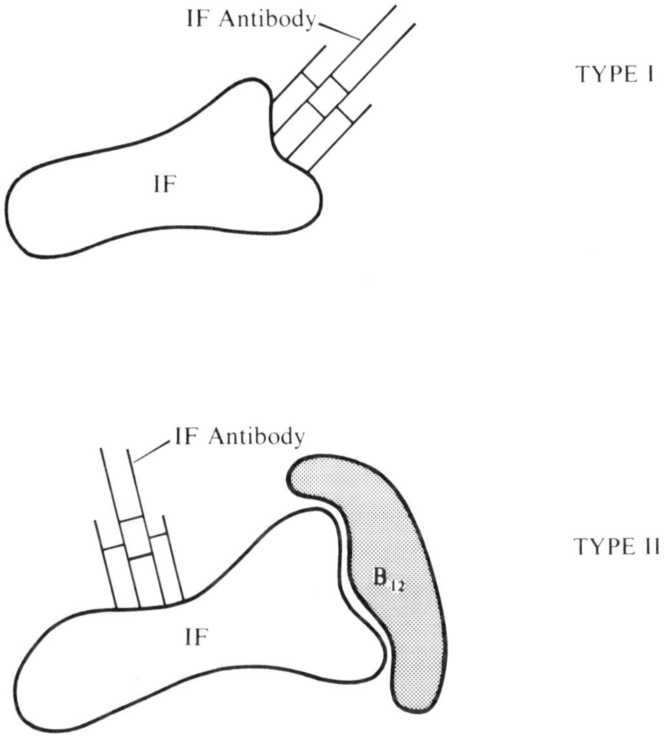

Figure 6.1. Mechanism of action of Type I and Type II antibody against IF in blocking absorption of B_{12}. Type I : blocks the binding of B_{12} to IF. Type II: this antibody can bind to the B_{12}-IF complex and thus inhibits absorption.

in patients under 60 years of age and rising to about 15 per cent in the elderly. Conversely, in very elderly pernicious anaemia patients the incidence of parietal cell antibody falls, perhaps due to disappearance of the autoantigen after lengthy disease. The parietal cell antibody is highly organ specific and will react with a subject's own intact parietal cells, and is thus a true autoantibody.

Antibodies against intrinsic factor (IF). There are two types of antibody directed against different sites on the IF molecule, and these may be found in the blood or gastric juice. Type I antibody, which is demonstrated by charcoal absorption of unbound B_{12} or by B_{12} uptake by guinea pig ileal homogenate, is the more common. It is found in serum and gastric juice in 50 to 60 per cent of pernicious anaemia cases. Type II 'binding' IF antibody, which reacts with IF or IF/B_{12} complex, is less common. It occurs in the serum of 35 to 40 per cent of pernicious anaemia cases and in the juice of 60 per cent of such subjects. It usually occurs along with type I antibody, and only rarely

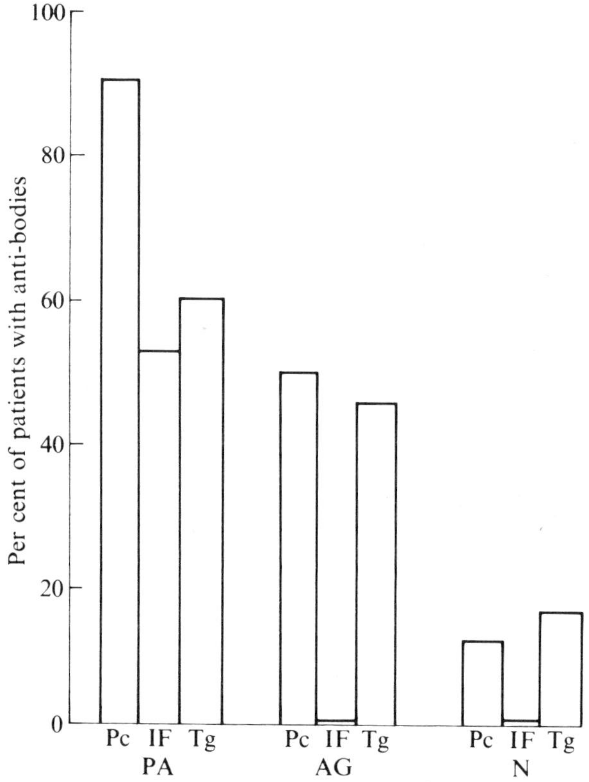

Figure 6.2. Incidence of autoantibodies in patients with pernicious anaemia (PA) and atrophic gastritis (AG) compared with normal controls (N). Pc = parietal cell antibody as detected by indirect immunofluorescence; IF = intrinsic factor antibody; Tg = thyroglobulin antibody as detected by haemagglutination.

alone. This can again be measured by B_{12} uptake by ileal homogenate or by immunodiffusion methods. These antibodies are usually of IgA class but are occasionally IgG. It seems likely that IF antibodies can inhibit IF activity and this could have a significant effect on B_{12} absorption, especially when secretion of IF is already minimal as in atrophic gastritis. If IF antibodies are present in both serum and gastric juice, it is likely that B_{12} absorption will be less than if the antibodies were absent. It is not clear whether serum antibodies alone have any effect on B_{12} absorption from the gut. It is of interest, also, that lymphocytes of about 85 per cent of pernicious anaemia patients show evidence of cell-mediated immunity against intrinsic factor.

By contrast with the situation in pernicious anaemia, where IF antibodies are present in some 60 per cent of patients, the serum of patients with chronic gastritis (who do not have pernicious anaemia) appears to be invariably negative for these antibodies as is the case in normal people. This striking difference would lend support to the idea that in the majority of cases the two groups of patients are distinct, and that pernicious anaemia is not usually a simple end result of chronic gastritis.

Thyroid autoantibodies. Thyroid autoantibodies occur more commonly in patients with pernicious anaemia, with or without overt thyroid disease, than in normal subjects. Similarly, in Hashimoto's disease and thyrotoxicosis an increased incidence of gastric autoantibodies is known to occur. These overlaps are not due to cross-reacting antibodies and the autoantigens involved are quite distinct. Thyroid autoantibodies may be demonstrated in 60 per cent of pernicious anaemia cases and in 40 to 50 per cent of chronic gastritis cases without pernicious anaemia, compared with 13 per cent in healthy controls.

In both pernicious anaemia and Hashimoto's disease there is a familial predisposition to the formation of gastric and thyroid autoantibodies, although these asymptomatic subjects may have some degree of chronic gastritis. Thus, in the case of the thyroid as well as the stomach, the incidence of autoantibodies has been shown to correlate with inflammatory lesions in the appropriate organ in symptomless subjects.

Use of immunological tests in the diagnosis of pernicious anaemia

In the case of classical Addisonian pernicious anaemia the combination of histamine fast achlorhydria, megaloblastic anaemia and impaired B_{12} absorption shown to be correctable in the Schilling test with oral IF make the diagnosis certain. Immunological tests are of a confirmatory nature. In elderly or fragile patients, where gastric intubation may be undesirable and B_{12} absorption studies are impracticable or unreliable, increased reliance may have to be placed upon antibody studies. Under these circumstances the finding of IF antibodies in the serum may be of considerable value since they do not occur in the normal population.

Apparent 'pernicious anaemia' may be encountered in a much younger age group than that normally associated with classical Addisonian PA. These patients can be classified into three main types:

1. Classical Addisonian PA occurring in a younger age group. These patients typically have a strong family history of thyroid or gastric disease and autoimmunity.
2. Those with near normal gastric acid production but vitamin B_{12} deficiency occurring because of the failure of absorption of the IF/B_{12} complex in the lower ileum.
3. Juvenile PA, where all immunological tests are negative and the condition probably represents a genetic failure of secretion of IF. These patients have a normal gastric mucosa and secretion of acid is unimpaired.

Coeliac Disease

Aetiology

The precise causation of coeliac disease has not been defined. While gluten intolerance may be a major factor, a primary aetiological role has yet to be convincingly demonstrated. Various other immunological phenomena have been described without providing firm clues as to aetiology. Antibodies to gluten have been shown both in the circulation and in the lumen of the bowel, and lymphocyte transformation studies have also shown positive results with gliadin fraction III. With immunofluorescent techniques, studies of the jejunal mucosa have shown some plasma cells directly secreting anti-gluten antibodies.

These findings suggest an immunological reaction to gluten without clearly demonstrating how the antigenic properties of this material bring about the disease. It has now been shown directly that in experimental challenge with gluten, histological changes consistent with inflammation, including complement fixation, occur in the mucosa within a matter of hours and the changes, initially at least, are confined principally to structures within the basement membrane and connective tissues, while epithelial damage occurs later. Within 12 hours eosinophils appear, as well as polymorphs and lymphocytes, and at 24 hours the mucosa itself is abnormal. By 48 hours the changes are regressing.

An antigen–antibody complex (incorporating gluten peptide(s)) could interact with complement and initiate the 'chain reaction' of complement activation—the later stages of this reaction involving direct tissue damage. Using an anticomplementary method it is possible to demonstrate immune complexes in the peripheral blood in a high proportion of patients with coeliac disease or dermatitis herpetiformis. In this disorder sensitivity to gluten and intestinal changes similar to those of coeliac disease are known to occur. In dermatitis herpetiformis it seems possible that immune complexes may be formed in the intestine in response to gluten and circulate thence to the skin, where they produce tissue damage. IgA deposits can be demonstrated in the unaffected skin in this condition, while at the sites of injury fibrin and complement are also seen.

Reticulin and autoantibody tests. When considered in relation to pathogenesis of the disorder, none of the techniques or observations are yet at the stage of established clinical diagnostic application. Approaching this status more closely, however, is the test for autoantibodies to reticulin, demonstrated by immunofluorescence. The antibody was first described in patients with adult coeliac disease, but is also now known to occur in other conditions (Table 6.2).

In patients with gluten-sensitive enteropathy (i.e. coeliac disease or dermatitis herpetiformis) there is a threefold greater incidence of reticulin antibodies in patients receiving a normal diet compared with those on a gluten-free diet. The presence of reticulin antibody would appear to be particularly helpful in diagnosing (hitherto untreated) cases of childhood coeliac disease where positive tests occur in over two-thirds of patients. In the context of differential diagnosis of bowel disorders it should also be noted that approximately a quarter of patients with Crohn's disease may have positive reticulin antibody tests as do occasional cases of tropical sprue. Colitis patients, other malabsorption states and alpha-chain disease patients do not appear to have these antibodies when sera are tested at 1 in 10 dilutions, but others have reported the antibodies in colitis when 1 in 5 dilutions were employed. Further analyses of larger series of different cases may clarify this situation.

In addition to the high incidence of the antibody in childhood coeliac disease compared with the adult form, high titre reactions are also more common in children (i.e. titres $>1:80$).

Table 6.2. Incidence of immunofluorescent reactions for reticulin antibodies in various disorders. Data of Rizzetto and Doniach, 1973.

Disease	Percentage positive reactions
Dermatitis herpetiformis	47
Coeliac disease	44
Chronic heroin addicts	20
Sjögren's syndrome	17
Myasthenia gravis	16
Vitiligo and alopecia	11
Rheumatoid arthritis/polyarthritis	10
Other collagen disorders (SLE/dermatomyositis/spondylitis/some indefinite)	7
Thyroid autoimmune disease (thyrotoxicosis, Hashimoto, myxoedema)	9
Thyroid non-autoimmune (all other goitres)	5
Autoimmune gastritis (PA/GPC + /B_{12} deficient)	4
Addison's disease	8
'Autoimmune' liver disease (PBC/CAH or crypto with autoantibodies)	3
Non-autoimmune liver disease	3
Drug hypersensitivity	6
Miscellaneous hospital patients	8
Healthy subjects	4

PBC = primary biliary cirrhosis; CAH = chronic active hepatitis; PA = pernicious anaemia; GPC = gastric parietal cell fluorescence.

Nature of reticulin antibodies. These may now be classified by differences in immunofluorescent staining reaction into five types reacting with distinct antigens of either intra- or extra-cellular components of the mesenchyme. Occurrence of the antibodies in patients with increased gut permeability and in heroin addicts suggests a relationship with bacterial (or nutritional) absorption. In this connection some staining similar to the reticulin pattern is seen in liver sections using experimental antistreptococcal sera. The exact origin, however, of reticulin antibodies is still far from clear. It seems likely that the antibodies represent anamnestic responses and not cross-reactions between gluten and reticulin.

There does not appear to be any relationship between the degree of intestinal abnormality in coeliac disease or dermatitis herpetiformis and the presence of reticulin antibody.

Serum immunoglobulin concentrations. The serum level of IgA tends to be elevated, in common with other inflammatory lesions of the gastro-intestinal tract. The rise probably results from an increased contribution of 7S IgA from the lamina propria of the bowel wall, although the number of plasma cells therein containing IgA is not always increased. Also, secretory 11S IgA is present in the serum of a significantly greater proportion of coeliac patients than normals (the same is also true of other inflammatory bowel disorders).

By contrast with the situation regarding serum IgA levels, IgM concentrations tend to be low in coeliac disease, and this appears to be due to decreased synthesis rather than increased loss into the bowel lumen. In the jejunal mucosa, however, there is an increased number of IgM-containing plasma cells while the number of IgA-containing plasma cells is relatively decreased, and the concentration of IgM is increased and of IgA relatively decreased in jejunal secretions in this disorder.

The intestinal mucosa of coeliac patients, if challenged with gluten, responds with a striking increase in synthesis of IgA and of IgM. How much of this reflects 'simple' formation of antibodies to gluten is uncertain. Similarly the relationship of these changes to pathogenesis of mucosal lesions is not clear. It may well be, however, that the intestinal mucosal damage in this disease may result from a local Arthus-type reaction, initiated by local excess of IgM-precipitating and complement fixing antibodies to gluten. It is of interest that complement and IgM are both found 'free' (on immunofluorescent staining) among the damaged mucosal and submucosal tissue elements. It is also of some interest that there appears to be a greater incidence of selective IgA deficiency in coeliac patients than in the general population.

Studies of IgG, IgD, and IgE immunoglobulin concentrations and of plasma cells containing these moieties have failed to show any characteristic pattern or abnormality in coeliac patients when compared with normals.

Dysgammaglobulinaemia and the Bowel

Congenital immunodeficiency syndrome

Combined immunodeficiency (Swiss type). Severe diarrhoea is the rule and is due to viral and bacterial infections. These patients have both a defect in antibody production and delayed hypersensitivity and are also prone to fungal infections.

Congenital agammaglobulinaemia (Bruton type). In this there is one intestinal form with diarrhoea perhaps due to bacterial infections and one with recurrent upper respiratory tract infections. These patients have a defect in antibody production but have normal delayed hypersensitivity.

Primary acquired hypogammaglobulinaemia

Here steatorrhoea is seen in 20 to 50 per cent of cases. The mucosa shows a striking lack of Ig-containing plasma cells, and sometimes there is nodular lymphoid hyperplasia of the intestine. Super-infection with *Giardia lamblia* may be of importance in these patients.

Secondary acquired dysgammaglobulinaemia

In malignant disease of the lymphoid system malabsorption may also occur, although it should be borne in mind that patients with long-standing coeliac disease may also themselves develop lymphoma.

Alpha-chain disease

The first case of alpha-chain disease was described in 1968, the clinical symptoms being steatorrhoea, weight loss and, especially noticeable, marked finger clubbing. It was initially thought that the disease was confined to the Mediterranean littoral, but it has now been shown to occur in a much wider

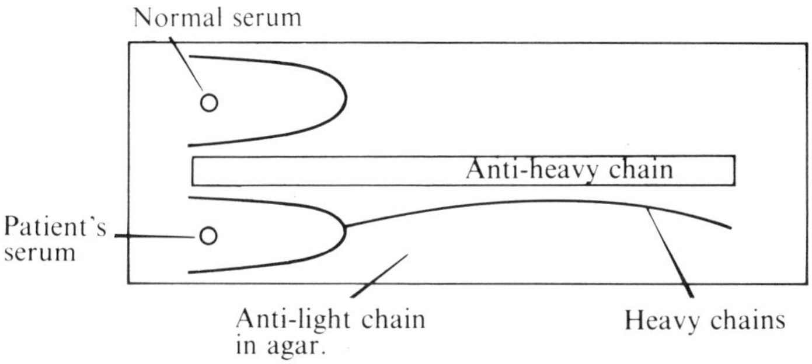

Figure 6.3. Immunoelectrophoresis of serum is performed in an 'immunoselection' plate containing anti-light chain antisera. In normal serum, all immunoglobulin will be precipitated by anti-light chain sera because light chains are attached to the heavy chains. Where *free* heavy chains occur they will travel further and undergo secondary precipitation with specific anti-heavy chain antisera.

geographical distribution. The characteristic finding in these patients is free alpha-chain (heavy chain of IgA) in the serum as well as marked plasma cell infiltration of the gut wall. Alpha-chains can also be detected in the urine, jejunal fluid and saliva. Most cases are associated with a malignant intestinal lymphoma.

The treatment for this condition is as for myeloma with Melphalan and corticosteroids. Some of the early cases responded to antibiotics alone, which led to the idea that intestinal infection might provide the initial stimulus for the proliferation of the plasma cells within the mucosa. To date no single constant pathogen has been demonstrated in patients with this disease.

Immunoelectrophoresis of serum is performed in an 'immunoselection' plate containing anti-light chain antisera. In normal serum all immunoglobulin will be precipitated by anti-light chain sera, because light chains are attached to the heavy chains. Where *free* heavy chains occur they will travel further and undergo secondary precipitation with specific anti-heavy chain antisera.

Protein-losing enteropathy

The best example of this disorder is idiopathic intestinal lymphangiectasia. There is often a deficiency of circulating immunoglobulin, while in some patients a significant lymphopenia also occurs. The immunological disturbances would appear to be secondary to the primary, anatomical disorder of the lymphatics.

The precise relationship of malabsorption to these various diseases characterised by immunoglobulin disturbances is not clear. The possible role of such auxiliary features as abnormal bowel flora, disturbed intestinal motility and lymphatic drainage, and possible impairment of hepatic or pancreatic function must all be borne in mind.

Ulcerative Colitis

Aetiology

Many theories have been advanced to explain the pathogenesis of idiopathic ulcerative colitis ranging from psychogenic factors to food allergy. Few are open to testing and can therefore neither be confirmed nor refuted. In recent years, however, antibodies reacting with human colon extracts have been demonstrated in the serum of patients with ulcerative colitis. The test antigen in the early experiments was adult human colon, which not only contained mucosal antigens but also a variety of gut bacteria. It is known that most human sera contain antibodies directed against gut flora, and the results could therefore be explained by normal antibodies directed against commensal organisms in the gut.

Colon antigen. Further experiments showed that antibody could also be demonstrated against fetal colon, both in haemagglutination and precipitation assays, and that the antibody was present in high titre in lymph nodes draining the colon. The lymphocytes of such patients also show cell-mediated reactions against colon cells as demonstrated by cytotoxicity and leucocyte migration inhibition. The question arises whether this immunological reactivity is primary or secondary to chronic inflammation. There is certainly no correlation between anti-colon antibody titres and the duration or severity of the disease. In other situations, however, where there is chronic inflammation of the gut due to other causes, such as coeliac disease or chronic gastro-intestinal infections, even when severe, anti-colon antibodies are only occasionally found.

E. coli 014. The colonic mucosal antigen in rat and human is a heat-stable mucopolysaccharide, chemically similar to blood group antigens but immunologically distinct from them. There is a chemical resemblance between the colon antigen and bacterial lipopolysaccharides and, in fact, haemagglutination with colon antigen-sensitised cells can be inhibited by an extract of *E. coli* 014, but not with other *E. coli* lipopolysaccharides. These results raise the interesting possibility that tolerance to colon can be broken by stimulation with cross-reacting bacterial antigens. However, can the actual lesions observed be directly related to these immunological observations? The killing of colon cells by patients' lymphocytes certainly occurs, and if peripheral blood leucocytes from colitis sufferers are injected into their own skin or rectal wall, a local inflammatory response results. However, all these systems are to a variable extent artificial and extrapolation of the findings to 'intact' adult sufferers with this disorder must be tentative.

Immune complexes. A further type of immunological reaction may be of importance in colitis. There is now evidence for circulating immune complexes in this condition, as detected by an anti-complementary method involving C1q fixation. Complexes have also been detected by their ability to block antibody-mediated cytotoxicity in vitro. Such inhibition by colitis sera parallels activity of the disease process. These tests for immune complexes are of theoretical interest, but as yet have no accepted part in the clinical investigation of colitis patients.

Occasionally an apparent idiopathic proctocolitis may be associated with other disorders, such as chronic active hepatitis or cirrhosis, and under these circumstances positive tests for ANA or even 'LE–cells' may occur. The exact connection between these observations is obscure. Coombs-positive haemolytic anaemia may also infrequently complicate idiopathic proctocolitis. Again the mechanism is unclear.

In ulcerative colitis the density of IgA-containing cells in the mucosa appears to be reduced and extra-cellular IgA may be seen to be increased on immunofluorescent staining. Serum immunoglobulin studies, however, have yielded no consistent pattern.

Milk allergy. (See also below). Favourable clinical response of a proportion of colitis patients to a milk-free diet is well known, and at time of relapse of such patients upon milk challenge high serum antibody titres to whole milk extract have been observed. Apart from this, however, there has been no convincing demonstration of abnormal immunological reactivity to milk constituents in colitic patients when compared with normals. The role of concurrent alactasia in producing milk-intolerance in colitis cannot be ignored.

Histocompatibility antigens. Recently it has been shown that the histocompatibility type HL-A 27 has a very high incidence in ankylosing spondylitis. Of relevant interest is an equivalent high incidence in patients with ulcerative colitis who also have sacroiliitis. This points to a genetic component in this interesting associated feature in ulcerative colitis. Other histocompatibility antigen studies have yielded somewhat conflicting results but have suggested increased frequency of HL-A 1 and -7, and reduced frequency of HL-A 3 in colitis.

Conclusion. Final comment must be made, however, that there are no routine immunological tests which need to be carried out in the investigation and management of colitis patients at the present time, although ANA and LE tests may be positive in one or two unusual instances as outlined above.

Milk Allergy

The observation that a diet excluding milk and milk products helps a proportion of patients with ulcerative colitis points to food being an important factor in some gastro-intestinal diseases. What is often not proven is whether this is related to enzyme deficiency (primary or secondary) or allergy. Unfortunately, evidence to support the diagnosis of food allergy is often difficult to obtain. Both skin tests and immunological investigations are often negative where the clinical history seems positive.

Clinical picture

A small group of patients react anaphylactically to cow's milk and it is such patients who do give a positive skin test to milk and also the relevant positive serology. Both IgE and complement fixing antibodies have been detected in these patients. In others, children especially, vomiting is a common feature in addition to colic and diarrhoea, being present in about one third of the patients. Projectile vomiting in milk allergic babies and young children can be stopped by substituting soya products for milk.

Crohn's Disease

Aetiology

It has recently proved possible to transmit granulomatous lesions to animals using a homogenate of human Crohn's tissue passed through a fine filter (0·2 μ). Changes were induced in some 75 per cent of animals following injection of this material into the wall of the ileum, but no such lesions were produced using normal human ileal homogenate. Similar findings have been obtained with foot pad injection and in this situation a second passage could be obtained. Whether such experiments indicate the presence of an aetiological agent is as yet unproven. The findings have not yet been independently confirmed.

Kveim antigen

Skin tests. By analogy with sarcoidosis, also a granulomatous condition, positive Kveim reactions on skin testing have been reported in 40 to 50 per cent of Crohn's patients. Similar positive findings have also been recorded in up to a quarter of ulcerative colitis patients and in a number of subjects with coeliac disease. The picture is further complicated by the finding of positive Kveim tests in patients with Hodgkins' disease. Reasons for positivity under these different circumstances is obscure. It is possible that certain special Kveim test antigen suspensions were responsible for these results.

Leucocyte migration test. When Kveim antigen is used in leucocyte migration inhibition tests in Crohn's patients a variable number of instances of inhibition can be recorded, but again similar findings have been reported by other workers in a few ulcerative colitis patients as well.

Delayed hypersensitivity

Skin tests. In certain granulomatous conditions, such as sarcoidosis as well as Crohn's disease, there is evidence of depression of delayed hypersensitivity as shown by skin testing with tuberculin or PPD. Further studies in this matter, however, have yielded conflicting results when skin tests employing other antigens, such as mumps, candida and trichophytin have been carried out.

Lymphocyte transformation. More direct parameters of cell-mediated immune competence in Crohn's patients have involved the use of the lymphocyte transformation test. Again, different workers have reported conflicting results but it seems likely that a proportion of patients have impaired lymphocyte responses to stimulation with phytohaemagglutinin (PHA) and also in the mixed lymphocyte reaction. Some experiments suggest that a serum factor plays a role in these impaired responses. The changes do not appear to correlate with disease activity, or to be more marked in immuno-suppressed individuals. They would appear to result from a relative reduction of T lymphocytes rather than an overall lymphopenia. One explanation would be that such lymphocytes are 'pre-empted' to the intestinal lesions. Indeed, a proportion of Crohn's patients do show a relative deficiency of T lymphocytes in peripheral blood as measured by the rosette test.

Primary sensitisation with dinitrochlorobenzene. Using a 'newly-encountered' antigen in the form of the contact-sensitising agent dinitrochlorobenzene (DNCB), depression of cutaneous reactions in Crohn's patients compared with controls has been reported, but again not confirmed by other workers using similar methods. Failure to react to this form of challenge may possibly be a non-specific effect of illness itself since depression can be demonstrated in a variety of chronic debilitating diseases, such as carcinomatosis or active tuberculosis.

Serology

Recent experiments studying complement consumption or employing a system involving inhibition of cytotoxicity have strongly suggested the presence of circulating immune complexes in Crohn's disease, although again their role in pathogenesis is not yet clear. C3 levels in the serum as measured by radialimmunodiffusion do not differ from normal. Serum levels of IgG tend to be slightly higher and of IgM slightly lower, on the whole, than in normals, but the differences are too slight to be of use in clinical practice.

Histocompatibility antigens

Reports have appeared of a reduced incidence of HL-A 9 and an increase of HL-A 3 in patients with Crohn's disease. These results require confirmation on larger series of patients.

Evidence for autoimmunity

There is no evidence for Crohn's disease being due to autoimmunisation and the incidence of organ-specific and non-organ specific autoantibodies is the same as in control subjects. Crohn's sera do not stain cells of ileal or colonic mucosa by immunofluorescence, and if such tissues are used in leucocyte migration inhibition experiments no differences from normals result. This contrasts with the situation in proctocolitis, where a significant proportion of subjects show positive inhibition of their leucocytes with these tissue extracts.

Conclusion. What emerges is the fact that the diagnosis of Crohn's disease is still made on clinical, radiological and histopathological grounds, other laboratory tests helping remarkably little.

Carcinoembryonic Antigen (CEA)

CEA in neoplastic disease

Serological methods are the major analytical tool for the study of cancer specific antigens, especially in the human, as they are applicable to the analysis of both soluble antigens and antibody in the serum. Gold was among the first to show that cells from a colonic adenocarcinoma contained an antigen not present in normal mucosa. It was then found that this so-called cancer specific antigen was also present in many adenocarcinomas of endodermal origin, such as stomach, small intestine, pancreas and liver, as well as in normal gut tissues from human embryos. It also occurs frequently in malignant neoplasms of the bronchus and breast and in neuroblastoma. There seems to be a progressive increase in the frequency of positive assays with spread of the neoplasia, e.g. in colon cancer the incidence of positive results increases from 48 per cent in Duke's stage A to 100 per cent in stage C. Also the quantity of CEA detected is greater when the cancer has metastasised. Higher values of CEA occur in poorly-differentiated growths. Both squamous cell carcinoma and adenocarcinoma of the female reproductive tract appear to be equally associated with raised CEA levels. CEA is probably a single substance, a glycoprotein of molecular weight around 200 000. It has β_1 electrophoretic mobility.

CEA in non-neoplastic disease

More recently CEA-like activity has been demonstrated in serum in various non-neoplastic diseases, particularly those of the pancreas, liver and intestine.

Pancreas. CEA is found in the serum of patients with both neoplastic and non-neoplastic diseases of the pancreas. With cancer of the pancreas, most patients have detectable levels of CEA in the serum (90 per cent) and of these about half have large amounts.

Liver. The incidence of CEA in liver disease varies with the type of disorder. In alcoholic cirrhosis approximately 9 out of 10 cases have positive results, whereas with active chronic hepatitis only 1 out of 5 shows this pattern. It is possible that the damaged liver synthesises an abnormal glycoprotein with CEA activity, or that it is deficient in removing such material produced elsewhere.

Crohn's disease and ulcerative colitis. The incidence here is between 25 and 50 per cent.

As assays become more sensitive and capable of detecting smaller amounts the discriminatory value diminishes. With sensitive techniques, such as radioimmunoassay, low levels of CEA-like activity can now be detected in healthy control subjects and in normal tissues. If a relatively insensitive method is used to detect CEA or a high titre is taken using a sensitive method, then the test will detect patients with either gut neoplasia or extensive liver disease. Distinguishing between these two possibilities, however, should present no great difficulty clinically. Values greater than 40 ng/ml are highly suggestive of the presence of a new-growth.

From what has been said, it can be seen that CEA or, substances cross-reacting with it, can be detected in many tissues from patients with both neoplastic and non-neoplastic disease (e.g. inflammatory bowel disease) and in small amounts in healthy subjects. There is yet a further complication in the interpretation of a positive CEA assay, which results from observations that stored blood, whether from cancerous or non-cancerous patients, contains more CEA than fresh specimens. It would seem that erythrocyte glycolipid and glycoprotein has similar characteristics to CEA and that 'immunologically defined CEA' may represent a family of related molecules. A more positive view of CEA is that it is a 'division antigen', which is a product of proliferating cells and will eventually be shown to be specific for each cell type. CEA may represent a large increase in production of a normal protein by cancer cells and may be a constituent of normal mucus.

Summary of uses and limitations of CEA testing

The tests are probably of no use in the screening of populations for cancer; early lesions show very little elevation of CEA levels—more extensive ones would present clinically in all probability. CEA levels in serum appear to relate directly to the size of the tumour and the degree of spread. For similar reasons, CEA tests are of little value in differential diagnosis of malignant and non-malignant disease of an organ (e.g. colon or pancreas) or in the differentiation of types or sites of origin of tumours.

On the positive side, these tests may be of value in studying prognosis. In follow-up studies of patients with 'resected' colorectal cancer, prognosis can be related to *initial* levels of CEA. It is possible that CEA tests may be of use in the monitoring of radio- or chemo-therapy for malignant disease. Recurrence of CEA may precede the appearance of clinical metastases.

Alpha-fetoprotein (AFP)

Alpha-fetoprotein (AFP) is produced by neoplastic cells or regenerating tissue, and is also present in all fetuses, constituting 40 per cent of fetal serum protein in the second trimester of pregnancy. It is a polypeptide appearing among the alpha globulins and of molecular weight 70 000, and has no relationship to immunoglobulin molecules. The exact mode of origin of this protein in the adult is unknown. It appears that the proteins in fetuses and in adults with hepatomas are identical.

In malignant disease there seems little doubt that alpha-fetoprotein is produced by tumour cells but not all the tumour cells carry out this process, and the proportion doing so may even be as low as 20 per cent. How the fetal gene becomes activated in the tumour cell is, however, unknown. AFP in the circulation has a half-life of about 5 days.

Methods of detection (Table 6.3)

The first method of detection of AFP described was by precipitation in agar which could detect as little as 5 μg/ml. With the use of counter-current electrophoresis, auto-radiography and finally radioimmunoassay levels of less than 1 ng/ml can now be detected.

With the less sensitive methods (precipitation) positive results are obtained in few clinical situations and then are almost diagnostic of those conditions, e.g. hepatocellular carcinoma, germinal tumours of the testis or ovary or tumours of entodermal origin. With increasingly sensitive assays more patients with non-neoplastic diseases are found to have circulating AFP.

Thus, it can be seen that as the methods for detecting AFP become more sensitive, smaller amounts can be detected in the serum and the diagnostic use of the test from the point of view of detecting malignancy diminishes accordingly. Levels of 2 to 16 ng/ml AFP are commonly detected in healthy adults. It seems likely that this protein is produced by some of the cells in the liver but it is not as yet known whether it is these particular cells which turn malignant if and when a hepatoma develops. Elevated levels of AFP in maternal serum are well recognised in cases of intrauterine fetal death or

Table 6.3. Methods of detecting AFP

Detection of AFP by:	precipitation in agar immunoautoradiography radio-immunoassay	
Detection by precipitation: >2 *μg/ml AFP found in:*		
	Hepatocellular cancer	Testicular cancer
	Choriocarcinoma	Occasional non-hepatic cancer
Detection by immunoautoradiography: 0·1 *μg/ml AFP found in:*		
	Acute viral hepatitis	Partial hepatectomy
	Obstructive jaundice	Pregnancy (normal or abnormal)
	in addition to the conditions listed in first method	
Detection by radioimmunoassay: <1 *ng/ml AFP found in:*		
	Other malignancies (e.g. stomach) Hepatic cirrhosis Normal serum	
	in addition to the conditions listed in first two methods	

when the fetus has neural tube defects but this topic is outside the scope of the present work. High levels have also been described in ataxiatelangiectasia and in some metabolic disorders of tyrosine metabolism occurring in children.

AFP in liver disease

In the context of differential diagnosis of liver disease, it is well recognised that small amounts of alpha-fetoprotein occur in various non-malignant disorders. Thus, testing by radio-immunoassay has revealed that over 90 per cent of patients with acute viral hepatitis have raised levels during the course of the illness. Increases are usually modest, but, in as many as a quarter, levels measurable by immunodiffusion methods may be recorded (i.e. >2 μg/ml). The mechanism of these elevations is obscure but possibilities include liver cell retrodifferentiation during regeneration, an acute-phase reaction to liver-cell injury or viral derepression of the genome controlling synthesis of AFP.

It appears that AFP is more likely to appear in hepatitis in children, in the recovery phase of the disease, or if HBAg tests are positive.

With immunodiffusion methods of detection, reported incidences of positivity in primary hepatocellular cancer have varied between 40 and 90 per cent. Kohn has used countercurrent immunoelectrophoresis in cellulose acetate and has reported 85 per cent positives in primary liver cell cancer and about 2 per cent positives in miscellaneous non-malignant hepatic disorders. Very high titres were noted in infantile hepatoblastomas. This screening method detects concentrations of about 200 ng/ml. Japanese reports suggest an incidence as high as 10 per cent in carcinoma of the stomach, but this requires confirmation. The high incidence in teratomas and genital tumours is beyond the scope of this chapter. In an attempt to increase sensitivity in diagnosis of hepatoma a recent study from Germany has employed a passive haemagglutination microtitre method coupling anti- α-fetoprotein-IgG with diazotised benzidine on fresh sheep erythrocytes. This undoubtedly gives a very high positivity rate in primary liver cell cancer, but 15 to 20 per cent of patients with cirrhosis are also positive with this method in the absence of malignant change in the liver. Increased incidences of AFP in cirrhosis, particularly that of the alcoholic, and Indian childhood cirrhosis, are well recognised.

LIVER

Immunological tests have been applied extensively to the study of chronic inflammatory disease of the liver and its pathogenesis, and have an accepted place in clinical diagnosis. They have been used particularly in the investigation of jaundice and cholestasis, in distinguishing the various types of cirrhosis and in their differentiation from more acute forms of hepatocellular disorder.

Greater understanding about the pathogenesis of acute and chronic inflammatory disease has resulted from the identification of the Australia antigen and recognition of its close association with the long-incubation period hepatitis virus B. Use of polytransfused sera has revealed a number of antigenic materials possibly connected with other viruses which may be implicated in the aetiology of different types of hepatitis, also, various specific sub-types of the Australia antigen (HBAg) are now recognised. Detailed examination of the virological tests, however, is outside the scope of this review and applications of such tests will only be mentioned insofar as they inter-relate with other immunological studies. Similarly, tests for cytomegalovirus (CMV) and Epstein–Barr virus (EBV) will not be considered as such, although their importance in the pathogenesis of certain instances of acute hepatic inflammation is recognised.

Chronic hepatitis: pathogenesis

Histological considerations. 'Chronic hepatitis' may arise from persistence of a viral infection or be of uncertain aetiology, in which case autoimmune mechanisms have been postulated. Yet other cases may be related to drug ingestion, e.g. oxyphenisatin, methyldopa, or alcohol, or may result from metabolic disturbances, as in Wilson's disease. Following discovery of the Australian antigen it is possible to use this test as a marker of infection with the long-incubation hepatitis virus and, hence, to separate off a proportion at least of 'chronic hepatitis' cases.

Chronic persistent hepatitis. This may follow on acute hepatitis and is more likely to occur after long-incubation virus infection than after endemic hepatitis. Histologically, there is expansion of portal triads and increased inflammatory infiltrate, but lobular architecture is preserved and fibrosis is slight. The changes may persist for months but the outcome is favourable, and progression to cirrhosis unusual. If, however, in acute viral hepatitis there is 'bridging necrosis' linking central veins and portal triads, the prognosis becomes much worse both with regard to development of chronic liver disease and cirrhosis, and to mortality.

Chronic active hepatitis (CAH). This may also follow on identifiable infection with the long-incubation hepatitis virus, but here the inflammatory cell infiltrate is heavy and consists chiefly of mononuclear cells. The degree of parenchymal necrosis is variable and the term 'piece-meal' necrosis has been used. There is isolation of individual liver cells and evidence of regeneration. Fibrosis is conspicuous and cirrhosis frequent. These histological features have given rise to the term 'chronic aggressive hepatitis', but this appearance is in itself not pathognomonic of the condition and it should be noted that it often occurs when positive proof of initial viral infection is lacking. Similar histological appearances have also been reported in some cases of Wilson's disease. The prognosis of chronic active hepatitis is poor, few patients surviving for more than 10 years.

These histological classifications of chronic hepatitis leave many questions unresolved. Thus, the aetiology of a fairly high proportion of both 'persistent' and 'aggressive' cases remains obscure (although improved sensitivity of tests for HBAg and further knowledge of its subtypes may clarify the situation to some degree). Factors determining resolution of the hepatitic process or its progression to 'persistent' or 'aggressive' types of chronicity are also largely obscure, but clearly of importance. Also, it is becoming apparent that there are several distinct subtypes of the 'chronic active hepatitis' syndrome, and some at least would appear not to be of viral origin (e.g. those due to drugs).

Immunoglobulin studies (see below) in chronic persistent and chronic aggressive hepatitis show that serum IgG levels are significantly higher in those cases who are HBAg negative, suggesting that a different pathogenetic mechanism might be in operation in these cases.

Serum globulin and immunoglobulin changes

Hyperglobulinaemia is seen in a variety of liver diseases, but its pathogenesis is uncertain. In acute inflammation, as in hepatitis due to either short-incubation or long-incubation viruses, or cholangitis, a modest increase occurs 7 to 14 days after the onset, but it returns to normal within a few weeks. Persistence of high levels may indicate transition to chronic liver disease and development of cirrhosis. In this condition, serum protein electrophoresis may show β–γ fusion due to increase in the faster globulins (γ_1) whereas a narrow distinct gamma peak is characteristic of chronic active hepatitis ('juvenile' cirrhosis) and consists essentially of slower γ_2 globulins.

In acute hepatitis a rapid rise in serum IgM level may be seen but return to normal usually occurs within several weeks while changes in IgA and IgG levels occur much less frequently and are seldom marked. It has been suggested that IgM elevations may be minimal in long-incubation hepatitis (associated with positive HBAg tests) but this has not been confirmed. Similar immunoglobulin changes occur in hepatitis due to infectious mononucleosis. Extreme hypergammaglobulinaemia is characteristically seen in the active phase of chronic active hepatitis and is often associated with a substantial increase in serum IgG concentration. IgA elevation has been described as typical of portal cirrhosis, particularly in association with chronic alcoholism. In primary biliary cirrhosis (PBC) IgM is usually raised and it has been claimed that isolated elevation of this immunoglobulin may be used in differentiation from

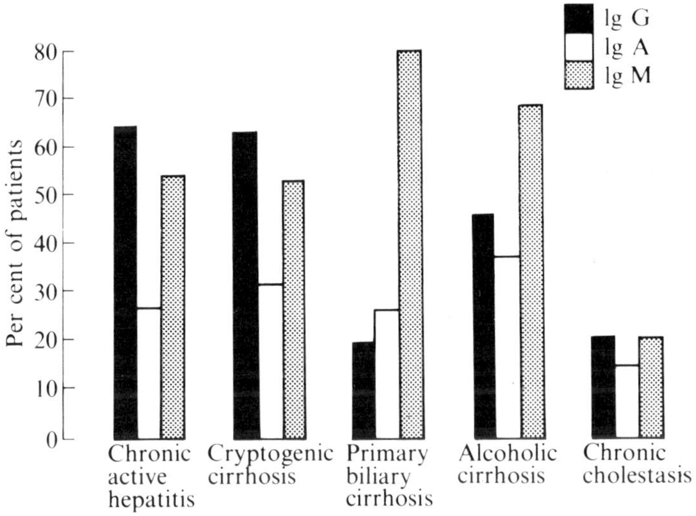

Figure 6.4. Incidence of raised immunoglobulin levels in chronic active hepatitis, cryptogenic cirrhosis, primary biliary cirrhosis, alcoholic cirrhosis and in chronic obstructive jaundice due to biliary strictures or stones. Data of Feizi (1968). By kind permission of the Editor of *Gut*.

secondary biliary and other forms of cirrhosis. However, in all types of cirrhosis the changes are rarely selective and varying degrees of elevation are found in each of the three major immunoglobulin classes (IgG, IgA and IgM). IgM levels are raised in about 80 per cent of PBC cases but elevations are also seen in some 20 per cent of patients with main bile-duct obstruction. The diagnostic value of immunoglobulin estimations in chronic liver diseases is thus very limited (see Figure 6.4). IgD levels appear to be normal in all the hepatic disorders so far studied, while IgE determinations have not as yet been reported in the context of liver disease.

In the majority of cases of hypergammaglobulinaemia the globulins are polyclonal. In a few isolated cases of cirrhosis M-bands with single light-chains, characteristic of monoclonal gammopathy, have been described. Immunoglobulins are not produced in the normal liver but in chronic hepatic disease they have been identified in lymphoid and plasma cells infiltrating portal areas and liver parenchyma. IgG appears to be the predominant immunoglobulin synthesised in the liver in chronic active hepatitis (CAH), while lymphoid aggregates around damaged bile ductules in PBC produce mainly IgM.

Mechanism of hyperglobulinaemia. The mechanism could be due to increased processing of antigen in the proliferating Küpffer cells, thus triggering antibody synthesis. Bacterial and viral antibodies are thought to be generally enhanced in hepatitis and cirrhosis, and high titres of antibodies to measles and rubella have been described in CAH. New information suggests that this applies particularly to enteric organisms and it is postulated that in these instances the diseased liver fails to sequester antigens absorbed from the gut and these then become available for stimulating antibody formation elsewhere, thus contributing to the observed hyperglobulinaemia. The distribution of antigen between liver and spleen may determine the magnitude of the immune response. In cirrhosis the increased production of antibody to both gut-derived and non-gut-derived antigen could be due to a reduction in capacity of the liver to trap antigen, which would result in more antigen reaching the spleen. Portocaval shunts further interfere with the Küpffer cell 'filter' and higher antibody titres are found after such operations. Pertinent to these remarks about by-passing of Küpffer cells are observations implicating the liver in the Chase–Sulzberger effect. It is known that animals given a hapten by mouth are subsequently resistant to sensitisation by that hapten. This specific immunological unresponsiveness induced by oral feeding may be prevented by portocaval shunt. This implies that prior circulation of antigen to the liver decreases the ability of immunologically competent cells elsewhere to recognise or react with antigen on subsequent contact.

Antibody studies in liver disease

The elevated serum immunoglobulin values in some cases of chronic liver disease are associated with circulating antibodies directed against various tissues and tissue components. Early studies and many later ones have shown that complement fixation tests (CFT) with crude liver or kidney homogenates are positive in viral hepatitis and in alcoholic and other types of cirrhosis. However, CFT with crude tissue homogenates show that three chronic liver disorders can be separated off as the reactions are present in very much higher titres. The conditions are PBC, CAH and cryptogenic cirrhosis. With the advent of immunofluorescent techniques it became apparent that high titres of other non-organ specific, non-species specific autoantibodies, namely those directed against nuclei, smooth muscle and mitochondria, are also restricted to these three conditions (with one or two special exceptions discussed below).

The concept of non-organ-specific autoimmune 'markers'

Most of the autoantibodies found in the serum of patients with liver disease are directed against sub-cellular organelles or soluble proteins, which occur not only in the liver but in other organs as well. The antibodies are not thought to be directly responsible for the progression of liver cell or bile duct destruction and their clinical importance is primarily diagnostic. They do not occur in cases of alcoholic cirrhosis or in diseases due to metabolic errors, such as haemochromatosis or Wilson's disease, where equally severe liver cell damage may nevertheless be present. Hence, they cannot be considered simply as epiphenomena occurring secondarily to liver cell injury. Since persistent titres are polarised to a small number of recognised clinical liver syndromes, it seems likely that in these cases the antibodies might represent markers of an underlying predisposition to autoimmunity.

Autoantibody Tests

Antinuclear antibodies (ANA). These are best detected by indirect immunofluorescence. The highest incidence (approximately 75 per cent) is seen in 'lupoid' hepatitis, where LE cell tests are positive, but high titres may also occur in CAH where LE cell tests are negative. In some instances it is possible that an inhibitor in the serum is responsible for the negative LE cell test. Chronic active hepatitis patients may, however, have ANA titres of only 10 or 20, with a positive LE cell test while rarely LE cells may be found without ANA fluorescence. The nuclear staining pattern is usually diffuse in CAH and the antibodies are predominantly IgG. In PBC and cryptogenic cirrhosis approximately 50 per cent of ANA positive cases show either speckled patterns or, more rarely, nucleolar antibodies. In all these conditions the serum may contain a mixture of ANA reacting with several nuclear constituents which show up by a change of pattern with increasing dilution or when using conjugates specific for single immunoglobulin classes.

ANA was the first 'marker' which was believed to distinguish 'autoimmune' cases of chronic hepatitis from prolonged cases of simple viral hepatitis. Among patients with an 'aggressive' liver histology, ANA tends to be positive in women, whereas Australia antigen is more frequent in males. However, the difficulty in using ANA as a marker of an innate autoimmune predisposition is that these antibodies can be stimulated by many drugs when they appear in a high proportion of subjects. ANA may be present in as many as 60 per cent of patients after procainamide treatment while SLE-like syndromes also occur after hydrallazine, methyldopa, isoniazid and penicillin. Reports have now appeared of CAH, sometimes with positive LE cells, developing in patients taking laxatives containing oxyphenisatin. The LE cells, ANA and hepatic inflammation apparently regress when the drugs are discontinued. Another diagnostic difficulty is that a positive ANA test is not uncommon in 'healthy' elderly subjects, while the antibodies also occur in collagen disorders and autoimmune diseases not affecting the liver.

The ANA test is positive in about 25 per cent of cases with PBC or cryptogenic cirrhosis. In the latter it may occur without any other evidence of autoimmunity, while in PBC it is of interest that it is found particularly in the small proportion of patients who have negative anti-mitochondrial antibody tests.

ANA is found only rarely in uncomplicated viral hepatitis, although well-authenticated cases of Australia antigen positive viral hepatitis can progress to a chronic stage with ANA and LE cells, and perhaps this arises in genetically predisposed individuals.

Smooth muscle antibody (SMA). This serum antibody is also detected using an immunofluorescent technique. The antigen is probably an actomyosin-like substance present near the cell membrane in many tissues. It is unstable, gradually losing potency in tissue kept frozen for several weeks. Sera must be tested at dilutions of at least 10, since even at that titre some 12 per cent of normal people show positive reactions.

In the context of differential diagnosis in liver disease, this 'marker' was once believed to be specific for CAH as titres greater than 80 were rarely found in viral hepatitis. Very occasionally the test is positive at higher dilutions in the presence of positive HBAg tests. Over 60 per cent of patients with viral hepatitis have a temporary trace of these antibodies, whereas in patients showing progressive liver involvement they may persist for many years. In acute viral hepatitis, the antibodies appear early, titres of 10 to 80 being most frequent in the first week of illness. Thereafter, the titres decline and most patients give negative results at 13 weeks. SMA shows no preference for the female sex or for older age groups. This is unlike the more familial types of autoimmunity. There is a correlation between serum bilirubin level and SMA titres suggesting that liver cell damage is the main stimulus to antibody formation under these particular circumstances.

In a recent study of SMA in various types of liver injury the highest titres of SMA occurred in HBAg negative cases. These patients frequently had positive tests for ANA and mitochondrial antibodies which were not found in HBAg positive cases. This suggests a different pathogenesis in the two groups. Approximately 45 per cent of PBC patients have some smooth muscle fluorescence but titres are low. The incidence in cryptogenic cirrhosis depends greatly on the selection of material; in cases with other evidence of autoimmunity it is around 40 per cent. Smooth muscle antibodies are not confined to liver diseases: a high incidence has been described in infectious mononucleosis without liver involvement and in the serum of patients with various tumours.

Mitochondrial antibodies (AMA). These antibodies have proved the most useful from a diagnostic point of view. They are also considered to be the most reliable 'markers' of autoimmune liver disease.

Incidence in liver diseases. About 90 per cent of PBC patients give positive immunofluorescence. In about a half, fluorescent titres are high, 200 to 6000, with a correspondingly high CFT. There is no correlation with the duration or stage of the disease and titres tend to remain unchanged on follow-up. The uncommon patients with verified primary biliary cirrhosis and a negative antibody test do not differ clinically or histologically from their antibody-positive counterparts. The antibodies are found in all three main immunoglobulin classes and bear no relation to the level of serum IgM, which is frequently raised in these patients. They do not appear in the bile. Treatment with corticosteroids or azathioprine does not inhibit their formation nor does orthotopic liver transplantation, although there is a temporary drop in titres following this procedure. Since the diseased liver is removed in these patients, continued synthesis of mitochondrial antibodies suggests there is a primary abnormality of the immune system resulting in autoimmunisation to mitochondria and that this is independent of changes in hepatic antigens. In CAH and cryptogenic cirrhosis the incidence of mitochondrial antibodies varies greatly according to diagnostic criteria and in different countries: the incidence is probably about 25 per cent in both syndromes. In other types of cirrhosis the antibodies do not occur.

In cryptogenic cirrhosis the patients who have these antibodies are usually middle-aged women, often with features of cholestasis and biopsies show resemblances to those in PBC. Similarly, some patients with CAH have these clinical and histological affinities with PBC and typical mitochondrial reactions of comparable titres.

It is preferable to test sera for AMA at 1:10 dilutions, since undiluted specimens may give non-specific fluorescence and occasionally strongly positive sera show prozone effects and appear negative until diluted. The use of mono-specific anti-IgG conjugate probably increases diagnostic accuracy for AMA but also reduces the number of positive PBC cases.

Previous claims that mitochondrial antibodies are present in a high proportion of patients with halothane jaundice have not been substantiated, and the incidence of AMA does not exceed two per cent in hepatic reactions due to other drugs, such as chlorpromazine. Negative results have been obtained in several series of infective hepatitis cases, which included HBAg positive and negative patients as well as jaundice due to infectious mononucleosis. A few cases of AMA do occur, however, in other diseases where disturbed immunological processes are known to exist and in association with a subclinical form of hepatitis. If patients without overt liver disease, but having persistently raised titres of mitochondrial antibodies in their serum, are studied closely, minor abnormalities of liver function tests (in particular the serum alkaline phosphatase level) may be observed, while liver biopsies show changes akin to both CAH and PBC. Thus, patchy necrosis of liver cells has been found in all cases biopsied while there is a variable incidence of aggressive hepatitis, bile ductular proliferation and intrahepatic granulomata. These patients also show a high incidence of SMA and ANA, while 'biological-false positive' tests for syphilis (BFP) and positive Latex agglutination tests (for antiglobulin factors) are not uncommon. Patients showing these interesting changes are almost invariably suffering from some form of collagenosis, arthritis, Sjögren's syndrome, thyroiditis or pernicious anaemia.

In addition, two SLE-like syndromes with AMA and without liver involvement have been identified. One shows a neuropathy resembling multiple sclerosis but with SLE-like serology and positive BFP. In these patients mitochondrial antibodies are usually of low titre, and of IgM class. More recently another SLE-like syndrome associated with mitochondrial antibodies has been described by German workers. The patients are mostly middle-aged women who present with recurrent fever, pleural effusions, joint or muscle pains and a high ESR. Unlike classical SLE there does not appear to be renal involvement or skin rashes and the patients tend to have a leucocytosis rather than leucopenia. Serologically they show high titres of AMA which are almost entirely confined to the IgG class, while LE cells and ANA are absent. Although liver function tests are mostly within normal limits about 10 per cent of these patients show periportal lymphoid infiltrates on liver biopsy and one third have raised serum IgM levels.

Incidence of AMA in normal populations and non-hepatic disease. The incidence in healthy people is 0·4 to 0·7 per cent. However, in non-hepatic autoimmune disorders, e.g. Hashimoto's thyroiditis, pernicious anaemia, Addison's disease and myasthenia gravis, the incidence is between 1·5 and 3 per cent. In collagen disorders the frequency is still higher (except in uncomplicated rheumatoid arthritis). In systemic lupus erythematosus it is about 5 per cent and in Sjögren's syndrome or systemic sclerosis approximately 8 per cent. These patients may have subclinical liver disease (see above). The highest incidence of mitochondrial antibodies apart from chronic liver disease patients, is found in chronic BFP reactors who have no evidence of liver dysfunction, although the mitochondrial fluorescence is usually of lower titre and confined to the IgM class. Some of these patients have rheumatoid arthritis, Sjögren's syndrome or SLE.

Practical implications of mitochondrial antibody tests. The primary value of tests for AMA is in the differentiation of extrahepatic ('surgical') obstruction of the main bile ducts from other forms of intrahepatic cholestasis. Under these circumstances, repeatable AMA tests in appreciable titre make the presence of surgical jaundice extremely unlikely, provided the patient is not suffering from one of the other diseases where AMA also occurs. It should also be remembered in this context that patients with primary biliary disease do have an increased incidence of gallstones, and the two conditions may therefore be present together. The accumulated experience of several published series shows that in main-duct biliary obstruction, even when a secondary biliary cirrhosis has developed, AMA tests remain negative. However, one group of workers have reported persistent high titres of AMA in prolonged cholestasis due to various causes, including main-duct obstruction, and these findings are contradictory to several published series spread over a nine year period. Others have studied certain difficult cases where there was evidence of extrahepatic main duct obstruction but where relief of the obstruction did not cause diminution of AMA production. In some of these patients, there was evidence of an underlying intrahepatic inflammatory process akin to PBC. A possible explanation for the reports of positive AMA in extrahepatic biliary disease may be found in the number of immunofluorescence patterns which may be produced when human sera are applied to the tissues of different species. Thus, at least six discrete and unrelated reactions may resemble those produced by mitochondrial antibodies on sections of rat kidney or stomach, and these tissues are frequently used for AMA tests.

The most important reaction to be differentiated from AMA is that produced by liver–kidney microsomal antibodies (LKM), which stain the third part of the proximal tubules in the rat kidney, whereas AMA produce their main reactions on distal tubules in the medulla. For a time it was mistakenly thought that this proximal tubular pattern was due to a 'second' mitochondrial antibody found in CAH, but this pattern has now been definitely identified as the liver/kidney microsomal (LKM) antibody.

Other patterns resembling those due to AMA are unconnected with liver disease. They include a ribosomal fluorescent antibody found in less than one per cent of SLE patients and which stains kidney tubules diffusely, and the so-called brush-border heterophile antibody which also reacts with rat gastric parietal cells and occurs in three per cent of normal people. Other antibodies which are known to cause confusion in inexperienced hands are the heterogeneous reticulin and vascular endothelial antibodies. Lastly, various other patterns may be seen by immunofluorescence on rat kidney sections due to antibodies that have not yet been properly investigated and whose clinical significance is obscure. An antibody which can be called 'mitochondrial', since it is directed against cardiolipin, is occasionally found in secondary syphilis and also in a few patients with monoclonal gammopathies and BFP reactions. This antibody produces a pattern similar to that caused by AMA but it can be absorbed out with cardiolipin. It is not associated with liver disease. The antigen reacting with PBC sera is also located in mitochondrial inner membranes but is chemically different and behaves like a lipoprotein.

The origin of mitochondrial antibodies is largely unexplained. There is, however, a familial predisposition to primary biliary cirrhosis and related disorders, while the symptomless relatives of PBC subjects show an AMA incidence of eight per cent. Despite the negative correlations with HBAg in primary biliary cirrhosis it is still quite possible that some other virus plays a causal role in the genesis of the disease and in formation of the autoantibodies. It is even conceivable that in primary biliary disease some phage-like organism invades the mitochondria in bile duct cells, since in a different context it has been suggested that mitochondria can become infected with virus derived nucleic acids. This, however, would fail to provide an explanation for persistence of autoantibody after transplantation of the liver.

Liver–kidney microsomal antibodies (LKM antibodies). These antibodies are directed against a membrane antigen of the rough endoplasmic reticulum, which is in the microsomal cytoplasmic fraction. They occur predominantly in CAH patients who appear, however, to be quite different from the subgroup showing mitochondrial antibodies. The sex incidence is approximately equal, the patients are much younger and cholestasis is not a feature. They also differ from patients with so-called 'lupoid' hepatitis in that they show little or no antinuclear (ANA) or smooth muscle (SMA) reactivity.

The LKM autoantibody is much less common than AMA, and has also been found in a number of cases of drug and viral hepatitis, in a few patients with hepatocellular carcinoma, 'subclinical hepatitis' (? analagous to that seen in association with AMA) and in various cases of thyroiditis, collagen disorder and BFP reactors.

Other autoantibodies. The 'bile duct' antibody described by Paronetto and co-workers requires an antigen present in newly regenerated ducts for its demonstration which may hence be technically difficult. A similar fluorescence pattern has been described using antistreptococcal antibodies and human liver. 'Bile canalicular' antibodies produce a characteristic fluorescent pattern of interrupted double lines between liver cells. They occur in 18 per cent of various liver disorders and in eight per cent of SLE cases. A 'hexagonal' immunofluorescent staining around liver cells has been observed in other cases and is thought to be partly due to smooth muscle actomyosin fibrils, but the pattern may be seen in the absence of smooth muscle fluorescence. Antibodies to contractile proteins associated with renal glomeruli are found in CAH and collagen disorders.

Further evaluation of the diagnostic and pathogenic significance of these less well-known markers is still in progress.

Pathogenesis of 'autoimmune' liver disease

Pending further development of the work on liver-specific proteins (see below) it is true to say that organ specific autoimmunity as a causative mechanism in the development and pathogenesis of chronic liver disease has not been demonstrated. There is no evidence to support any direct cause and effect relationship between the non-organ specific autoantibodies which appear in the serum and the chronic destructive processes going on in the liver. Could cell-mediated immune mechanisms provide the 'missing link'?

Studies of cellular immunity to liver homogenates have been carried out in man, utilising the lymphocyte transformation test in CAH and various types of cirrhosis in response to challenge with liver biopsy tissue. Human fetal liver homogenate has also been used in the migration inhibition test. Positive results were obtained in about half of CAH and PBC patients and as a temporary phenomenon in viral hepatitis but not in normal controls or in extrahepatic biliary obstruction. The organ-specificity of these reactions is not yet clear as some patients' lymphocytes react also with salivary gland or kidney extracts, this being particularly common in Sjögren's syndrome or renal tubular acidosis, both of which are very commonly found in association with primary biliary disease. Correlation between the presence of serum autoantibodies and positive tests for cell-mediated immunity is imperfect. In patients with primary biliary cirrhosis and a positive serum mitochondrial antibody test, migration inhibition of leucocytes by rat liver mitochondria (as antigen) has been demonstrated in about half the cases. Surprisingly, however, similar inhibition can also be identified in some two-thirds of patients with Hashimoto's thyroiditis.

Positive results using mitochondria as antigen in the leucocyte migration inhibition test (LMT) occur in a wide spectrum of autoimmune diseases and can also develop after tissue injury as seen following myocardial infarction or surgical operation. The exact significance of these tests is unclear.

In the pathogenesis of 'autoimmune' liver disease an interplay of three factors may be postulated, namely: a genetic predisposition to liver disease, a tendency to autoimmunity and (an) external factor(s)—in all probability the hepatitis virus(es). Predisposition of persons with certain tissue types and blood groups to develop chronic active hepatitis is also now appearing, and this again highlights the importance of genetic factors. Other evidence supporting a selective 'autoimmune' nature for these patients' diseases consists of the strong female sex incidence and evidence of multisystem involvement.

Liver specific autoimmunity. Evidence supporting this concept has been imperfect in the past, as older studies were based on complement fixation tests employing crude liver homogenates and can be discounted since recently Meyer zum Buschenfelde and co-workers have isolated two liver specific antigens from fresh human post-mortem material. One is a microsomal protein and the other an unstable lipoprotein derived from the liver cell membrane. Using a mixture of these two antigens in a passive haemagglutination reaction positive results were obtained in a proportion of cases of

Table 6.4. Chronic active hepatitis viewed as a syndrome

Subgroup	Salient features				
	Sex	Age	Serum HBAg	Serum autoantibodies	Serum IgS
1 Wilson's disease	M ≃ F	5–30	–	–	variable
2. Drug-induced[a] (e.g. oxyphenisatin, methyldopa)	M ≃ F	variable	–	transient ANA, SMA; occasional LE cells +	variable
3. HBAg+[b]	M > F	variable	+	–	IgG+
4. 'Lupoid'[c]	F > M	20±	–	ANA++ LE cells± SMA+	IgG++
5. PBC-related[d]	F > M	50±	–	AMA+	IgM+
6. Microsomal (LKM)+	M ≃ F	20± variable	– (occasionally +)	LKM+ ANA± SMA–	variable
7. Undefined	M ≃ F	variable	–	ANA± SMA±	variable

[a] May be reversible
[b] Cell-mediated immunity may be deficient in this group
[c] Increased incidence of HL-A 8 tissue type
[d] Raised serum alkaline phosphatase and pruritus common.

ANA: Antinuclear antibody
AMA: Antimitochondrial antibody
LKM: Liver/kidney microsomal antibody
SMA: Antismooth muscle antibody.

aggressive hepatitis with hypergammaglobulinaemia. Antisera made in rabbits against these antigens reacted with sera of patients with acute massive liver necrosis, thus suggesting that the liver proteins are released into the circulation following severe cell damage. Studies on cell-mediated immunity to the liver specific protein (LPII) are in progress at the present time.

Chronic active hepatitis—a syndrome

Despite failure to demonstrate a clear pathogenetic mechanism for autoimmune liver disease, or indeed to prove conclusively that the latter exists as a primary disorder per se, serological and autoantibody studies in particular have permitted a tentative classification of the syndrome of chronic active hepatitis, the basis for which appears in Table 6.4. It should be appreciated, however, that this classification is merely an attempt to categorise broad sub-groups and that in each atypical features may be present in individual cases and, as a result, some degree of overlap between the sub-groups is inevitable.

References

General review articles

Dausset, J. (1972) Correlation between histocompatibility antigens and susceptibility to illness. In *Progress in Clinical Immunology*, ed. R. S. Schwartz, p. 183. New York: Grune & Stratton.

Doe, W. (1972) The secretory immune system of the intestine. *Gut*, **13**, 572.

Doniach, D. & Walker, G. (1972) Immunopathology of liver disease. In *Progress in Liver Diseases*, Vol. IV), ed. Popper, H. & Schaffner, F., p. 381. New York: Grune & Stratton.

Immunology of the Liver (1971) Proceedings of an International Meeting held at King's College Hospital Medical School, London, 6th and 7th July, 1970, ed. Smith, M. & Williams, R., 314 pp. London: Heinemann.

Jones, E. A. (1972) Immunoglobulins and the gut. *Gut*, **13**, 825.

Paronetto, F. (1970) Immunologic aspects of liver diseases. In *Progress in Liver Diseases*, (Vol. III), eds. Popper, H. & Schaffner, F., p. 299. London: Heinemann.

Shearman, D. J. C., Parkin, D. M. & McClelland, D. B. L. (1972) The demonstration and function of antibodies in the gastrointestinal tract. *Gut*, **13**, 483.

Taylor, K. B. (1972) Immune mechanisms and diseases of the gastrointestinal tract. In *Recent Advances in Gastroenterology*, ed. Badenoch, J. & Brooke, B. N. p. 1. Edinburgh and London: Churchill Livingstone.

Wright, R. (1973) Immunology of gastrointestinal and liver disease. *British Journal of Hospital Medicine*, **9**, 33.

Mouth-aphthous ulcers

Lehner, T. (1974) Immunological aspects of oral diseases. In *Clinical Aspects of Immunology*, ed. Gell, P. G. H., Coombs, R. R. A. & Lachmann, P. (in press). 3rd edition. Oxford: Blackwell.

Sjögren's syndrome

Whaley, K., Webb, J., McAvoy, B. A., Hughes, G. R. V., Lee, P., MacSween, R. N. M. & Buchanan, W. W. (1973) Sjögren's syndrome: II. Clinical associations and immunologic phenomena. *Quarterly Journal of Medicine*, **42**, 513.

Whaley, K., Williamson, J., Chisolm, D. M., Webb, J., Mason, D. K. & Buchanan, W. W. (1973) Sjögren's syndrome: I. Sicca components. *Quarterly Journal of Medicine*, **42**, 279.

Oesophagus–post-cricoid web

Chisolm, M., Ardran, G. M., Callender, S. T. & Wright, R. (1971) Iron deficiency and autoimmunity in post-cricoid webs. *Quarterly Journal of Medicine*, **40**, 421.

Pancreas

Anderson, J. R. (1968) Auto-allergy in diseases of the liver, adrenal, pancreas and prostate. In *Clinical Aspects of Immunology*, ed. Gell, P. G. H. & Coombs, R. R. A. p. 1095. Oxford: Blackwell.

Stomach and pernicious anaemia

Ardeman, S. & Chanarin, I. (1963) A method for assay of human gastric intrinsic factor and the detection and titration of antibodies against intrinsic factor. *Lancet*, **ii,** 1350.

Bardhan, K. D., Hall, I. R., Spray, G. H. & Callender, S. T. E. (1968) Blocking and binding autoantibody to intrinsic factor. *Lancet*, **i,** 62.

Chanarin, I. & James, D. (1974) Humoral and cell-mediated intrinsic-factor antibody in pernicious anaemia. *Lancet*, **i,** 1078.

Coghill, N. F., Doniach, D., Roitt, I. M., Mollin, D. L. & Wyn Williams, A. (1965) Autoantibodies in simple atrophic gastritis. *Gut*, **6,** 48.

Fisher, J. M., Mackay, I. R., Taylor, K. B. & Ongar, B. (1967) An immunological study of categories of gastritis. *Lancet*, **i,** 176.

Fisher, J. M., Rees, C. & Taylor, K. B. (1965) Antibodies in gastric juice. *Science*, **150,** 1467.

Fisher, J. M., Rees, C. & Taylor, K. B. (1966) Intrinsic factor antibodies in gastric juice of pernicious anaemia patients. *Lancet*, **ii,** 88.

Garrido-Pinson, G. C., Turner, M. D., Crokston, J. H., Samloff, J. M., Miller, L. L. & Segal, H. L. (1966) Studies of human intrinsic factor autoantibodies. *Journal of Immunology*, **97,** 897.

Samloff, I. M. & Barnett, E. V. (1965) Identification of intrinsic factor autoantibody and intrinsic factor in man by radioimmunodiffusion and radioimmunoelectrophoresis. *Journal of Immunology*, **95,** 536.

Schade, S. G., Feick, P., Muckerheide, M. & Schilling, R. F. (1966) Occurrence in gastric juice of antibody to a complex of intrinsic factor and vitamin B_{12}. *New England Journal of Medicine*, **275,** 528.

Strickland, R. G., Baur, S., Ashworth, L. A. E. & Taylor, K. B. (1971) A correlative study of immunological phenomena in pernicious anaemia. *Clinical and Experimental Immunology*, **8,** 25.

Taylor, K. B., Roitt, I. M., Doniach, D., Couchman, K. G. & Shapland, C. (1962) Autoimmune phenomena in pernicious anaemia: gastric antibodies. *British Medical Journal*, **ii.** 1347.

Coeliac disease, dysgammaglobulinaemia and the bowel

Alp, M. H. & Wright, R. (1971) Autoantibodies to reticulin in patients with idiopathic steatorrhoea, coeliac disease and Crohn's disease, and their relation to immunoglobulins and dietary antibodies. *Lancet*, **ii,** 682.

Bonomo, L., Dammacco, F., Marano, R. & Bonomo, G. M. (1972) Abdominal lymphoma and alpha chain disease: report of three cases. *American Journal of Medicine*, **52,** 73.

Rambaud, J. C., Bognel, C., Prost, A., Bernier, J. J., Le Quintrec, Y., Lambling, A., Danon, F., Hurez, D. & Seligmann, M. (1968) Clinicopathological study of a patient with 'Mediterranean' type of abdominal lymphoma and a new type of IgA abnormality (alpha chain disease). *Digestion*, **1,** 321.

Rizzetto, M. & Doniach, D. (1973) Types of 'reticulin' antibodies detected in human sera by immunofluorescence. *Journal of Clinical Pathology*, **26,** 841.

Seah, P. P., Fry, L., Holborow, E. J., Rossiter, M. A., Doe, W. F., Magathaes, A. F. & Hoffbrand, A. V. (1973) Antireticulin antibody: incidence and diagnostic significance. *Gut*, **14,** 311.

Shiner, M. (1973) Ultrastructural changes suggestive of immune reactions in the jejunal mucosa of coeliac children following gluten challenge. *Gut*, **14,** 1.

Taylor, K. B. (1972) Dysgammaglobulinaemia and intestinal dysfunction. In *Recent. Advances in Gastroenterology*, ed. Badenoch, J. & Brooke, B. N. p. 24. Edinburgh and London: Churchill Livingstone.

Ulcerative colitis and Crohn's disease

Asquith, P., Mackintosh, P., Stokes, P. L., Holmes, G. K. T. & Cooke, W. T. (1974) Histocompatibility antigens in patients with inflammatory bowel disease. *Lancet*, **i,** 113.

Jewell, D. P. & MacLennan, I. C. M. (1973) Circulating immune complexes in inflammatory bowel disease. *Clinical and Experimental Immunology*, **14,** 219.

Kraft, S. C. (1971) Cellular immunity in Crohn's disease. *Gastroenterology*, **61,** 545.

Kraft, S. C. & Kirsner, J. B. (1966) Present status of immunological mechanisms in ulcerative colitis. *Gastroenterology*, **51,** 788.

Lagercrantz, R., Hammarström, S., Perlmann, P. & Gustafsson, B. E. (1966) Immunological studies in ulcerative colitis. III. Incidence of antibodies to colon-antigen in ulcerative colitis and other gastro-intestinal diseases. *Clinical and Experimental Immunology*, **1,** 263.

Lagercrantz, R., Hammarström, S., Perlmann, P. & Gustafsson, B. E. (1968) Immunological studies in ulcerative colitis. IV. Origin of autoantibodies. *Journal of Experimental Medicine*, **128,** 1339.

Lennard-Jones, J. E. (1970) Crohn's disease. In *Modern Trends in Gastroenterology*, 4, eds. Card, W. I. & Creamer, B. p. 273. London: Butterworths.

Perlmann, P., Hammarström, S., Lagercrantz, R. & Campbell, D. (1967) Autoantibodies to colon in rats and human ulcerative colitis: cross reactivity with Escherichia coli 0:14 antigen. *Proceedings of the Society for Experimental Biology and Medicine*, **125,** 975.

Thayer, W. R. (1971) The Kveim test in Crohn's disease. *Gastroenterology*, **60,** 612.

Watson, D. W. (1969) The lymphocyte and ulcerative colitis. *Gastroenterology*, **56,** 385.

Weeke, B. & Bendixen, G. (1969) Serum immunoglobulins and organ-specific, cellular hypersensitivity in ulcerative colitis and Crohn's disease. *Acta Medica Scandinavica*, **186,** 87.

Wright, R. (1970) Ulcerative colitis. *Gastroenterology*, **58,** 875.

Wright, R. & Truelove, S. (1966) Auto-immune reactions in ulcerative colitis. *Gut*, **7,** 32.

Milk allergy

Frankland, A. W. (1970) Food allergies. *Royal Society of Health Journal*, **90,** 243.

Freier, S. & Kletter, B. (1970) Milk allergy in infants and young children: current knowledge. *Clinical Paediatrics*, **9,** 449.

Carcinoembryonic antigen (CEA)

Dykes, P. W. & Ring, J. (1972) Carcinoembryonic antigen (CEA). *Gut*, **13,** 1000.

Hunt, P. S. & Mackay, I. R. (1973) Studies of carcinoembryonic antigen of whole and extracted serum in ulcerative colitis. *Gut*, **14,** 545.

Khoo, S. K., Hunt, P. S. & Mackay, I. R. (1973) Studies of carcinoembryonic antigen activity of whole and extracted serum in ulcerative colitis. *Gut*, **14,** 545.

Khoo, S. K. & Mackay, I. R. (1973) Carcinoembryonic antigen in serum in diseases of liver and pancreas. *Journal of Clinical Pathology*, **26,** 470.

MacSween, J. M., Warner, N. L. & Mackay, I. R. (1973) The detection of carcinoembryonic antigen in whole serum from patients with malignant and non-malignant disease. *Clinical Immunology and Immunopathology*, **1,** 330.

Rule, A. H., Goleski-Reilly, C., Sachar, D. B., Vandevoorde, J. & Janowitz, H. D. (1973) Circulating CEA: relationship to clinical status of patients with inflammatory bowel disease. *Gut*, **14,** 880.

Zamcheck, N., Moore, T. L., Dhar, P. & Kupchile, H. (1972) Immunological diagnosis and prognosis of human digestive tract cancer: carcinoembryonic antigens. *New England Journal of Medicine*, **286,** 83.

Alpha-fetoprotein

Abelev, G. I. (1971) Alpha-fetoprotein in autogenesis and its association with malignant tumours. *Advances in Cancer Research*, **14,** 295.

Alpert, E. (1974) Alpha-fetoprotein: need for quantitative assays. *New England Journal of Medicine*, **290,** 568.

Edynak, E. M., Old, L. J., Vrania, M., Michael, P. & Lardis, M. P. (1972) Fetal antigen associated with human neoplasia. *New England Journal of Medicine*, **286,** 1178.

Florin-Christensen, A. & Arana, R. M. (1973) $Alpha_1$ fetoprotein and $antialpha_1$ fetoprotein in acute viral hepatitis. *British Medical Journal*, **ii,** 94.

Kew, M. C., Dos Santos, H. A. & Sherlock, S. (1971) Diagnosis of primary cancer of the liver. *British Medical Journal*, **iv,** 408.

Kew, M. C., Purves, L. R. & Bersohn, I. (1973) Serum alpha-fetoprotein levels in acute viral hepatitis. *Gut*, **14,** 939.

Kohn, J. & Weaver, P. C. (1974) Serum $alpha_1$-fetoprotein in hepatocellular carcinoma. *Lancet*, **ii,** 334.

Ruoslahti, E. & Seppälä, M. (1972) Normal and increased alphafetoprotein in neoplastic and non-neoplastic liver disease. *Lancet*, **ii,** 278

Liver

Doniach, D., Roitt, I. M., Walker, J. G. & Sherlock, S. (1966) Tissue antibodies in primary biliary cirrhosis, active chronic (lupoid) hepatitis, cryptogenic cirrhosis and other liver diseases and their clinical implications. *Clinical and Experimental Immunology*, **1,** 237.

Doniach, D. & Walker, J. G. (1969) A unified concept of autoimmune hepatitis. *Lancet*, **i,** 813.

Doniach, D. & Walker, G. (1974) Progress report—mitochondrial antibodies. *Gut*, **15,** in press.

Gold, P. & Freedman, S. O. (1965) Demonstration of tumor-specific antigens in human colonic carcinomata by immunological and absorption techniques. *Journal of Experimental Medicine*, **121,** 439.

Holborow, E. J. (1972) Smooth-muscle autoantibodies, viral infections and malignant disease. *Proceedings of the Royal Society of Medicine*, **65,** 481.

Johnson, G. D., Holborow, E. J. & Glynn, L. E. (1965) Antibody to smooth muscle in patients with liver disease. *Lancet*, **ii,** 788

Sherlock, S. (1970) The immunology of liver disease. *American Journal of Medicine*, **49,** 693.

Smith, M. G. M., Williams, R., Walker, G., Rizzeto, M. & Doniach, D. (1974) Hepatic disorders associated with liver kidney microsomal antibodies. *British Medical Journal*, **ii,** 80.

Triger, D. R. & Wright, R. (1973) Hyperglobulinaemia in liver disease. *Lancet*, **i,** 1494.

Walker, G. (1974) The immunology of liver disorders. *Proceedings of the Royal Society of Medicine*, **67,** 566.

Walker, J. G., Doniach, D., Roitt, I. M. & Sherlock, S. (1965) Serological tests in diagnosis of primary biliary cirrhosis. *Lancet*, **i,** 827.

7. Immunology of Renal Disease

N. P. MALLICK

For a number of reasons, renal disease has been an interesting subject for immunological study. The well-known sequence of acute renal damage following a streptococcal throat infection stimulated a search for a relationship between the renal disease and an immunological reaction to streptococcal components, and this continues. During the past decade, the more general involvement of immune mechanisms in glomerular disease has become clear. Study of renal biopsy specimens has shown immunoglobulins and products of the complement cascade in the glomeruli in a variety of conditions, usually unassociated with evidence of previous streptococcal infection. In patients suffering from histologically different forms of glomerular disease modern techniques have shown that the complement system is intimately involved and that there are distinctive changes in the levels of circulating complement components. Workers have also reported that cell-mediated immunity (CMI) to renal and other antigens can be detected in some glomerular diseases, and have attempted to relate these findings to the varying natural history of the different forms of glomerulonephritis. Finally, biopsy study of technically successful renal homografts has thrown light on the early changes in the kidney in those cases in which the original renal disease recurs.

The study of basic immunological mechanisms has been facilitated by the ease with which glomerular damage can be induced experimentally. There are two ways of doing this. One is to prepare an antibody against glomerular tissue and to inject it into a suitable experiment animal. The antibody can then be identified in host glomeruli severely damaged by an inflammatory reaction involving complement components and intraglomerular fibrin deposition, which appears to induce glomerular crescent formation. The other method is to produce glomerular damage by inducing the formation of circulating immune complexes, for example, by injecting bovine serum albumin (BSA), which forms BSA/anti-BSA complexes of an appropriate size. These lodge in (are filtered by) the glomerular capillary bed, and induce an inflammatory reaction which also involves the complement and coagulation systems. The development of these experimental models has been of particular interest since it is now recognised that glomerular damage in man is often due either to autoantibody directed against components of the glomerular basement membrane (GBM) or, much more commonly, to a reaction to circulating immune complexes deposited in the glomeruli.

The coincidence of the experimental and clinical approaches to the study of glomerulonephritis has resulted in major developments in the understanding of the immunological mechanisms involved and this chapter deals in the main with those points which have particular clinical relevance. There are also a number of studies on the role of the immune system in chronic pyelonephritis and there has been increasing recognition that the general principle underlying the development of many renal disorders is an inherited or acquired failure of elements of normal immune competence which predispose individuals to develop such diseases. These points are also covered briefly.

MECHANISMS FOR IMMUNOLOGICAL DAMAGE TO THE KIDNEY

The concept of 'glomerular basement membrane antigen'

Each glomerulus is a specialised capillary bed, lying between its afferent and efferent arterioles. Glomeruli can be isolated from kidney tissue by sieving techniques and glomerular chemistry and ultrastructure have been examined. Kefalides (1971) has suggested that the basement membrane is composed of a distinctive collagen rich in hexose sugars linked to two non-collagen glycoproteins with different molecular weights. However, the precise number of protein or peptide fractions isolated from GBM depends on the chemical methods used to dissect it, and the enzymes used to do this may themselves affect the antigenicity of the fractions (Misra, 1973). GBM is physically altered in glomerular diseases and there is increasing awareness that its chemical composition alters also, but the details of both physical and chemical changes are not yet complete. GBM is important in health since it determines what passes into and what is excluded from the glomerular filtrate. Damaged GBM may impede filtration so that glomerular filtration rate (GFR) is reduced or may permit protein leakage from the plasma. Electronmicroscopic studies have suggested that the normal GBM has 'holes' in it, which in disease may be altered and allow protein leakage; other workers consider that GBM is a continuous structure and attribute the protein leakage to undefined chemical changes.

Both cellular and humoral immunity have been demonstrated to GBM components in glomerular disease. GBM collagen and each of the associated non-collagen glycoproteins is antigenic when tested separately (Kefalides, 1971) and GBM solubilised by collagenase contains at least seven antigens when tested immunochemically against rabbit anti-GBM antiserum (Marquardt, Wilson and Dixon, 1973).

In glomerular disease it is probable that immunity develops to more than one of the antigens present in normal GBM. There have been conflicting reports as to the identity of the antigen(s) which stimulate the production of circulating antibody in 'anti-glomerular basement membrane antibody nephritis'. In a recent study, Marquardt, Wilson and Dixon (1973) suggest that this is within the non-collagen glycoproteins and Misra (1973) provides evidence that it is a sialoglycoprotein. Earlier workers (Mahieu, Dardenne and Bach, 1971) had suggested that the antigen was part of the collagen itself. These reports may not be mutually exclusive, since diseased GBM is altered both structurally and chemically. If the antigenic collagen fraction is normally covered by the non-collagen glycoprotein it may be exposed when there is GBM damage. It is also possible that antigens which are not found in normal GBM may form in diseased GBM as a result of changes in the chemical structure. Antibody directed to such antigens might not be detected readily. These considerations should leave no doubt that the concept of a single entity 'the GBM antigen' is not sufficiently precise.

GBM contains antigenic specificities which cross-react with antigens in the lung alveolar septal membrane, and in some group A (β-haemolytic) streptococci. This cross-reactivity can be detected in tests for both humoral and cellular immunity. In anti-GBM antibody-induced glomerulonephritis the shared immunogenicity of lung and kidney tissues is thought to be important in the pathogenesis of the disease, but the significance of the cross-reactivity between streptococcal antigen and GBM in post-streptococcal glomerulonephritis is less clear. It is generally thought that post-streptococcal glomerulonephritis is caused by immune complex deposition on the GBM, the antigen in the complexes arising from circulating streptococcal protein, and it is unnecessary to postulate antigenic cross-reactivity between GBM and a streptococcal component for such immune complexes to induce glomerular damage.

Cell-mediated immunity (CMI) to GBM and other renal antigens

There are several reports of CMI in different glomerular diseases, but neither the techniques used to demonstrate CMI nor the antigen preparations derived from the kidney have always been precisely characterised. Using the one-stage leucocyte migration test, we (Mallick et al, 1972) and others (Mahieu, Dardenne and Bach, 1972 and Macanovic, Evans and Peters, 1972) have detected CMI in patients with glomerulonephritis associated with immune complex deposition. Rocklin, Lewis and David (1970) using the two-stage test to demonstrate the release of migration inhibition factor detected CMI in anti-GBM antibody nephritis. Even in steroid-sensitive no light microscopic change nephrotic syndrome, CMI may be found (Mallick et al, 1972; Eyres et al, 1974). It has been pointed out that CMI to streptococcal/GBM cross-reacting antigen occurs in a number of cases of progressive glomerulonephritis, and this has prompted speculation that CMI to this antigen may play a role in perpetuating streptococcus-induced glomerular damage (see Zabriskie, 1973). The recognition that CMI may occur to some antigens in glomerular diseases is a recent development. However, the results obtained so far are sufficiently concordant to show that CMI as measured by the techniques used is sometimes detected, and so may have a pathogenic role.

Circulating anti-GBM antibodies

These are IgG immunoglobulins and have usually been detected in serum by layering it on to sections of normal kidney tissue and observing linear fluorescence when a fluorescein-labelled anti-IgG preparation is superimposed. However, not all normal kidney tissue binds anti-GBM antibodies, and the method is difficult to quantitate. Newer techniques utilise soluble well-characterised GBM antigens either coated onto red blood cells (passive haemagglutination method) or radio-labelled (radioimmunoassay). These methods should prove sensitive and reliable, and permit quantitative analysis.

Soluble immune complex formation and glomerular damage

In many patients with glomerulonephritis, indirect immunofluorescence techniques show that immunoglobulins—usually subclasses of IgG—form granular deposits on the epithelial aspect of the GBM or in the mesangium.

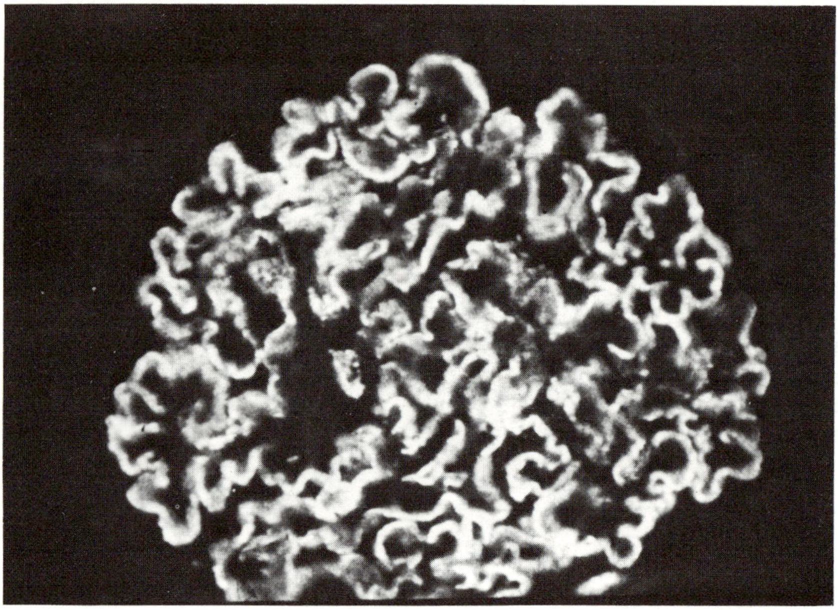

Figure 7.1. Diffuse granular IgG deposition along GBM; epimembranous glomerular disease. UV microscopy ×350.

Similar deposits occur in the experimental animal after induction of circulating soluble immune complexes, for example, by the regular injection of bovine serum albumin. Both antigen and immunoglobulin can be identified in the GBM deposits in such a model. Chronic viral infections induce immune complex formation in some animals; for example, some strains of mice infected by lymphocytic choriomeningitis virus develop immune-complex induced glomerular damage, and both antigen and antibody have been identified in the complexes.

On the basis of such experimental evidence it has been assumed that the granular deposits seen in the glomeruli in human renal disease are immune complexes. The immunoglobulin moiety can be identified, the antigen is usually unknown, although several nucleoproteins have been identified as antigens in the GBM deposits found in systemic lupus erythematosus (SLE), and antigen derived from *Plasmodium malariae* has been found in the GBM deposits of malaria-associated nephrotic syndrome. From these and other reports identifying the antigen in human immune complex disease it seems probable that much glomerular disease in man is caused by this mechanism.

It must be pointed out that there is equally convincing evidence of immune complex deposition in association with different histological categories of glomerulonephritis (diffuse proliferative with or without crescent formation, focal proliferative, mesangiocapillary, epi-membranous). The factors which determine the histological findings may depend on the phlogistic responses produced by the particular immune complex concerned. These responses may or may not involve the complement system and may or may not involve intraglomerular coagulation with fibrin deposition.

Attention has been paid to the mechanism of immune complex induced glomerular injury. Circulating soluble immune complexes form in the presence of plasma antigen excess which may be achieved if there is continued release of antigen or if the antigen derives from an actively replicating virus. Complexes formed by 'avid antibody' appear to be rapidly removed and it has been suggested that complexes of a critical size are necessary in order to produce vascular damage. It follows that an antigen which forms a lattice with several immunoglobulin molecules will create complexes of the necessary size and some antigens may be particularly likely to do this. The host immune response is also important. Only some animals on challenge with a given antigenic stimulus will produce soluble immune complexes and the characteristics of the immunoglobulin produced (subclass, amount, avidity) will determine whether appropriately sized complexes occur. These characteristics may be genetically determined, or may be affected by intercurrent disease. Such considerations are of obvious importance when considering the production of immune complex disease in man, but have not yet been studied in detail.

Once formed, the immune complexes are thought to promote the release of vasoactive amines from platelets and also to cause platelet clumping. The amines may facilitate the deposition of complexes on the GBM and platelet aggregates around deposited complexes may stimulate the complement cascade.

The deposited immune complexes may bind the early complement component C1q and so initiate the classical complement reaction, or may activate the complement system by the 'alternate pathway' mechanism. In either case, leucotactic factors are released and immune adherence of neutrophil leucocytes to the complexes via C3 may occur. The neutrophils release tissue-damaging enzymes which, with GBM fragments, may appear in the urine.

It is of interest that when the fate of radio-labelled bovine serum albumin (BSA) is followed during the induction in the rabbit of persistent BSA/anti-BSA immune complex glomerulonephritis, the complexes are first found in the glomerular mesangium and only later on the GBM. This suggests that at first the mesangial cells (a part of the reticulo-endothelial system) are active in removing the complexes, later becoming less effective in this respect so that complexes persist in the GBM. In the development of immune-complex induced glomerulonephritis, therefore, the mesangial cells may have an important role, a balance being struck between deposition of the immune complexes and removal of them by these reticulo-endothelial elements of the glomerulus. The histological counterpart of this activity is the increased number ('proliferation') of mesangial cells commonly seen in immune complex disease. Electronmicroscopy reveals that such cells are very active metabolically.

THE CLASSIFICATION OF HUMAN GLOMERULAR DISEASE

The older description of glomerular disease by Ellis into types I and II glomerulonephritis was essentially clinical. Type I had an acute onset. There was haematuria, weight gain with facial swelling and moderate oedema, proteinuria and raised blood pressure. GFR was reduced with a raised blood urea. The syndrome was studied in detail and thought usually to follow a β-haemolytic streptococcal infection. It was considered to have a good prognosis and it was claimed that 80 to 90 per cent of cases recovered. By contrast, type II disease had an insidious onset, characterised by increasing oedema with heavy proteinuria and hypoalbuminaemia; the BP and blood urea were usually normal. The prognosis was uncertain, many cases proceeding over years to die in renal failure.

During the last fifteen years, renal biopsy studies have produced a classification of glomerular disease based on the histopathology of the diseased kidney rather than on the clinical features of the illness. It was soon agreed that glomerular lesions could be grouped under three main headings, '*minimal change*', in which the glomeruli were essentially normal by light microscopy, '*membranous*', in which there as a thickening of the GBM (later recognised as a combination of immune complex deposition and intervening extention of the GBM) and '*proliferative*' in which there was proliferation of one or more of the cellular elements of the glomerulus. (In these lesions too, immune complexes appear to be involved and the immunoglobulin moieity has been identified by immunofluorescent techniques.) An important area of agreement between histopathologists who studied serial biopsies was that it was rare for lesions to change with time from one category to another.

The confusion which arose because of difficulties in marrying the older (clinical) and newer (histological) classifications of glomerular disease is still being resolved, but it seems clear that the Ellis classification should be replaced. The clinical syndrome of acute glomerulonephritis of course occurs, and bacteriological studies confirm that it may follow some streptococcal infections. However, no such association can be detected in other cases and an identical syndrome may occur in some connective tissue disorders. Furthermore, the renal lesion is not always the same histologically. It is usually 'proliferative', but shows distinctive subpatterns within this group. For example, in post-streptococcal glomerulonephritis (APSGN) there is endothelial and mesangial, and sometimes epithelial cell proliferation, whereas a number of patients who present with an identical clinical illness without evidence of streptococcal involvement have typical changes of mesangio-capillary disease (q.v.) with extension of mesangial tissue along the GBM. When the clinical features of Ellis 'type II' disease occur, the renal histology is even more varied, and any

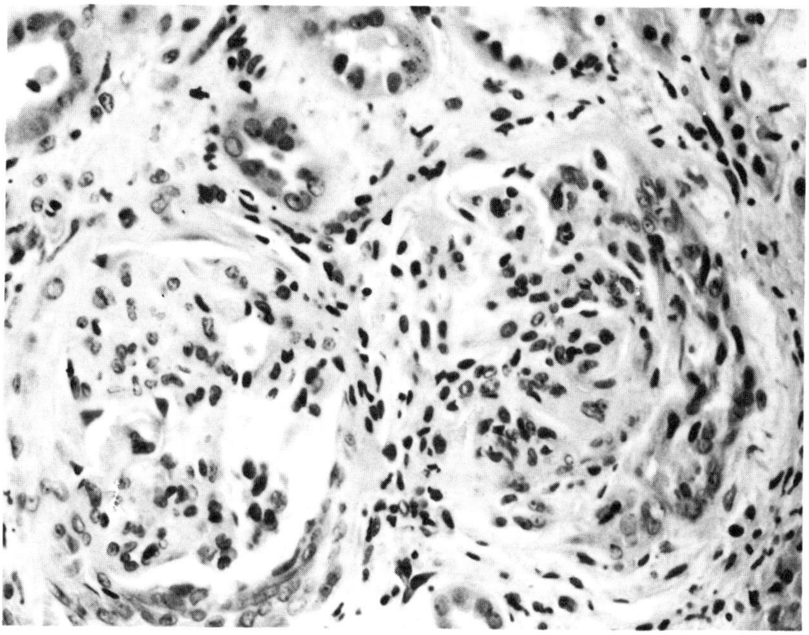

Figure 7.2. Diffuse glomerular cell proliferation with epithelial crescent formation. H & E. ×350.

of the histological patterns mentioned may be found. Because of these difficulties it has become customary in clinical practice to speak of 'the acute nephritic syndrome' and 'the nephrotic syndrome', to identify the elements of the Ellis classification, and to use the histological findings to classify the underlying lesion.

The steadily increasing recognition that glomerular disease is commonly the result of immunological damage has led to many studies of the immune system in such patients. Sufficient data are now available for some lesions to be classified by clinical, histological and immunological criteria. This is an on-going process, and some points of general agreement are listed in Table 7.1.

Table 7.1. Classification of glomerular disease by clinical, histological and immunological criteria

Category	Histology	Immunology	Clinical	Prognosis
Minimal change	No significant changes on light microscopy. No consistent immunohistological changes.	None generally accepted. Reports of involvement of complement as shown by raised immunoconglutinin and of CMI to renal antigen.	Nephrotic syndrome	Good. Disease is recurrent but renal failure rarely, if ever occurs.
Membranous	Changes confined to GBM epimembranous deposition of C3 and IgG in granular fashion on immunohistology. GBM thickened by these deposits, and intervening spikes of GBM material; later uniform GBM thickening and less obvious deposits of C3 or IgG.	C3 levels normal. Little evidence of intraglomular coagulation.	Asymptomatic proteinuria. Nephrotic syndrome.	About 25% recover within 5 years and another 25% die. The remaining patients have continuing proteinuria and may eventually develop renal failure.
Diffuse cellular proliferation	Deposition of IgG and C3 in mesangium (early) and at GBM. Polymorphs in capillary loops. Fibrin deposition in glomeruli. Epithelial cell crescent formation.	Low C4 and C3 levels if disease has acute onset. C3 convertase detected in acute phase and also cryoglobulinaemia.	Acute nephritic syndrome. Nephrotic syndrome. Asymptomatic proteinuria.	Not a single disease. May follow β-haemolytic streptococcal infection. Prognosis in doubt.
Mesangio-capillary	Mesangial proliferation encroaching onto endothelial aspect of GBM. IgG and (often dense C3) deposition in mesangium and on GBM.	C3 convertase (C3 NeF) and persisting hypocomplementaemia occur, but not in all cases.	Acute nephritic syndrome. Nephrotic syndrome. Asymptomatic proteinuria. Overt haematuria.	Up to 33% die within 5 years.

IMMUNE INVOLVEMENT IN SPECIFIC HUMAN RENAL DISEASES

Anti-glomerular antibody induced glomerulonephritis

In a small proportion (probably three to five per cent) of patients with glomerulonephritis, anti-GBM antibody is found in the plasma and is deposited in linear fashion along the endothelial surface of the GBM. In a number of these patients, but not in all, there is intra-pulmonary haemorrhage, causing haemoptysis, and linear immunoglobulin deposition is found along the alveolar septal membrane. Antibodies eluted from kidney or lung in such cases have been shown to cross-react immunochemically.

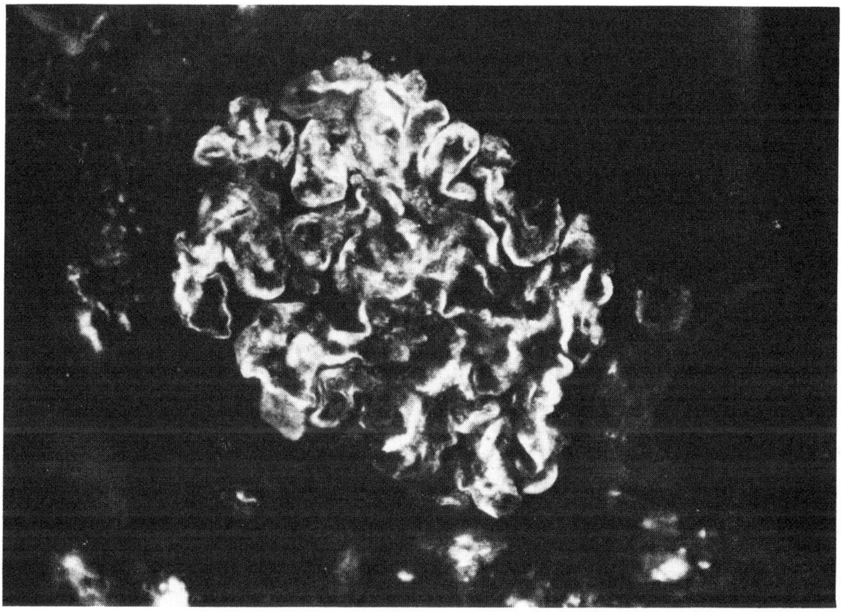

Figure 7.3. Linear immunoglobulin deposition along GBM; UV microscopy ×350.

This syndrome of pulmonary alveolar haemorrhage and glomerulonephritis associated with cross-reacting antibody directed against antigen contained in alveolar and glomerular tissue is often termed 'Goodpasture's syndrome', since Goodpasture (1919) described the post-mortem findings in a young man who died during the influenza pandemic of acute haemorrhagic pneumonia and associated glomerulonephritis. The eponymous term should be avoided, however, as the syndrome may occur in connective tissue disorders, in association with cryoglobulinaemia, and with immune complexes rather than linear anti-GBM antibody deposited in the kidney.

The experimental counterpart of this syndrome is the Masugi model, in which anti-GBM immunoglobulin injected into an animal forms linear deposits on the GBM in the host kidney and produces glomerulonephritis.

This immunoglobulin is complement binding and neutrophil leucocytes, attracted by leucotactic products of the complement cascade or attaching directly to the deposited immunoglobulin, release enzymes which produce glomerular inflammation. This model provides an understandable sequence of events to explain human anti-GBM induced antibody disease. However, in a small proportion of patients with severe glomerulonephritis and deposited anti-GBM antibody there is no evidence of complement utilisation nor is complement found in the glomeruli by the indirect immunofluorescent technique. These cases do not fit the Masugi model and appear to be produced by anti-GBM antibodies which do not bind complement, yet remain capable of inducing tissue damage. The mechanisms involved in such reactions are as yet poorly understood.

There is good evidence that anti-GBM antibody is the prime pathogenic mechanism in so-called anti-GBM antibody-induced glomerulonephritis. In the experimental model, antibody eluted from the kidney will cause glomerulonephritis when injected into another animal; monkeys develop glomerulonephritis when injected with antibody eluted from human kidneys; anti-GBM glomerulonephritis may develop in a renal allograft following transplantation in patients with proven anti-GBM antibody glomerulonephritis, providing that circulating antibody is present at the time of transplantation. It is noteworthy that recurrence of this form of glomerulonephritis is unlikely if transplantation is delayed after bilateral nephrectomy until circulating anti-GBM antibody is no longer detected by indirect immunofluorescence on normal kidney tissue. This takes several months (1 to 25, average 8 months, Wilson and Dixon, 1973) during which time maintenance by regular dialysis therapy is required.

There is no acceptable solution to the problem of why anti-GBM antibody arises in the first place, but there are a number of possibilities. It has been suggested that the antibody may be primarily directed against viral protein, or that following bacterial or viral pulmonary infection, pulmonary alveolar membrane proteins may be exposed or released stimulating the production of the cross-reacting antibody. A small number of cases of anti-GBM antibody-induced glomerulonephritis have been reported after chronic exposure to solvent hydrocarbons: these or other chemical agents may damage lung or glomerular basement membrane and exposure or release the necessary antigenic stimulus for the development of damaging antibody. Finally, antigens cross-reacting with anti-GBM antibody are present in normal urine, and may induce glomerulonephritis when injected into an experimental animal. Such antigens whether derived from the kidney or formed as part of body glycopeptide metabolism and filtered by the glomerulus, are a potential source of autoantibody in susceptible subjects.

An authoritative review of anti-GBM antibody induced glomerulonephritis has recently been published (Wilson and Dixon, 1973).

Acute post-streptococcal glomerulonephritis (APSGN)

It is accepted that an acute glomerulonephritis follows throat (or skin) infection with certain group A streptococci, for example types 1, 4, 12 and 49 (Red Lake). By light microscopy, renal biopsy specimens show diffuse endothelial and mesangial cell proliferation, and discrete deposits containing IgG and C3 have been identified on the epithelial surface of the GBM by immunofluorescent techniques. APSGN has therefore been taken to be an immune complex disease (Michael et al, 1966), but it has proved difficult to identify streptococcal protein in the glomerulus. Tresor et al (1970) reported that streptococcal membrane antigen was detectable either on the GBM or in the mesangium in biopsies taken within a few days after clinical onset of the disease; other workers have reported mesangial, but not GBM deposition of similar antigens (e.g. Michael et al, 1966). The initial cause of glomerular damage remains uncertain therefore and it may be that a streptococcal toxin or perhaps a fibrinogen-streptococcal complex are involved (see Zabriskie, 1973). However, the weight of present evidence favours the view that APSGN is caused by circulating immune complexes, whose presence is suggested by the finding of cryoglobulins in early APSGN (Adam, Morel-Maroger and Richet, 1973).

The complement system has been studied in APSGN by several groups. C3 levels are low in the first few weeks and serum levels of early complement components (e.g. C4) may be low at this time, indicating complement activation by the classical pathway. In addition, Williams et al (1972, 1973) have identified a C3 activation factor in 44 per cent of cases examined which was capable of breaking down C3 in normal human serum in vitro by the alternate pathway, which bypasses C1 and C42. After about two months C3 levels return to normal, and neither cryoglobulins nor the complement activation factor are found in healing APSGN, indicating that these changes are associated with the active phase of the disease.

Circulating anti-streptococcal membrane antibody has been identified in APSGN and shown to cross-react in vitro with GBM, but its role in the disease is uncertain. Zabriskie and colleagues (1973) and other workers (e.g. Macanovic, Evans and Peters, 1972) have demonstrated CMI to streptococcal membrane antigens cross-reacting with GBM antigens in APSGN and in patients with chronic proliferative glomerulonephritis (CPGN). This raises the questions: does APSGN lead on to CPGN (and if it does so what proportion of patients with CPGN have developed the disease as a result of streptococcal infection) and does CMI play a part in such a pathogenesis? The finding of CMI to such cross-reacting antigens in patients with CPGN who have no history of previous APSGN can be taken to support the hypothesis that subclinical, perhaps repeated, APSGN has nevertheless been the underlying basis for the CPGN. The role of CMI may be that once it has developed to antigen derived from infecting streptococci the fortuitous cross-reactions of such antigen with GBM leads to a persisting autoimmune glomerular disease. These concepts might receive support if there was consistent data on the natural history of overt APSGN to show that it frequently resulted in CPGN. However, this is not available, and recent authorities have made such differing statements as 'It is probable that, at least in children, chronic disease is never seen as a result of typical APSGN' (Cameron, 1973) and '. . . irreversible renal damage, which is probably progressive, occurs in the majority of patients with post-streptococcal glomerulonephritis' (Baldwin, 1972). Baldwin's statement is based on a personal study of well-documented cases. Cameron, while drawing on his own experience, points to the difficulty in assessing the older literature since relatively few reports have considered the long-term outcome of bacteriologically and biopsy proven APSGN. It is clear that further studies are urgently needed to clarify the natural history of APSGN and the relation of immunological events to the observed pattern of disease.

Systemic lupus erythematosus (SLE)

It is recognised that SLE is an immune disorder and that renal involvement is an important feature of the disease, being a major cause of death. The renal lesion may relapse and remit along with other manifestations of the syndrome, or separately from any of them. Severe SLE may (uncommonly) involve many other systems and spare the kidney, or the renal involvement may occur in isolation preceding any other evidence of the disease. Clinically, renal SLE may be very mild, there being only microscopic haematuria and a little proteinuria, or it may be severe with a nephrotic syndrome or an acute, even fulminating, glomerulonephritic illness with hypertension and uraemia.

There have been a number of descriptive studies of renal histology in SLE and the findings are not easily summarised. Membranous changes, diffuse or focal endothelial and epithelial cell proliferation occur; the histological category usually remains constant in a given patient and either progression or healing may be observed in sequential biopsies. The severity of glomerular damage is reflected in the clinical findings. Diffuse proliferative lesions with crescent formation are associated with a severe illness, whereas microscopic haematuria and mild proteinuria without hypoalbuminuria, hypertension and uraemia occur where the glomeruli show only focal mesangial and endothelial cell proliferation.

SLE is characterised by the finding of circulating antibodies to nuclear components and sometimes also to red blood cells and platelets and to factors involved in the coagulation cascade. In a series of studies Kunkel and his associates (see Agnello, Koffler and Kunkel, 1973) report that antibody to native or double stranded DNA (NDNA) occurs uniquely in SLE, and that circulating NDNA/anti-NDNA complexes occur which can be detected at the glomerular basement membrane during activity of the underlying disease. In the glomeruli these complexes are associated with C3, and occur along with evidence of clinical renal involvement. Single stranded DNA (SDNA) complexed with DNA antibody may also occur in the glomeruli. More than one form of circulating complex may occur at the same time, each composed of nuclear elements and appropriate antibody. The close relation (and multiplicity) of circulating immune complexes to the renal element of SLE is extended by the observation that an entirely different 'compound' complex containing an IgG-unknown antigen complex itself associated with IgM having anti-IgG specificity, occurs in active SLE and can sometimes be identified as a cryoprecipitate in the serum (cryoglobulin) and as heavy deposits in the glomerular basement membrane. These studies are contributing to understanding of renal involvement in SLE, and are of special importance since they also serve as examples of the way in which different immune complexes cause different types of glomerular damage.

Focal glomerulonephritis (benign recurrent haematuria), and renal involvement in non-thrombocytopenic purpura and connective tissue disorders

The term 'focal glomerulonephritis' best refers to a clinical entity in which there is recurrent macroscopic haematuria without hypertension, heavy proteinuria or oedema. The condition occurs principally in children and young adults, and may be associated with upper respiratory tract infections. During the acute phase, there may be some proteinuria and urinary casts

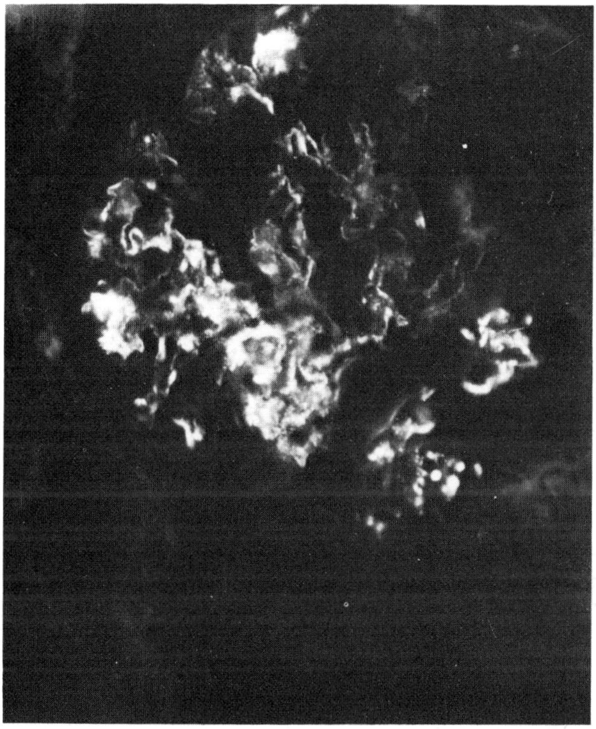

Figure 7.4. Focal IgA deposition in mesangium and on GBM; Henoch-Schönlein syndrome. UV microscopy ×350.

are often present; microscopic haematuria and mild proteinuria may persist between attacks. It is considered unusual for progressive renal damage to occur and the condition is sometimes known as 'benign recurrent haematuria'.

On renal biopsy, changes are seen in the glomerular mesangium and characteristically involve only a segment of any one glomerulus, although there may be diffuse glomerular damage and even small epithelial crescents. Berger et al (1967), Berger, Yaneva and Hinglais (1968) showed by indirect immunofluorescent techniques that there is mesangial deposition of IgA and IgG. Properdin has also been identified (Evans et al, 1973), which suggests that the alternate complement pathway is involved. There is no evidence of complement activation by the classical pathway, C4 is absent from the glomeruli, and the serum levels of haemolytic complement and early complement components are within the normal range. The aetiology is uncertain, but a persuasive case exists, a priori, for aggregated viral/IgA complexes within the glomerular mesangium to trigger the alternate complement pathway and for the C3 so activated to produce glomerular inflammation.

By definition focal glomerulonephritis (benign recurrent haematuria) is not associated with any evidence of systemic disease. However, segmental glomerular inflammation is seen in the renal manifestation of a number of connective tissue disorders, in sub-acute bacterial endocarditis (SABE), and in association with non-thrombocytopenic purpura (Henoch–Schönlein disease). Confusion arises when these renal complications are referred to as focal glomerulonephritis.

Renal histology in non-thrombocytopenic purpura resembles that in benign recurrent haematuria. IgA, IgG and C3 may be found in the glomerular mesangium, and properdin, but not C1q, can also be detected (Evans et al, 1973). The prognosis is less favourable in this syndrome, however, and a proportion of cases progress to renal failure.

In connective tissue disorders or SABE, however, the location and type of immunoglobulin deposition may differ from that in benign recurrent haematuria and there is sometimes evidence of classical complement pathway activation. Furthermore, steroid and immunosuppressive agents may be helpful in the connective tissue disorders, whereas those drugs have no proven role in benign recurrent haematuria, and an uncertain place in the treatment of non-thrombocytopenic purpura with renal involvement.

Mesangio-capillary (membrano-proliferative) glomerulonephritis (MCGN)

This is a recently defined entity in which there is mesangial cell proliferation and encroachment of mesangial matrix onto the sub-endothelial aspect of the basement membrane. In silver-stained preparations, this produces a characteristic 'double-line' effect on the glomerular capillary loops. On immunofluorescence, C3 is regularly found, and may be much more prominent than any immunoglobulin. It is distributed along the basement membrane in granular fashion and also present in the mesangium. In some cases, IgG is also found in granular deposit along the basement membrane, the predominantly peripheral depositions giving a characteristic immunofluorescent appearance. Sub-endothelial deposits are found which may be large and dense on EM. Some authors (e.g. Habib et al, 1973) consider that clinically significant subvarieties of mesangio-capillary glomerulonephritis can be distinguished on morphological grounds.

The histological appearances suggest that MCGN is an immune-complex disease. The clinical presentation varies, and the presenting illness may be an 'acute glomerulonephritis', with haematuria, proteinuria and hypertension. This may progress to a nephrotic syndrome, which may also develop without a preceding overt 'nephritic illness'. Less commonly, the diagnosis is made after the chance findings of symptomless proteinuria without hypertension or oedema, or in a patient presenting with overt haematuria (see Cameron et al, 1970).

In MCGN the characteristic renal biopsy appearances are associated with very low levels of circulating C3, about 80 per cent of patients demonstrating this phenomenon at some stage of the disease. The C3 level may remain low over months or years, or may fluctuate and at times be within the normal range. The serum of patients with MCGN who show hypocomplementaemia contains a factor which causes C3 activation by the 'alternate pathway', early complement components C1, C2 and C4 being present in normal concentration, while later components such as C5 and perhaps C6 and C7 which enter the complement cascade after C3, are reduced. The circulating factor which produces the C3 activation, originally described by Spitzer et al (1969) and termed C3 nephritic factor or C3 NeF has not been characterised precisely but may be an immune complex or an IgG3 antibody.

The evidence that increased C3 utilisation occurs in MCGN is convincing (see West et al, 1973). It is not yet clear whether impaired C3 synthesis also contributes to the low serum C3 level. Originally, observations of the fractional catabolic rate of C3 using a radiolabelled marker suggested that there was impaired C3 synthesis. In the patients studied C3 levels were low, and it is now recognised that C3 NeF activation of C3 proceeds only slowly if the serum C3 level is already low.

West et al (1973), pointing out this difficulty, suggested that if the C3 level was first raised towards the normal range by injection of unlabelled C3, the radiolabelled marker should reflect the increased C3 utilisation via C3 NeF. Nevertheless, the persistent hypocomplementaemia which occurs in many patients must reflect a homeostatic situation in which C3 synthesis never *rises* to compensate for the increased C3 utilisation by C3 NeF, as might be expected, and the reason for this failure is not clear.

The observation that C3 NeF causes little or no C3 utilisation if the serum C3 level is very low has led to the recognition that C3b, a degradation product of C3 is a required cofactor. (Indeed C3b appears to be essential for any activation of the alternate pathway of C3 utilisation). Sufficient C3b to activate the pathway cannot be produced if the C3 level is already very low (Williams et al, 1973).

While the *mechanisms* which underlie the hypocomplementaemia of MCGN are becoming clear, the *significance* of these changes is undetermined. C3 NeF is not produced in the kidney since it is still detected in patients on regular dialysis therapy who have undergone bilateral nephrectomy. The initial or subsequent level of C3 and the presence or absence of C3 NeF (which shows an inverse correlation with the C3 level) do not appear to influence the prognosis of MCGN. Cameron et al (1973) have shown in a series of 73 patients that the actuarial survival rate was not influenced by the initial complement level and that 5 of 11 patients in whom the serum C3 level was never found to be less that 80 mg/100 ml were dead within six years of diagnosis. Since approximately two-thirds of all their patients with MCGN survived for five to six years the normocomplementaemic group actually fared worst. It is noteworthy that in the same series the *clinical* severity of the disease was a reasonably good guide to prognosis. Patients who had only recurrent haematuria or persistent proteinuria showed a better survival rate than those who developed the nephrotic syndrome.

Peters et al (1973) have studied three patients with partial lipodystrophy and glomerulonephritis and have shown that the glomerulonephritis was of the MCGN type with hypocomplementaemia and that C3 NeF could be detected. Pointing out that Alper, Block and Rosen (1973) have described a case of partial lipodystrophy with the same pattern of complement system abnormalities but without MCGN (the patient suffered from recurrent infections), these workers propose that the development of a C3 activator may precede MCGN and predispose to it. There is some evidence that other complement deficiency states may be associated with immune complex disease; and it has been suggested that modified immune competence (poor antibody avidity) may predispose individuals to develop immune complexes. The suggestion of Peters et al therefore brings forward the unifying concept that immune complex induced glomerulonephritis in general may arise because of one or more defects in immune competence whether congenital or acquired. MCGN would then be the variant which arises when a complement activator is the cause of the altered immune competence. Since measles may be associated with partial lipodystrophy, the possibility of an initial viral illness which induced the complement activator must be considered.

It is recognised that MCGN may recur after transplantation. Typical glomerular changes may be found within four months with heavy proteinuria and alternate pathway activation of the complement system (low C3 and properdin, normal C4). Berthoux et al (1974) suggest that MCGN recurs in one-third to one-half of cases within 18 months of transplantation. It may be that if hypocomplementaemia persists and C3 NeF is present, patients with MCGN should remain on regular dialysis therapy and be transplanted only when these abnormalities remit.

The 'minimal change' lesion

The commonest cause of heavy proteinuria in young children and one which accounts for about 30 per cent of nephrotic syndrome in adults is a glomerular lesion unassociated with any specific change on light microscopy, and with no consistent deposition of immunoglobulin or complement as judged from indirect immunofluorescent techniques (although some workers have reported that IgE may be identified at the GBM). The lesion responds to steroid therapy in almost all cases, and cyclophosphamide may be effective as an adjunct, or in the few cases where steroids do not produce a response. The condition commonly runs a relapsing course. The ultimate prognosis is favourable, although during relapse there may be the considerable loss of body protein and infection will be poorly resisted. Death may also occur from ischaemic heart disease, or veno-occlusive complications, but uraemia rarely, if ever, results.

There are no accepted associations between this lesion and other diseases, but some workers have suggested that there is an increased incidence in patients with an atopic diathesis and we have noted the lesion in patients with psoriasis and with connective tissue disorders. Interest has been directed to the clear therapeutic effect of anti-inflammatory and immunosuppressive agents, but evidence of immunological activity has been hard to find. Ngu, Barratt and Soothill (1970) described changes in immunoconglutinin, suggesting that the complement system may be activated in relapses, and we (Eyres et al, 1974) have noted CMI to renal antigens in patients who undoubtedly have this steroid/cyclophosphamide sensitive renal lesion. The renal lesion is similar to that produced experimentally by aminonucleoside injection; however, there is no evidence at present that the relapsing course of the human diseases results from repeated exposure to an exogenous toxin.

Immune competence in renal failure

It is recognised that uraemic patients are prone to infection and they may respond poorly to an immunogenic challenge. The many reports of persisting asymptomatic infectivity of the hepatitis viruses in patients in regular dialysis units and the discovery in such patients of active infection with 'opportunist' organisms such as cytomegalovirus and of unsuspected disseminated tuberculosis are good examples. The rejection of skin grafts is delayed in severe uraemia, which also modifies rejection in clinical and experimental renal transplantation.

All the findings point to defects in immune competence in chronic renal failure, but there are few detailed systematic studies. We (Byron, 1973; Byron, Mallick and Taylor, 1974) have investigated humoral and cellular immune responses in subjects with different degrees of renal failure, all established on selected high biological value protein/high calorie diets, the nitrogen content of which has varied according to the GFR and in whom hypoproteinaemia was not observed. The serum level of each of the major immunoglobulin subclasses was within the normal range even when the GFR was less than 5 ml/minute. However, both the IgG and IgM responses to an immunogenic challenge, normal when the GFR was > 15 ml/minute, were progressively weaker as the GFR fell below that level. A group of patients who were first investigated when in very severe renal failure (GFR < 5 ml/minute) were subsequently re-tested after being established on regular dialysis therapy for at least three months and the IgG and IgM responses remained depressed.

In the same study there was evidence that cell-mediated immunity, measured by the local response to inunction of DNCB or intradermal injection of antigen, followed the same pattern in renal failure as did the humoral responses already mentioned, being normal at GFR > 15 ml/minute and decreasing as the GFR fell. However, these cell-mediated responses improved (but were still subnormal) in those patients retested after the period of regular dialysis therapy.

Although the effects of regular dialysis therapy on immune competence have not yet been reported from other centres, workers studying the responses in renal failure (e.g. Boulton-Jones, Cameron and Vick, 1972) have produced results of a similar fall off in immune competence with increasing renal failure.

It is not clear exactly how these effects on the immune system are produced. It has been suggested that macrophage function is depressed, and Souhami (1971) produced evidence that the uraemic rat is incapable of processing soluble protein antigen. While there is scope for further study it seems probable that there are multiple defects of immune competence in renal failure, possibly involving both the afferent and efferent arms of the immune response. Our work does not support a major role for protein malnutrition in producing these defects, and it seems unlikely that a single dialysable toxin is alone responsible in view of the remaining immune incompetence of the dialysis patient. The results of studies to date are obviously of significance in considering the role of immunosuppressive drug therapy in renal transplantation, and the question of effective vaccination against the hepatitis virus in patients with chronic renal failure.

Chronic pyelonephritis

The last decade has brought a much greater understanding of this condition. It is now recognised that mechanical and infective factors play a predominant role in the development of the scarred contracted kidney. For a number of reasons, the interaction of immune mechanisms has seemed possible. For example, the kidneys are most easily damaged by ascending infection in the neonatal animal, in which immune competence is not yet fully developed. Epidemiological studies suggest that in man most renal scarring occurs in early life; also, the incidence of lower urinary tract infection, which is the common precursor of parenchymal infection, is increased when immune competence is depressed as by the use of immunosuppressive drugs.

Antibody specific to organisms infecting the renal parenchyma may be detected in the plasma, and may 'coat' the organisms but experimental studies have so far failed to show that these antibodies have any protective role. Nor does the presence or absence of thymic tissue affect the way in which experimentally induced ascending urinary tract infection causes renal damage in neonatal animals, suggesting no protective role for T-lymphocyte function.

Although these studies have not shown as yet a specific role for the immune system in protecting the kidney from invading organisms or in contributing to the renal damage which follows infection, studies of immune mechanisms in the lower urinary tract have shown that IgG, IgA and IgM antibodies are generated locally, and the studies suggest that T-lymphocyte involvement or cooperation also occurs. Secretory IgA, and locally produced IgM may have particular relevance in combating active lower urinary tract infection. A review of these factors is given by Spencer and Fairhead (1972).

References

Adam, C., Morel-Maroger, L. & Richet, J. (1973) Cryoglobulins in glomerulonephritis not related to systemic disease. *Kidney International*, **3**, 334–341.

Agnello, V., Koffler, D. & Kunkel, H. J. (1973) Immune complex systems in the nephritis of systemic lupus erythematosus. *Kidney International*, **3**, 90–99.

Alper, C. A., Block, K. J. & Rosen, F. S. (1973) Increased susceptibility to infection in a patient with type II essential hypercatabolism of C3. *New England Journal of Medicine*, **288**, 601–606.

Baldwin, D. S. (1972) Natural history of post-streptococcal glomerulonephritis. *5th International Congress of Nephrology, Abstracts of Plenary Sessions*. p. 45.

Berger, J., Neuveu, T., Morel-Maroger, L. & Antoine, B. (1967) Localisation des immunoglobulines et du fibrogène dans les lésions glomérulaires. *Act. Néphrol. Hôp. Necker*, 1 vol. Paris. Ed. Méd. Flammarion, p. 161.

Berger, J., Yaneva, H. & Hinglais, N. (1968) Les glomérulonephrites focales, *Act. Néphrol. Hôp. Necker*, 1 vol. Paris. Ed. Méd. Flammarion, 1. 141.

Berthoux, F. C., Touraine, J. L., Blanc, N., Colon, S., Revillard, J. P., Zech, P. Y. & Traeger, J. (1974) High incidence of recurrence of mesangioproliferative glomerulonephritis after transplantation: Studies of complement and properdin systems. *Abstracts European Society of Clinical Investigation*, **219**, 137.

Byron, P. R. (1973) *The Quantitation of Immune Potential in Uraemic Subjects*. Ph.D. Thesis, University of Manchester.

Byron, P. R., Mallick, N. P. & Taylor, G. (1974) *Unpublished.*

Boulton-Jones, J. M., Cameron, J. S. & Vick, R. (1972) Immune responses in uraemia. *Kidney International*, **2**, 179.

Cameron, J. S. (1973) The natural history of glomerulonephritis. In *Renal Disease* ed. D. A. K. Black. London: Blackwell. p. 313.

Cameron, J. S., Glasgow, E. F., Ogg, C. S. & White, R. H. R. (1970) Membranoproliferative glomerulonephritis and hypocomplementaemia. *British Medical Journal*, **iv**, 7–14.

Cameron, J. S., Ogg, C. S., White, R. H. R. & Glasgow, E. F. (1973) The clinical features and prognosis of patients with normocomplementaemic mesangio-capillary glomerulonephritis. *Clinical Nephrology*, **1**, 8–13.

Evans, D. J., Williams, D. G., Sissons, J. G. P., Boulton-Jones, J. M., Ogg, C. S., Cameron, J. S. & Hoffbrand, B. I. (1973) Glomerular deposition of properdin in Henoch–Schönlein syndrome and idiopathic focal nephritis. *British Medical Journal*, **3**, 326–328.

Eyres, K., Mallick, N. P., Taylor, G. & Williams, G. (1974) *Unpublished.*

Goodpasture, E. W. (1919) The significance of certain pulmonary lesions in relation to the pathology of influenza. *American Journal of Medical Science*, **158**, 863.

Habib, R., Kleinkrecht, C., Gubler, M. C. & Levy, M. (1973) Idiopathic membranoproliferative glomerulonephritis in children. Report of 105 cases. *Clinical Nephrology*, **1**, 194–214.

Kefalides, N. (1971) Chemical properties of basement membranes. *International Review of Experimental Pathology*, **10**, 1–39.

Macanovic, M., Evans, D. J. & Peters, D. K. (1972) Allergic response to glomerular basement membrane in patients with glomerulonephritis. *Lancet*, **ii**, 207–210.

Mahieu, P., Dardenne, M. & Bach, J. F. (1971) Isolation of glycopeptide antigenic site from kidney basement membrane. *Lancet*, **ii**, 314.

Mahieu, P., Dardenne, M. & Bach, J. F. (1972) Detection of humoral and cell-mediated immunity to kidney basement membranes in human renal diseases. *American Journal of Medicine*, **53**, 185–192.

Mallick, N. P., Williams, R. J., McFarlane, H., Orr, W.McN., Taylor, G. & Williams, G. (1972) Cell-mediated immunity in nephrotic syndrome. *Lancet*, **i**, 507.

Marquardt, H., Wilson, C. B. & Dixon, F. J. (1973) Isolation and immunological characterization of human glomerular basement membrane antigens. *Kidney International*, **3**, 57–65.

Michael, A. F., Drummond, K. M., Good, R. A. & Vernier, R. L. (1966) Acute poststreptococcal glomerulonephritis: immune deposit disease. *Journal of Clinical Investigation*, **45**, 237.

Misra, R. P. (1973) Glomerular basement membrane antigens of Masugi nephritis. *Immunology*, **25**, 967–980.

Ngu, J. L., Barratt, T. M. & Soothill, J. F. (1970) Immunoconglutinin and complement changes in steroid sensitive relapsing nephrotic syndrome of children. *Clinical and Experimental Immunology*, **6**, 109–116.

Peters, D. K., Williams, D. G., Charlesworth, J. A., Boulton-Jones, J. M., Sissons, J. G. P., Evans, D. J., Kourilsky, O. & Morel-Maroger, L. (1973) Mesangiocapillary glomerulonephritis, partial lipodystrophy and hypocomplementaemia. *Lancet*, **ii**, 535–538.

Rocklin, E. R., Lewis, E. J. & David, J. R. (1970) In vitro evidence for cellular hypersensitivity to glomerular basement membrane antigens in human glomerulonephritis. *New England Journal of Medicine*, **283**, 497.

Souhami, R. L. (1971) Antibody production in uraemic mice. *Clinical Science*, **40,** 11.
Soothill, J. F. & Steward, M. W. (1971) The immunopathological significance of the heterogeneity of antibody affinity. *Clinical and Experimental Immunology*, **9,** 193–199.
Spencer, A. G. & Fairhead, A. P. (1972) The cellular immune response in pyelonephritis and the effects of immunization. In Brumfitt and Asscher. *Proceedings of 2nd National Symposium on Urinary Trace Infection.* Oxford: Oxford University Press.
Spitzer, R. E., Vallota, E. H., Forristal, J., Sudora, E., Stitzel, A., Davis, N. C. & West, C. D. (1969) Serum C3 lytic system in patients with glomerulonephritis. *Science*, **164,** 436–437.
Tresor, G., Semar, M., Ty, A., Sagel, I., Franklin, M. A. & Lange, K. (1970) Partial characterization of antigenic streptococcal membrane components in acute glomerulonephritis. *Journal of Clinical Investigation*, **49,** 762–768.
West, C. D., Ruley, E., Forristal, J. & Davis, N. C. (1973) Mechanisms of hypocomplementaemia in glomerulonephritis. *Kidney International*, **3,** 116–125.
Williams, D. G., Kourilsky, O., Morel-Maroger, L. & Peters, D. K. (1972) C3 breakdown by serum from patients with acute post-streptococcal nephritis. *Lancet*, **ii,** 360–361.
Williams, D. G., Charlesworth, J. A., Evans, D. J., Peters, D. K., Morel-Maroger, L., Kourilsky, O., Adam, C., Richet, G., Cameron, J. S. & Ogg, C. S. (1973) Complement studies in acute glomerulonephritis. *Kidney International*, **4,** 243.
Wilson, C. B. & Dixon, F. J. (1973) Anti-glomerular basement membrane antibody-induced glomerulonephritis. *Kidney International*, **3,** 74–89.
Zabriskie, J. (1973) Streptococcus-related glomerulonephritis. *Kidney International*, **3,** 100–104.

8. Immunology of Pulmonary Disease

FREDERICK E. HARGREAVE

JERRY DOLOVICH

The lung is so situated that there is exposure to large quantities of antigen. There is perfusion by the entire blood flow and ventilation by about 10 000 litres of air each day. A variety of defence mechanisms, both non-specific and specific, have evolved to preserve the integrity of the respiratory system (Green, 1970). The tortuous upper airways and the branching, narrowing bronchi influence the patterns of delivery of airborne substances to the airways and lungs. The anatomical characteristics of these airways including the lining mucociliary system provide for the efficient filtration and clearance of foreign substances. The local production of lysozyme and interferon are additional non-immunological defences which contribute to the control of microorganisms. Alpha 1-antitrypsin is a naturally occurring plasma proteinase inhibitor; the occurrence of panlobular emphysema in persons with hereditary deficiencies of alpha 1-antitrypsin has illustrated the requirement of this inhibitor for the protection of the lung from the effects of proteolytic enzymes. Alveolar macrophages protect the outer reaches of the air passages through phagocytosis and microbial killing.

The lung functions as a complex lymphoid organ which provides an immunological defence and, at the same time, a potential for involvement in immunological diseases. Exposure to airborne antigens stimulates immune responses both locally and systemically. Antibodies of the IgA class are produced in the lamina propria of the airways mucosa in disproportionately large quantities. IgA is transported into the luminal mucus by a specialised secretory process involving the addition of a secretory piece to the IgA molecules (Tomasi and Bienenstock, 1968). In addition, there is synthesis in the airways mucosa and regional lymph nodes of relatively large quantities of IgE (Tada and Ishizaka, 1970). Antibodies of the IgE class are present in respiratory secretions in relatively larger quantities than in the blood; however, there is no known specialised secretory system comparable to that for IgA. In addition, the lung can be the portal of entry of antigen which induces a systemic response. There may be serum antibodies of the various immunoglobulin classes to inhaled antigen. The occurrence of serum precipitins to inhaled antigen is evidence of a vigorous systemic immune response. Cell-mediated immunity may result from antigens deposited in the lung and find expression in both local and generalised delayed hypersensitivity reactions. With the deposition of poorly metabolised particles in the lung, local granulomatous reactions can develop, determined at least in part by immune responses of the host. Thus, inhaled antigens can elicit the various forms of immune responses in the lungs and the corresponding forms of hypersensitivity are similarly represented.

Diseases of the respiratory tract resulting from immunological reactions depend upon factors relating to the responsible allergens and to the immunological status of the host. The most important immunological diseases induced by inhaled allergens are asthma and extrinsic allergic alveolitis. Both asthma and alveolitis are features of allergic broncho-pulmonary aspergillosis. In a variety of other diseases of the lungs with immunological features, the reactants are not as well defined.

ALLERGENS

Allergens which are inhaled have received most study, are the best understood and seem to be most important in pulmonary diseases (Muir, 1972). By contrast, little is known about blood-borne allergens including assimilated foods, drugs and parasites. Nevertheless, it is clear that the role of ingested foods in allergic lung diseases has been grossly overemphasised in some quarters.

The allergens which originate outdoors consist chiefly of atmospheric pollens and fungal spores. These airborne particles are derived from the local vegetation within a radius of about 10 miles and the numbers are greatly affected by weather. There are also geographical, seasonal and diurnal variations The actual counts and their seasonal variations in Cardiff, Wales, are. shown in Table 8.1 and Figure 8.1 (Hyde, 1972). The most common particles are tree and grass pollen, the fungal spores of *Cladosporium*, *Alternaria*, *Penicillium*/*Aspergillus* types and a number of *Basidiomycetes*, and *Ascomycetes*. The pollens have short and relatively well-defined seasons. Tree pollen is more localised, and the counts tend to be more variable from place to place and lower than counts of grass pollen. However, tree pollens are sometimes very important allergens, as with birch pollen in Sweden. In other areas, other types of pollen may be most abundant. For example, ragweed pollen is one of the most important pollen allergens in North America (Figure 8.2) but is absent from Europe. Fungal spores outnumber pollen in Cardiff by about 60 to one; however, this is not an expression of the relative importance of fungal spores and pollens as allergens. Like pollen, certain fungal spores may be more abundant in some places than in others. The fungal spores of *Alternaria* are found in especially high counts in the crop-growing areas of central North America. There are diurnal fluctuations in counts due to diurnal changes in the weather. Thus those particles released in dry air such as pollen (Figure 8.3) and fungal spores of *Cladosporium* and *Alternaria*,

Table 8.1. Fungus spores and pollen grains at Cardiff: daily mean concentrations averaged for the year in particles per cubic metre, 1 January 1958 to 31 December 1961 (reproduced from Hyde, 1972, with permission of the publisher)

Fungi		
1. Phycometes		2·0
2. Ascomycetes		
Erysiphe	4·2	
Ascospores (coloured)	76·1	
Ascospores (hyaline)	468·0	548·3
3. Basidiomycetes		
(a) Agaricales (coloured)	224·4	
Agaricales (hyaline)	539·4	
(b) Lycoperdales (puff balls)	0·5	
(c) Sporobolomyceteae		
Sporobolomyces	271·2	
Tilletiopsis	18·5	
(d) Uredinales (rusts)	6·6	
(e) Ustilaginales (smuts)	85·0	1145·6
4. Fungi imperfecti		
(a) *Alternaria*	8·0	
(b) *Botrytis*	29·2	
(c) *Cladosporium*	1204·2	
(d) *Epicoccum*	15·4	
(e) Aspergillaceae	49·8	
(f) *Polythrincium*	7·6	
(g) *Pullularia*	27·5	
(h) *Torula*	8·7	
(i) Others	11·0	1361·4
5. Undetermined		24·7
Total fungus spores		3082·0

Spermaphyta		
1. Gramineae (grasses)		16·68
2. Trees		
(a) *Ulmus* (elm)	5·05	
(b) *Betula* (birch)	2·53	
(c) *Fraxinus* (ash)	2·06	
(d) *Quercus* (oak)	1·58	
(e) *Taxus* (yew)	1·11	
(f) *Alnus* (alder)	0·95	
(g) *Corylus* (hazel)	0·63	
(h) *Castanea* (chestnut)	0·62	
(i) *Pinus* (pine)	0·61	
(j) Others	1·14	
Total trees		16·28
3. Miscellaneous herbs (weeds)		
(a) *Urtica* (nettle)	8·41	
(b) *Plantago* (plantain)	0·92	
(c) *Rumex* (sorrel and dock)	0·70	
(d) *Artemisia* (mugwort)	0·25	
(e) Compositae (excl. *Artemisia*)	0·12	
(f) Chenopodiaceae	0·09	
(g) Others	0·12	
Total weeds		10·61
Other pollens (determinate)		0·77
4. Other pollens (unknown)		3·52
Total pollen grains		48·04

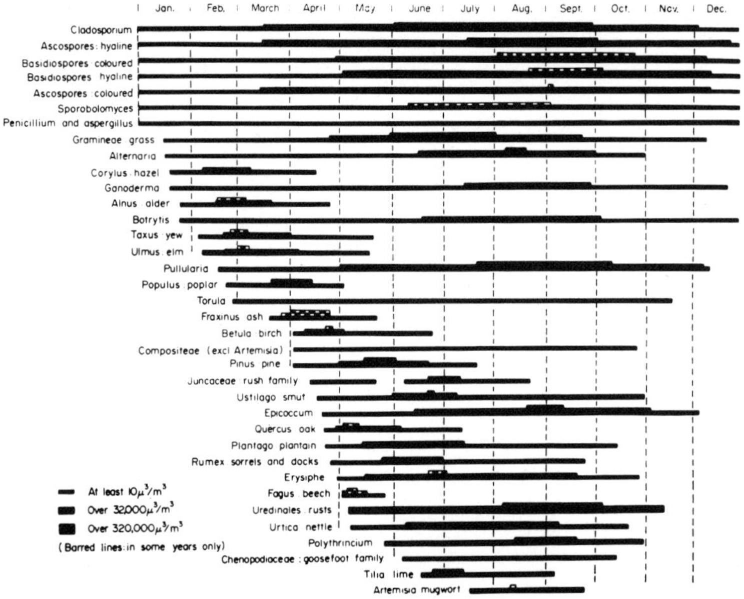

Figure 8.1. Pollen and spore calendar, Cardiff, Wales (reproduced from Hyde, 1972, with permission of the publisher).

have highest counts during the day. By contrast, those which are released in wet air such as basidiospores and ascospores tend to be most numerous at night or in the daytime after a rain.

Atmospheric pollen and fungal spores were initially counted by gravity samplers. These relied upon the sedimentation of particles by gravity and failed to collect representative samples. They were influenced by wind

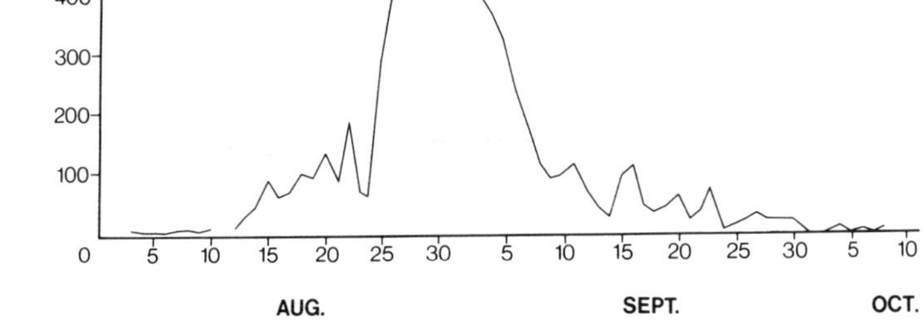

Figure 8.2. Seasonal incidence of ragweed pollen in Hamilton, Ontario, Canada.

velocity and favoured the trapping of large particles. Suction traps now in use have overcome these disadvantages. For example, the Hirst automatic volumetric spore trap catches particles between 3 and 100 μ with equal efficiency. It operates continuously in all weather and is unaffected by wind. The counts are expressed per cubic metre of air, being roughly the amount of air inhaled in one hour.

Airborne allergens encountered indoors in the home include house dust with its contained mites, especially *Dermatophagoides* sp. The mites are world-wide in distribution but are apparently less important in North America than in other regions of the world. This can probably be attributed to low levels of humidity characteristic of North American homes due to central heating

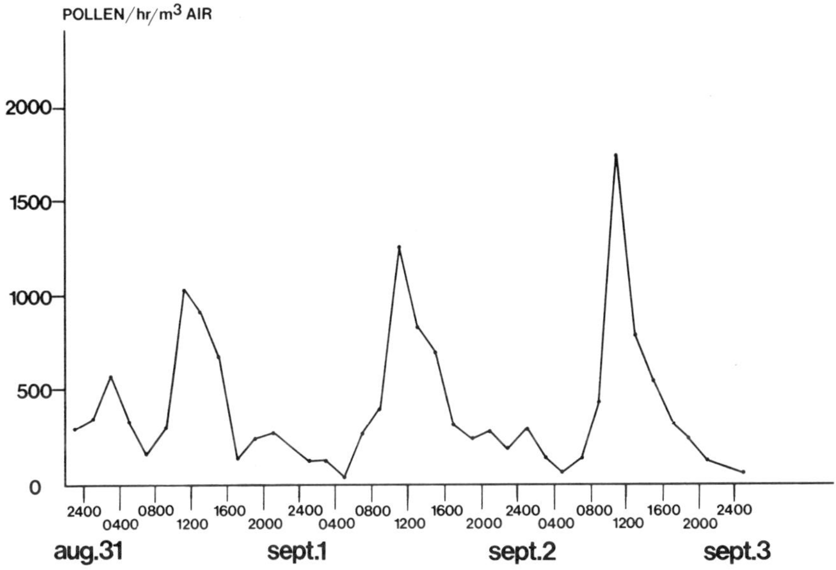

Figure 8.3. Diurnal variation of ragweed pollen in Hamilton, Ontario, Canada.

systems. The products of animals and birds are also important indoor allergens in the home. Pollen and fungal spores in the air indoors are largely representative of those occurring outdoors but are generally less numerous. There may be local sources of fungal spores in the home such as dry rot or contamination of humidifiers or air-conditioners by thermophylic actinomycetes. Many types of airborne allergens are characteristic of particular work environments. These include the spores of thermophylic actinomycetes on farms, wood dusts in wood-handling industries, tolylene diisocyanate used in polyurethane production, fumes of aminoethylethanolamine in certain fluxes used in welding and *Bacillus subtilis* enzyme products in the non-soap detergent industry. Allergens which originate indoors often have a seasonal variation with the highest concentrations during the winter months when ventilation is reduced.

There is a direct relationship between the intensity of exposure to inhaled allergens and the probability of disease. Occupational asthma from sensitisation to *B. subtilis* enzyme products occurs most frequently in the workers with the heaviest exposure. Extrinsic allergic alveolitis seems to require a more intense exposure to inhaled allergens than asthma. In this respect, extrinsic allergic alveolitis has been compared with serum sickness; in the latter, as the dose of heterologous serum increases, the frequency of disease approaches 100 per cent. The generation of antigen in situ in the airways as with the saprophytic growth of *Aspergillus fumigatus* appears to lead to an unusually heavy exposure to antigen.

Allergens are reputed to vary in their tendency to sensitise. This appears to be a function of the general immunogenicity of the substances and the exposure dose. For example, hypersensitivity is readily induced by exposure to products of *Ascaris* and castor beans. Grass and ragweed pollen seem to induce sensitivity more frequently than fungal spores despite the vastly greater numbers of airborne fungal spores inhaled. Pigeons and budgies produce extrinsic allergic alveolitis more frequently than poultry.

Table 8.2. Particle size of common pollen and fungal spores

Pollen	Approximate dimensions (microns)	Fungal spores	Approximate dimensions (microns)
Birch	19 × 23	*Cladosporium*	5–29 × 2·5–7
Pine	50 × 78	*Alternaria*	35–95 × 18–26
Grass	28–32	*Aspergillus*	5–9
Ragweed	20	*Coprinus*	7–9 × 3–4·5
		Thermophilic actinomycetes	2

The size of airborne particles determines their depth of penetration into the respiratory tract and, thereby, the type of disease which may result. Table 8.2 illustrates the size of some of the common pollen and fungal spores. Large particles do not enter the lower respiratory tract. During nasal breathing, most of these impact in the nasal airways. Particles down to about 6 μ in diameter can penetrate into the airways but do not reach the peripheral respiratory tissues; they may provoke asthma but not alveolitis. Particles less than 6 μ in diameter can penetrate to the peripheral respiratory tissues and thereby have the potential to provoke alveolitis as well as asthma.

ATOPY

Coca and Cooke introduced the term atopy in 1923 to refer to a form of 'abnormal hypersensitiveness' (Coca and Cooke, 1923). Through the years, the term has undergone subtle changes in usage. At the present time, it is most commonly used to refer to the presence of IgE-dependent sensitivity or the capacity to develop such sensitivity. The atopic status of individuals is commonly assessed by the use of allergy skin tests with a series of extracts of common allergens to which the subject is exposed. A positive test is indicated by a weal and flare response. The number and sizes of responses to a group of common allergens provides a rough basis for grading the degree of atopy. The highly atopic subject shows large responses to many allergens and the mildly atopic individual has responses, possibly smaller in size, to only one or two allergens. There is a close relationship between this type of grading of skin responses to commonly encountered allergens and the serum concentrations of IgE. An atopic status is indicated by the presence of infantile eczema, allergic rhinitis, food allergy and extrinsic asthma. There is an increased risk of atopy when these conditions are present in members of the family. However, it should be remembered that eczema, asthma, chronic rhinitis and food intolerance can occur by mechanisms other than IgE-dependent reactions and are, therefore, not necessarily an indication of atopy.

The serum level of IgE is, at least in part, under hereditary control (Bazaral, Orgel and Hamburger, 1971). Nevertheless, while illnesses such as allergic rhinitis and food allergy are familial, there is no simple hereditary pattern to their acquisition.

A variety of factors influence the development of allergy. For example, it has been demonstrated that immunisation by topical administration of allergen to the nasal mucosa but not subcutaneous administration is associated with a high rate of sensitisation in the atopic but not the normal individual (Leskowitz, Salvaggio and Schwartz, 1972). A high rate of sensitisation from immunisation at the level of the mucosal surface is not unexpected since IgE-forming plasma cells have a disproportionately high representation in the lamina propria of the mucosa of the airways and gastrointestinal tract and in the lymphoid tissues draining these areas (Tada and Ishizaka, 1970). The observation that absolute deficiency of IgA is associated with an increased risk of allergic sensitisation is probably a related finding. The suggestion is that, under normal circumstances, the secretory IgA system provides a mucosal barrier reducing the quantity of potential allergen passing through the mucosal surface thereby reducing the possibility of sensitisation. This observation has been extended to an examination of the potential relevance of the rate of development of the IgA system in infants. An observed relative lag in the appearance of serum IgA in infants who manifest allergy has been taken to indicate that this slow development of the IgA system may be a predisposing factor in the acquisition of allergy (Taylor et al, 1973).

It has been customary to regard the atopic status as one in which there is a more or less non-selective tendency to develop one or other of the diseases associated with atopy. Similarly, it has been assumed that there is simply a predisposition to become sensitised with no particular antigen preference. However, recent data suggest that sensitisation to particular antigens may be, at least in part, genetically determined. For example, a close link has been demonstrated between inherited histo-compatibility types and sensitisation to a particular ragweed allergen (Marsh et al, 1973).

Atopy appears to be an important influence determining whether inhaled small particles will provoke asthma or alveolitis. In the atopic subject, the inhalation of relatively small quantities of allergen may induce asthma. The acute response to a small dose of allergen strictly limits the amount that can be tolerated. In this situation, only a limited quantity of inhaled allergen can penetrate to the peripheral respiratory tissues. In the non-atopic subject, there is a greater opportunity for heavy exposure and deeper penetration of particles in the lung, thereby creating a risk of extrinsic allergic alveolitis which is due to mechanisms which do not involve IgE-dependent reactions.

ASTHMA

Asthma was known to the ancients such as Hippocrates (460 to 370 BC) and Areteaus (2nd to 3rd century AD). It is of interest to note that 2000 years later there is still no satisfactory definition. The Ciba Foundation Guest Symposium (Scadding, 1971a) failed to arrive at a definition; however, an earlier symposium (the Ciba Foundation Guest Symposium, 1959) produced a reasonable working definition. Asthma was defined as the "condition of subjects with widespread narrowing of the bronchial airways, which changes in severity over short periods of time either spontaneously or under treatment, and is not due to cardiovascular disease". The definition is of limited value in the demarcation of asthma as a disease entity for a number of reasons. There is no single aetiologic factor. There is a heterogeneity in clinical presentations. In addition, asthma can closely resemble chronic bronchitis in that there also may be some reversibility of airways obstruction in the latter condition. Moreover, asthma can coexist with other diseases of the airways.

Asthma is an important cause of morbidity and it may be fatal. It restricts activity, disrupts family and social life and causes loss of school and work. According to one estimate, 4 per cent of the population of the United States is suffering from asthma and 7 per cent have had it at some time (Davis, 1972). The prevalence is probably greatest in childhood but it can be present and indeed may start at any age.

Clinical features

Asthma presenting classically with well-defined attacks of dyspnoea with wheezing is easy to recognise. However, occasionally the dyspnoea may be continuous and wheezing may not be evident. Furthermore, in some patients the presenting symptoms are cough and the production of sputum. The diagnosis is more commonly missed in the very young and where the onset is in older age groups. In the very young, episodes of asthma can be exclusively a part of febrile illnesses presumed to be viral in origin. There results an erroneous preoccupation with the febrile, apparently infectious, component with inadequate treatment of the airways obstruction. In older age groups, continuous symptoms sometimes suggest chronic bronchitis or emphysema and the possibility of asthma may not initially be considered.

The classification introduced by Rackemann in 1940 divided asthma into two types, extrinsic and intrinsic (Rackemann, 1940). Extrinsic implies that asthma is due to allergy to substances originating extrinsic to the body. The term intrinsic implies that allergy to extrinsic substances is not responsible; by exclusion, the cause must be intrinsic. It would be more appropriate to refer to idiopathic asthma rather than intrinsic asthma. Many people are highly allergic with hay fever symptoms and never wheeze so that those who do have asthma provoked by allergic reactions appear to have an additional constitutional susceptibility in the form of bronchial hyper-reactivity. In many persons with allergy and asthma, allergic reactions are often not the only provoking factor so that in extrinsic asthma it is not only allergy that is involved. In some allergic individuals, the pattern may nevertheless be predominantly intrinsic. Thus, there are problems in the use of the terms extrinsic and intrinsic to classify asthma. However, extrinsic and intrinsic asthma in their characteristic forms are sufficiently distinct to merit their separate description.

People with extrinsic asthma are atopic and typically have a past history of infantile eczema, allergic rhinitis or gastrointestinal food intolerance. Symptoms usually start in childhood. Experience has demonstrated that inhaled allergens can initiate asthmatic attacks. There are immediate skin responses to extracts of several of the common allergens and the results correspond to provoking factors described in the history. Serum IgE concentrations are elevated. Occasionally, extrinsic asthma occurs in association with a low atopic status where there was no disease in childhood. In these persons, skin tests are positive to a limited number of common allergens such as an animal or a pollen to which there is current exposure. Serum IgE concentrations are normal. It is important to identify this latter type of patient since the disease can sometimes be completely reversed when exposure to the offending allergen is stopped.

Intrinsic asthma is typically not preceded by a history of atopy. Symptoms usually begin in adult life. Perennial non-allergic rhinitis and nasal polyps may be present. There is no relationship between wheezing and exposure to common allergens. Allergy skin tests are negative and serum IgE concentrations are normal. The asthma often begins with an illness suggesting infection and there may be apparent respiratory infection from time to time but this is not the cause of the persisting symptoms. Airborne irritants and exercise can aggravate the situation, but symptoms do not depend upon these inciting factors. Aspirin may provoke severe airways responses in up to 20 per cent of these patients but aspirin is not the cause of the continued symptoms. Such reactions to aspirin which involve the airways and not the skin are due to idiosyncrasy and not to allergy. In addition, there are persons who react to aspirin with angioedema and urticaria; in these cases, antibodies to aspirin are demonstrable and the reaction is apparently allergic (Phills, Pearlmutter and Liakopoulou, 1972). In intrinsic asthma, blood eosinophil counts are elevated, generally 1000 to 2000/mm^3, despite the absence of detectable allergic reactions. Some patients have a history of rhinitis or asthma in young life which was associated with reactions to inhaled allergens with improvement over the years, followed by the development in adult life of severe, continuous asthma unassociated with inhaled allergens and characteristic of intrinsic asthma.

The physical examination in asthma may be normal between attacks or there may be audible wheezes, prolongation of forced expiratory time and rhonchi on auscultation. When the airways obstruction is chronic and severe, other signs may be present such as an increased anterior–posterior diameter of the chest, a shortened neck, taut sternomastoid muscles and inspiratory indrawing of the supraclavicular fossi and lower costal margins.

The chest radiograph may be normal or show transient bronchial wall thickening and evidence of hyperinflation including low flat diaphragms.

Spirometry may be normal or show airways obstruction which improves after inhalation of isoprenaline. If the airways obstruction is severe, there may be little effect by isoprenaline but marked improvement following a course of treatment with adrenal corticosteroids.

Eosinophilia of the blood and sputum are almost invariable in asthma. In the older child or adult who is having chest symptoms, the absence of eosinophilia on repeated examinations of the blood or sputum which cannot be attributed to either steroid therapy or bacterial infection strongly suggests a diagnosis other than asthma (Lowell, 1967).

Pathology

Most descriptions of the pathology of asthma have been derived from fatal cases and, as a result, the changes may not be representative of all stages of the disease. The most prominent feature is the obstruction of the airways which has various components including viscous mucus plugs, smooth muscle constriction and inflammatory swelling of the bronchial mucosa (Dunnill, 1971). The smooth muscle is greatly increased. Mucous glands may be enlarged. The basement membrane of the mucosa shows marked thickening. There is infiltration by eosinophils. Mast cells may be few in number and have few granules. The secretions are composed of mucous and serous components and contain eosinophils and the remnants of eosinophils, the Charcot–Leyden crystals. There may be clumps of columnar ciliated cells (Creola bodies) which represent strips of airway epithelium which have become detached. There is a notable and consistent absence of destructive emphysema.

Autonomic mechanisms

The basic abnormality in asthma is a widespread but reversible narrowing of the airways. An increased reactivity of the airways appears to be fundamental to the disease. Hyperventilation, exercise, infection and the inhalation of cold air and irritants, which have little effect in normal individuals, induce narrowing of the airways of most asthmatics. The experimental inhalation of appropriate concentrations of aerosols of histamine or methacholine usually elicits bronchial constriction in asthmatics but not in normals; this procedure is useful in diagnosis. Allergic reactions are potent stimuli of asthmatic responses but these responses are most likely to be elicited when bronchial hyper-reactivity is present.

The status of the airways is under the continuing influence of the autonomic nervous system (Figure 8.4) and is greatly affected by changes in activity of the component parts of this system (Middleton, 1972; Reed, 1974). Parasympathetic stimulation induces bronchial constriction and increased bronchial glandular secretions. These effects are mimicked by the inhalation of methacholine. Bronchial constriction may result from stimulation of receptors in the airways by the experimental inhalation of histamine or by naturally occurring stimuli including hyperventilation, cough, cold air or irritant particles or fumes. There is a reflex bronchial constriction which can be blocked by atropine.

The effects of sympathetic stimulation of the airways appears to be more complex. Stimulation of alpha-sympathetic receptors leads to smooth muscle contraction but the significance of these receptors in the airways is not entirely clear and their effects are certainly not predominant. Stimulation of beta receptors produces bronchial relaxation and cardiac stimulation. The latter is a familiar response to the potent adrenergic stimulant, isoprenaline. The development of agents which are selectively active upon the heart or upon the bronchi illustrates that the beta receptors of these organs differ. The receptors of the heart have been designated beta-1 receptors and those of the bronchi, beta-2 receptors. Bronchodilators such as salbutamol are highly

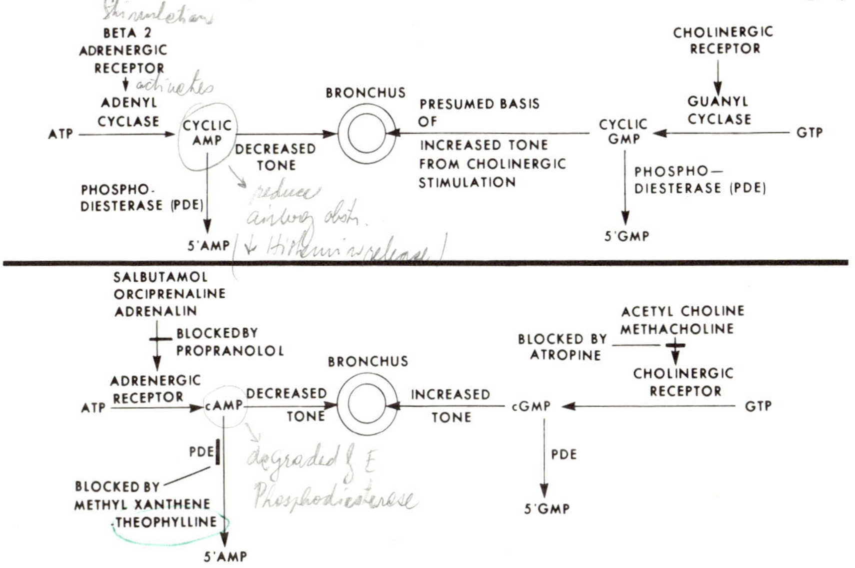

Figure 8.4. Autonomic stimulation of the bronchial airways.

selective beta-2 agonists so that a potent bronchodilator effect can be obtained with little or no effect on the heart. The selectivity of these agents is further enhanced in therapy by the local delivery to the airways by administration by inhalation.

Stimulation of beta receptors by a hormone such as epinephrine activates the enzyme adenyl cyclase. This catalyses the transformation of ATP to cyclic AMP thereby increasing the cellular level of cyclic AMP which influences a vast number of cellular functions. In the airways, there is a decrease in the tone of bronchial muscles. Cyclic AMP inhibits the release of chemical mediators such as histamine and slow-reacting substance of anaphylaxis (SRS-A) from basophils and mast cells. Thus, adrenergic stimuli which increase cellular levels of cyclic AMP may reduce the airways obstruction of asthma. Cyclic AMP is normally degraded by the enzyme phosphodiesterase. Theophylline inhibits this enzyme; this favours the preservation of cellular cyclic AMP and appears to explain the therapeutic value of this drug in asthma. Cholinergic stimulation leads to a cellular accumulation of cyclic GMP. The cellular effects of cyclic GMP are antagonistic to those of cyclic AMP. An increase in cyclic GMP would probably increase bronchial muscle tone and favour the release of histamine and SRS-A.

The blockade of beta receptors by propranolol induces broncho-constriction in asthma. A naturally occurring partial blockade or reduced responsiveness to beta-adrenergic stimulation would similarly be expected to alter the balance between beta adrenergic and cholinergic activity and predispose to asthma. The concept has arisen that a process of this type is responsible for the underlying bronchial hyper-reactivity of asthma (Reed, 1974). The presence of such a blockade is supported by a variety of studies including observations on the actions of adrenaline in asthmatic and normal subjects. In asthmatics, responses to adrenaline such as the elevation of blood glucose, fall in blood eosinophil counts and rise of urinary cyclic AMP which depend upon beta receptor stimulation are less than in the normal.

The view that autonomic alterations may be basic to asthma is supported by some animal models. For example, some types of hypothalamic ablation or stimulation can lead to asthma-like responses. The rodent treated with *Bordetella pertussis* has many features resembling atopy in man and is considered to have altered responses as a result of beta-adrenergic blockade; many features of this altered responsiveness can be mimicked by propranolol treatment.

Allergic mechanisms

Allergic reactions are a potent stimulus of asthmatic responses. Allergen inhalation tests in allergic asthmatic individuals may elicit early, dual (early followed by late) or late asthmatic responses (Hargreave et al, 1974). The early asthmatic response (Figure 8.5) begins within 10 minutes, reaches a maximum within 30 minutes and clears spontaneously within 1 to 3 hours.

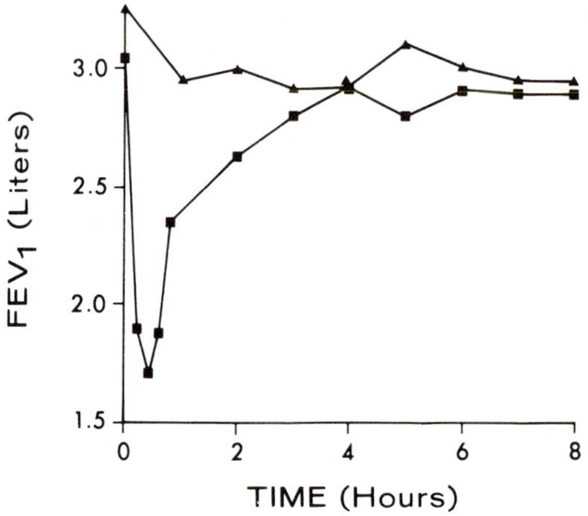

Figure 8.5. Allergen inhalation test with ragweed pollen extract; early (immediate) asthmatic response.

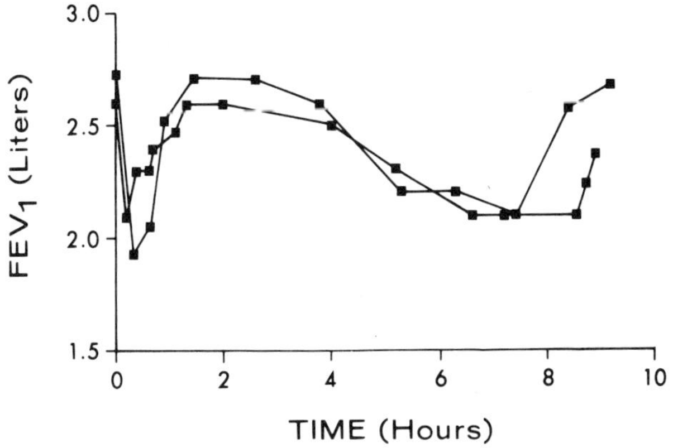

Figure 8.6. Allergen inhalation test with ragweed pollen extract; dual asthmatic response.

It is inhibited by disodium cromoglycate administered before the allergen challenge, is reversed by inhaled isoprenaline and is virtually unaffected by antihistamines and corticosteroids. In the dual asthmatic response (Figure 8.6) the early response clears spontaneously before the onset of the late response. The late response usually begins after 4 to 6 hours, reaches a peak at 8 to 12 hours and clears in one or more days. The late response is more prolonged than the early response and is often more severe. A late asthmatic response not preceded by an early asthmatic response is shown in Figure 8.7. Its timing is similar to the late components of the dual asthmatic response. Late asthmatic

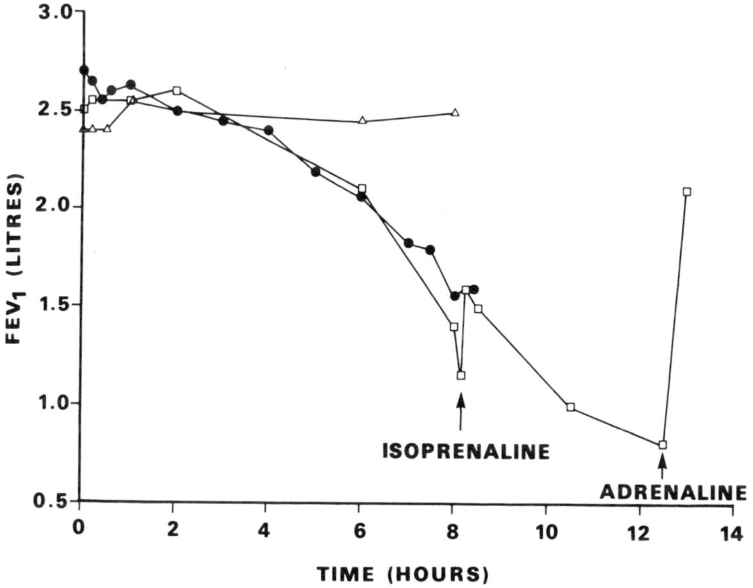

Figure 8.7. Allergen inhalation test with ragweed pollen extract; late asthmatic response.

responses may be inhibited by disodium cromoglycate or by corticosteroids administered prior to allergen challenge. When mild, they are reversed, at least for a time, by isoprenaline, but when more severe they respond poorly to isoprenaline, adrenaline and aminophylline.

Early asthmatic responses, either in isolation or as a part of dual responses, are typically elicited in persons with type 1 sensitivity. They can be induced by the inhalation of various common allergens to which there is sensitisation including pollen, house dust and animal products. They seem to depend upon processes similar to those involved in early weal and flare responses in the skin. Antibodies of the IgE class specific for the particular allergen are bound to the plasma membranes of mast cells in the airways or in the skin thereby sensitising these organs. In addition, there is now evidence that antigen-induced asthmatic responses can result from reactions with antibodies which differ from IgE insofar that they exhibit greater resistance to heat and a shorter period between the introduction of the antibody and the actual sensitisation (Bryant, Burns and Lazarus, 1973). These 'short latency' antibodies probably belong to the IgG class. Interaction of sensitising antibody with antigen results in the rapid release of pharmacologically active substances including histamine, SRS-A and eosinophil chemotactic factor (ECF-A). Histamine predominates in the production of the weal and flare skin response. SRS-A is a potent stimulus of smooth muscle contraction and is believed to be important in the bronchoconstriction of asthma. ECF-A accounts for the accumulation of eosinophils at the site of the reactions. Eosinophil infiltration is also a feature of intrinsic asthma in which type 1 sensitivity to environmental antigens cannot be demonstrated, suggesting the possibility that intrinsic asthma may have a final common pathway with allergic reactions. Eosinophils are capable of phagocytosis of a variety of substances including immune complexes. There is apparently a preferential phagocytosis of immune complexes in which the antibody is of the IgE class. Eosinophils have been shown to produce a product or products which inhibit the antigen-induced release of histamine (Hubscher and Eisen, 1973). Thus, eosinophils in the allergic reaction may have a kind of negative biological feedback function. It is now evident that the prostoglandins PGE_2 and $PGF_{2\alpha}$ are produced in the lungs and could be involved in asthma. $PGF_{2\alpha}$ causes bronchial smooth muscle contraction (Parker and Snider, 1973). These substances also probably have effects upon the pulmonary vascular bed.

Late asthmatic responses may occur as a part of dual responses or in isolation. They have been considered to be due to type 3 or Arthus reactions involving the airways. There is a presumed involvement of serum antibodies of the IgG and/or IgM classes which interact with the first component of complement thereby sequentially activating the entire complement system. Products of the complement system and of leucocytes which are attracted to the site produce the inflammatory response. The observed deposition of β1c (C3) in tissues undergoing late cutaneous responses induced by grass pollen extracts lends support to this putative involvement of the complement system in these responses (Taylor and Shivalkar, 1971). In the skin, a late allergic response is seldom elicited without a preceding early allergic response and it has been suggested that the vascular permeability produced by the early response allows a diffusion of antibodies into the tissues, thereby creating the conditions appropriate for the interactions of components involved in Arthus or type 3 reactions. Regardless, it needs to be recognised that late responses are a relatively common sequel to early allergic responses. In subjects sensitive to pollen, a sufficiently large early cutaneous allergic response to an intracutaneous antigen injection is almost invariably followed by a late cutaneous response at the site (Robertson et al, 1974). Initially, there is a weal and flare maximal at about 10 minutes. After about 1 hour, the flare fades and the weal loses its sharp margin. If there is to be a late response, a small swelling persists and gradually increases in diameter to become maximum at about 6 to 12 hours and clear within 24 to 48 hours. The late swelling is ill-defined, erythematous or pale, soft and often tender to tapping. Histologically, there is oedema and infiltration with eosinophils and neutrophils and fewer mononuclear cells. Degranulation of mast cells is observed. Similar cutaneous responses in man are observed in passively sensitised skin sites challenged with antigen. Early followed by late cutaneous allergic responses are also observed in reactions induced by the injection of antiserum to human IgE (Dolovich et al, 1973). These latter observations introduce the possibility that IgE-dependent reactions in man may initiate events that give rise to both the early weal and flare and the late allergic responses. Similar considerations with respect to mechanisms apply to late asthmatic responses which, particularly as a part of dual responses, are relatively common following allergen inhalation tests in asthmatic individuals with type 1 sensitivity to common allergens.

Early, dual and late asthmatic responses are also provoked by the inhalation of a variety of additional airborne substances like tolylene diisocyanate, aminoethylethanolamine, cotton products, western red cedar and complex salts of platinum. In instances such as these, there is little or no information on the characteristics of the associated immune responses. Nevertheless, it seems likely that in most instances there is an involvement of immune mechanisms similar to those which have been discussed.

Other allergic mechanisms could well be involved in the pathogenesis of asthma. The pathogenesis of intrinsic asthma remains undefined. A deposition of various immunoglobulins and beta 1c in the thickened basement membrane has been observed. Cell-mediated immunity might influence asthmatic responses to pollen allergens. There is evidence of delayed hypersensitivity in some persons with type 1 allergy to pollen. The production of macrophage inhibition factor by lymphoid cells stimulated with pollen allergen has been described. It has recently been observed that an accumulation of basophils may be a function of cell-mediated immunity; this could represent a process through which type 4 reactions inter-relate with IgE-dependent sensitivity.

Diagnosis and investigation

In the clinical assessment of asthma, it is necessary to establish the correct diagnosis, the severity of the illness and the identity of provoking factors. It should be remembered that troublesome asthma can be present despite a normal physical examination and spirometry at the time the person is seen. The diagnosis of asthma should be considered in any patient with airways obstruction including those with apparent chronic bronchitis or emphysema.

Where the diagnosis is not obvious, supporting evidence is provided by blood or sputum eosinophilia and by the provocation of asthma by exercise, histamine or methacholine. The demonstration of a major reversal of airways obstruction by bronchodilator or adrenal corticosteroid treatment confirms the diagnosis. The assessment of severity is essential for proper management and is made from the history, physical examination and spirometry. Provoking factors can include specific allergens and non-specific stimuli such as airborne irritants, exercise, hyperventilation, infection, changes in the weather and emotional upset. Further consideration here will be limited to allergens as provoking factors.

The history is the most useful single method to elicit the possible relevance of allergenic stimuli in asthma. It is necessary to be aware of seasonal variations of the local atmospheric pollens and fungal spores and the potential allergens in the patient's home, work, school and hobby environments. Particular attention should be given to intermittent exposure to animals, birds, house dust, industrial dusts, industrial fumes and drugs, particularly aspirin, and any relationship of the exposure to symptoms. Useful ancillary evidence of the relevance of airborne allergens is provided by a history of nasal or eye symptoms typical of allergy associated with particular exposures. Some aspects of the history can be misleading. For example, symptoms induced by inhaled substances may result from irritation. Sometimes the relationship of exposure to symptoms may not be recognised because their responses develop insidiously as the dose of inhaled allergen gradually increases or because symptoms are due mainly to late asthmatic responses which begin 4 to 6 hours after the exposure.

Allergy skin tests for type 1 hypersensitivity together with the history provide a quite reliable indication of the potential relevance of airborne allergens in disease. Tests are performed with a series of extracts of common allergens with the addition of particular allergens relevant to the environment of the patient. Common airborne allergens include house dust, *Dermatophagoides* sp., tree and grass pollen and, in North America, ragweed pollen. Additional common airborne allergens are derived from cat, dog, horse, birds and the fungal spores of *Cladosporium*, *Alternaria* and *A. fumigatus*. Of the three methods of skin tests, prick, scratch and intracutaneous, the prick test is preferred for routine testing. It is performed by lifting the skin gently with a sharp needle through a drop of the allergen extract. The method requires little experience, is rapid and causes little trauma, thus minimising dermographism. The small doses introduced are most unlikely to cause systemic responses. A positive test is indicated by a weal and flare response maximal at about 10 minutes. This early or type 1 response demonstrates the presence of sensitising antibody in the skin but does not necessarily indicate a relevance of the allergen to symptoms. Negative skin tests indicate a lack of sensitising antibodies or a weak antigen preparation. False negative tests may be produced by the ingestion of antihistamines but not by adrenal corticosteroids. Early cutaneous allergic responses may evolve into late cutaneous allergic responses, particularly with intracutaneous tests. Late responses were initially observed and examined in detail in patients with allergic bronchopulmonary aspergillosis and extrinsic allergic alveolitis. It is now apparent that any sufficiently intense allergic skin response to any allergen can evolve into a late response.

Serological tests are not essential for the usual assessment of asthma but they may sometimes be helpful. Skin tests are a sensitive indicator of type 1 sensitisation and there is a direct relationship between the number and intensity of immediate skin test responses and the serum concentration of IgE. Moreover, the skin tests demonstrate the specific antigens to which there is sensitivity. Assay of the serum IgE concentration has the advantage of a numerical result. The normal serum IgE concentration is very low with values of less than one microgram per ml. The IgE level may be elevated in extrinsic asthma but is normal in intrinsic asthma. IgE levels can also be elevated in persons with hay fever or eczema without asthma and in parasitic infestations and liver disease.

A number of in vitro biological and immunochemical procedures have been developed to quantitate sensitivity to specific antigens. The radio-allergosorbent test (RAST), designed to measure specific IgE antibodies immunochemically, has gained widespread acceptance in research due to the accuracy and the ease of performing large numbers of tests. For clinical purposes, the RAST test has not replaced allergy skin tests, which, if used judiciously, are safe, simple, versatile and provide quick answers.

Allergen inhalation tests have been used extensively in research and, to some extent, in diagnosis. An aerosol of the allergen extract is inhaled under controlled conditions and responses of the airways are carefully monitored. Patients should be well at the time of study, physically and mentally at rest, not smoking and preferably not on medication. They should attend the hospital for the day so that they are in a known environment where frequent observations can be made for 9 to 12 hours. The aerosol may be delivered through a face mask and inhaled by normal breathing through the mouth. Only one test extract is administered on one day. A graded increase in dose is provided. This can be accomplished by administration of the aerosol for 30 seconds, 60 seconds and 2 minutes at intervals of 10 minutes between the inhalations. The patient should be unaware of the contents of the aerosol so as to minimise any subjective effects. On the first day, a control buffer solution is administered by aerosol so as to exclude non-specific early responses and to examine any naturally occurring diurnal variation. On the second and subsequent days, aerosols of the allergen are carefully administered starting with weak solutions. In patients with asthma and positive allergy skin tests, the starting strength of the test solution may be determined by allergy skin test by the prick method. It is safe to begin with a solution which causes small early weals 2 to 3 mm in diameter. If no respiratory response occurs within 10 minutes after inhalation of the aerosol for a total of 3·5 minutes, a solution with a 10-fold higher antigen concentration is used and the sequence of inhalation is repeated. Investigation prior to inhalation should include a symptom inquiry, chest auscultation, oral temperature, spirometry, and WBC and differential and total eosinophil counts. After the inhalation, the symptoms and spirometry at 10, 20, 30, 45 and 60 minutes and at one or two hourly intervals are recorded. Oral temperatures at one or two hourly intervals and chest findings and blood counts after 8 to 12 hours are determined. Additional indices of responses can be included according to the objectives of the procedure.

Allergen inhalation tests in research have demonstrated the different patterns of asthmatic responses and permitted the investigation of some of the mechanisms involved. They have been used to determine the effects of drugs and allergen injection treatment on asthmatic responses. In the diagnosis of respiratory allergy, they generally have little advantage over careful history, skin tests and clinical trials of avoidance of exposure. When the history indicates that an exposure to an allergen induces symptoms and the skin test with that allergen is positive, the inhalation test is usually positive. When the history is negative and the skin test is positive, the inhalation test is sometimes positive. When the history is positive or negative and the skin test is negative, the inhalation test is usually negative. An important exception to the latter situation occurs in some instances where late bronchial responses are elicited despite a negative skin test. In addition, shortly after initial exposure to an allergen, skin tests are sometimes temporarily negative despite the presence of allergen-induced allergic respiratory symptoms. In instances such as these allergen inhalation tests may confirm the sensitisation.

Management

Asthma has been a common cause of chronic disability; however, improved understanding and new modalities of treatment have greatly improved the outlook. In asthma, subtle changes in the extent of bronchial narrowing affect function and are quickly noticed. Whilst this contributes to the disability, it can also be used to enlist the patient as an effective collaborator in the treatment. Good results require that the patient learns the objectives and principles of treatment and how to respond to changes in the intensity of the airway problem. An optimistic outlook can legitimately be cultivated. In this regard, there are numerous reassuring points which should be presented to the patient in one way or another. For example, it is now evident that asthma is not, in the first instance, due to emotions. The affected individual cannot be held at fault or blamed for the disease. It does not cause permanent damage to the heart or lungs. It does not cause emphysema. It is a reversible and controllable type of disease. Most of the medicines for asthma, even if used daily for many years, are harmless. With good therapy, the risk of death from asthma is extremely small.

The symptom pattern and peak flow rate, FEV_1 and vital capacity determinations provide relatively sensitive indices of the activity of the disease and the efficacy of the treatment regimen. The objectives of treatment are to maintain normal or nearly normal function of the individual and to prevent severe attacks of asthma.

The best treatment of allergic reactions is to avoid the offending allergens; in some instances, this may be all that is required as when there is isolated sensitivity to animals in the home or to allergens encountered only in an occupational environment. In many instances, it is possible to reduce but not entirely eliminate exposure to offending allergens. In homes, the use of mechanical air-cleaners and frequent vacuuming of items including mattresses with a good vacuum cleaner can reduce exposure to dust and the contained house dust mites. With air conditioners, windows can be kept closed during the summer months thereby isolating the indoor environment from allergenic particles such as fungal spores and pollen grains which originate outdoors.

The bronchial hyper-reactivity which is basic to asthma is expressed by the narrowing of the airways in response to a variety of stimuli. Irritants such as tobacco smoke, fumes, perfumes and dusts can aggravate symptoms and should be avoided where possible. The airways obstruction induced by such irritants can be inhibited by the inhalation of atropine. However, the airways obstruction appears to be more effectively countered by sympathomimetic and xanthene bronchodilators and atropine is not used in practice.

The most widely used medicines for asthma are the various bronchodilators. Sympathomimetic or xanthene bronchodilators or both are generally chosen as the initial form of treatment. The choice of sympathomimetic agent for use in treatment is governed largely by the effort to avoid undesired side effects. The oral ephedrine in aminophylline preparations is often responsible for dose-related side effects which are distressing and which reduce the amount of aminophylline that can be used. Oral sympathomimetic bronchodilators in general have disappointing therapeutic results at dosage levels below those which induce side effects. Inhaled sympathomimetic bronchodilators, particularly isoprenaline, have been frequently over-used in the past, sometimes with fatal results (Speizer, Doll and Heaf, 1968). The development of selective bronchodilators such as salbutamol and orciprenaline represents a significant advance in asthma treatment. Inhalation of these agents can produce effective bronchodilation from 4 to 6 hours through stimulation of bronchial beta-2 receptors; there is relatively less stimulation of beta-1 receptors of the heart and cardiovascular effects are thereby minimised. This type of treatment is sufficient to reverse mild episodes of asthma and often prevents asthmatic responses from a variety of stimuli including exercise, hyperventilation and irritants. It is necessary to place rigorous upper limits on the dose of inhaled sympathomimetic agents to avoid overdosage. A usual recommendation is that the maximum dose from a pressurised container should be no more than two sprays 6 times per day in the adult and one spray 6 times per day in children above the age of 6 years.

Theophylline-containing preparations can be used orally or intravenously. Theophylline, like sympathomimetic bronchodilators, increases the cellular concentration of cyclic AMP and, as a result, the two drugs are probably synergistic in therapeutic effects. Theophylline is safe at all ages if used in appropriate doses. Toxic effects in children in the past could be attributed to overdosage. There is a danger of duplicating dosage if there is administration by various routes.

Disodium cromoglycate (DSCG) represents a major advance in the treatment of asthma. There is inhibition of the antigen-induced release of mediators from mast cells. The mechanism by which this is accomplished has not yet been determined. The medicine is used as a powder inhaled from a capsule placed in a so-called spinhaler. There is increasing benefit with increasing dosage up to four capsules daily. More than four capsules per day can be used safely but in most cases, there is probably no additional therapeutic benefit. The inhalation of DSCG prior to an inhalation of allergen prevents the asthmatic response. It is not effective when used after the exposure to allergen so that it is a preventative agent. Nevertheless, it is reasonable to begin treatment as early as possible so as to avoid delay in achieving a therapeutic effect. DSCG may also inhibit asthmatic responses from inhaled irritants including histamine and from alcohol ingestion, hyperventilation, cold air and exercise. There is a high rate of success in the treatment of young people with extrinsic asthma. There are no known side effects apart from a mild local irritation. Inhaled sympathomimetic bronchodilator taken 5 or 10 minutes before the DSCG may improve the delivery of the DSCG to the airways and reduce the effects of irritation.

The airways obstruction in asthma involves not only spasm but a variety of changes including inflammatory oedema of the bronchial mucosa and thickened tenacious sputum. The obstruction, if prolonged or severe, is often relatively unresponsive to agents such as aminophylline and sympathomimetic bronchodilators. In this situation, it is necessary to add corticosteroids. Steroids, in sufficient dosage and after sufficient time, invariably exert a beneficial effect. Prednisone or prednisolone by mouth or hydrocortisone or methylprednisolone intravenously are the medications of choice. If oral adrenal corticosteroid is required on a long-term basis, it is best administered on an alternate-day-basis with a single minimum required dosage taken after breakfast every second day. If it is not possible to establish this regimen in any particular patient, then it is best to use a single sufficiently large dose after breakfast every day. The use of additional medication including bronchodilators and DSCG is indicated in order to assure that the dose of steroid used is the lowest possible which is sufficient to control the asthma. In life-threatening asthma, large pharmacological doses, even up to gram quantities of hydrocortisone or the equivalent, should be administered as often as once per hour until a therapeutic response is achieved.

The introduction of beclomethasone diproprionate for use by inhalation permits the local delivery of steroid and the avoidance of systemic side effects. With this agent, it is often possible to reduce or discontinue the use of oral steroid in patients who have previously required it on a long-term basis (Clark, 1972).

Allergen injection treatment is known to be beneficial in allergic rhinitis induced by a variety of allergens including pollen and house dust but not animal danders. It has been shown to reduce the bronchial reactivity to the particular allergen and there is some evidence of a symptomatic benefit in the treatment of asthma. If a trial of allergen injection treatment is started, it should be discontinued after about two years if there has been no benefit. In some instances, there is aggravation of asthma with each injection; if this occurs, the dose should be decreased or the injection treatment discontinued. It is the view of the authors that improvements in the treatment of asthma, particularly with newer pharmacological agents such as DSCG, selective beta-2 agonists and locally administered adrenal corticosteroid, have greatly reduced the indication for allergen injection treatment of asthma.

Bacterial or viral infections sometimes aggravate the airways obstruction of asthma. When this occurs, it is necessary to increase the level of treatment with the medications used for asthma. If the infection is bacterial, appropriate antibiotic treatment is also indicated.

ALVEOLITIS

'Alveolitis' is an inflammatory process in the peripheral gas-exchanging part of the lung, beyond terminal bronchioles, affecting principally alveolar walls. In some cases it develops in response to inhaled airborne particles which induce a hypersensitivity reaction in the gas-exchanging tissues, and is called 'extrinsic allergic alveolitis'. In the majority, however, the cause is unknown and the disease is called 'cryptogenic fibrosing alveolitis'. In a third group the process follows ingestion of toxic substances, foods or drugs which reach the lungs by the blood stream. In all of these situations there is a tendency for the reaction to progress to a fibrosis of the alveolar walls. Widespread fibrosis may also occur following certain infections, in association with mineral dust pneumoconioses, and in certain systemic diseases of unknown cause including sarcoidosis, histiocytosis X, and tuberose sclerosis.

Extrinsic Allergic Alveolitis

This group of diseases have also been called 'hypersensitivity pneumonitis', 'interstitial granulomatous pneumonitis' and 'extrinsic allergic pneumonia'. The first example recognised was farmer's lung, in which the airborne allergens are small thermophilic actinomycetes derived from mouldy hay and mouldy vegetable produce. Since then disease induced by an increasing number of

Table 8.3. Causes of extrinsic allergic alveolitis

Antigen particles	Sources of particles	Disease synonyms
Micropolyspora faeni *Thermoactinomyces vulgaris*	Mouldy hay	Farmer's lung
T. sacchari	Mouldy bagasse	Bagassosis
T. vulgaris	Contaminated air conditioner	
M. faeni, T. vulgaris	Contaminated humidifier	
Post-spawning compost *M. faeni, T. vulgaris*	Mushroom post-spawning compost	Mushroom worker's lung
Mouldy cork dust *Penicillium frequentans*	Mouldy cork dust	Suberosis
Cryptostroma corticale	Infected maple bark	Maple bark pneumonitis
Aspergillus fumigatus *A. clavatus*	Mouldy barley, malt	Malt worker's lung
Graphium, Pullalaria pullulans	Mouldy sawdust	Sequiosis
Penicillium casei	Mouldy cheese	Cheese-washer's lung
Alternaria	Wood-room of paper mill	Wood-pulp worker's disease
Sitophilus granarius	Infested wheat flour	Wheat weevil disease
Bird proteins and droppings	Budgie, pigeon, parrot, hen	Bird fancier's lung
Bovine and porcine protein and pituitary antigens	Bovine and porcine pituitary snuff	Pituitary snuff taker's lung
Fish meal	Animal food factory	Fishmeal worker's lung
Rat proteins	Rats	

other inhaled organic allergens from a variety of sources has been recognised (Table 8.3) (Pepys, 1959; Villar, Avila and Telles de Araujo, 1973). Similar disease may be provoked by inorganic particles such as copper sulphate neutralised by hydrated lime ('vineyard sprayer's lung'), but, in these cases, it is not yet known whether immunological mechanisms are involved.

Clinical features

The clinical features are determined by the intensity of exposure, the site of reaction in the peripheral respiratory tissues and by the immunopathological mechanisms involved.

The symptoms are systemic and respiratory. Systemic symptoms include episodes of fever, malaise and anorexia, and weight loss. The respiratory

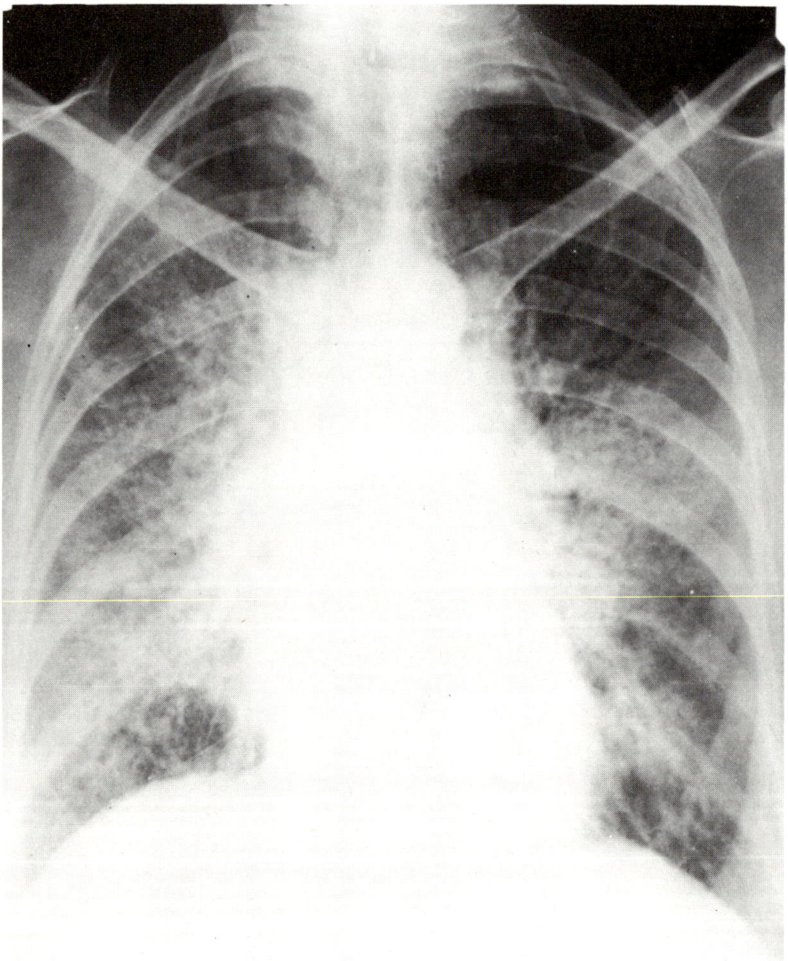

Figure 8.8. Radiograph of a woman with extrinsic allergic alveolitis associated with exposure to a budgie showing widespread small nodular shadows.

symptoms include dyspnoea without wheezing, and cough without much sputum. The types of symptoms are determined by the pattern of exposure. When the exposure to the responsible airborne allergen is intense and brief, e.g. in pigeon fanciers, the presentation is 'acute'. Febrile episodes with respiratory symptoms begin 5 or 6 hours or so following exposure and clear within 24 to 48 hours providing they are not too severe. When there is inhalation of smaller amounts of allergen over longer periods of time, such as to the

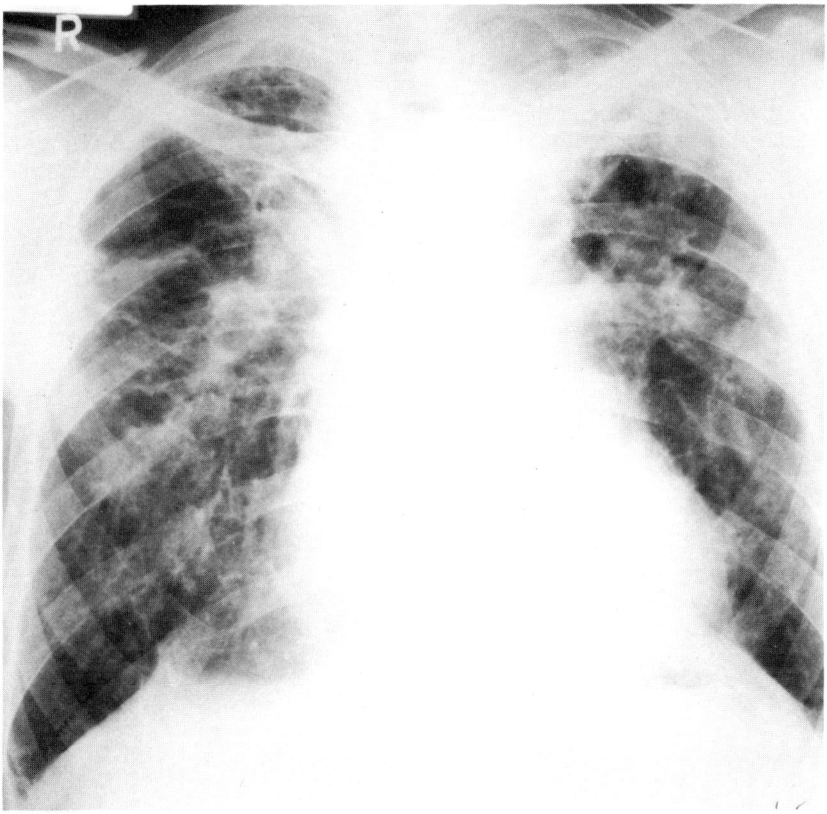

Figure 8.9. Radiograph of a man with extrinsic allergic alveolitis associated with budgie contact to illustrate the later predominant involvement and shrinkage of the upper lobes.

dust originating from a budgie in the home, the presentation is 'insidious'. The chief features are progressive dyspnoea, cough, malaise and weight loss. Febrile episodes are absent or mild and less clearly related to exposure. The insidious presentation leads to the most severe disease because there is a gradual progression to a late stage of the disease before the help of a physician is sought. Moreover, the relationship of symptoms to exposure is less clearly defined, and the diagnosis is more easily missed.

On examination it is noteworthy that physical signs are often few in spite of troublesome symptoms. In the early stages crepitant rales may be heard at the bases or throughout the lung fields. Later, tachypnoea may be present and tracheal displacement and flattening of the anterior chest may suggest underlying lung shrinkage. Clubbing is usually absent.

The earliest changes on the chest radiograph are nodular shadows which are usually pinpoint to 2 mm in diameter (Figure 8.8). These may be initially observed in any particular zone, but when more pronounced, they are widely distributed in keeping with the wide distribution of inhaled particles. In later stages of the disease honeycomb shadows and lung shrinkage occur particularly affecting the upper lobes (Figure 8.9).

Physiological studies classically show a non-obstructive (restrictive) ventilatory defect with impairment in lung compliance and gas exchange. In addition, some patients have airways obstruction.

Haemoglobin and WBC are usually normal. ESR tends to be moderately elevated in the range of 20 to 60 mm in one hour. The serum IgA and IgG levels may be raised. Serum non-organ specific antibodies like rheumatoid factors and antinuclear factor may be present in the early stages, but not usually in the chronic stages.

Pathology

The peripheral respiratory tissues are involved in an inflammatory reaction with a cellular infiltration progressing to fibrosis (Figure 8.10) (Hinson, 1970). This infiltration is chiefly in and around the walls of bronchioles and small bronchi, but it is also seen in alveolar walls. The cells are mainly histiocytes, lymphocytes and plasma cells. Little desquamation occurs within alveolar spaces but when present it may contain foamy mononuclear cells. Accumu-

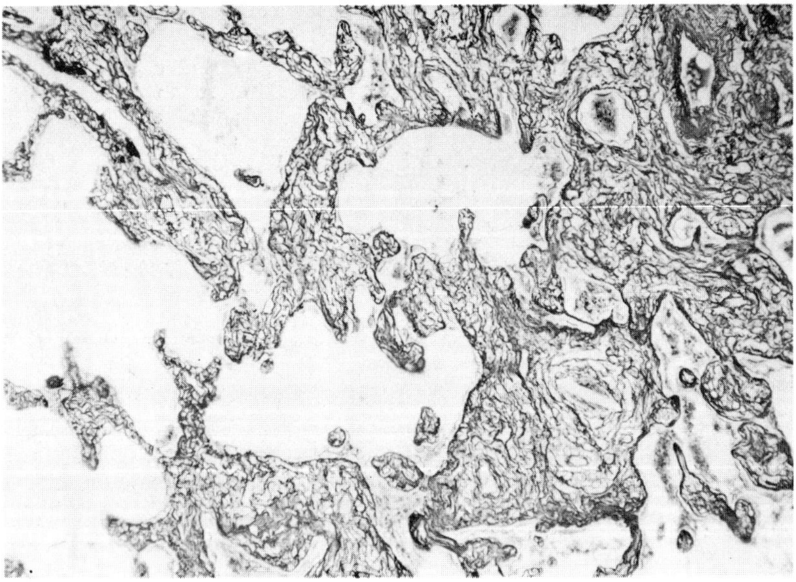

Figure 8.10. Lung biopsy from a patient with extrinsic allergic alveolitis showing patchy thickening of alveolar walls (by courtesy of Dr. K. Shier).

lations of epithelioid cells with a few giant cells forming granulomatous lesions occur especially in the earlier stages of disease (Figure 8.11). The giant cells sometimes have clefts which are characteristic but not diagnostic. Similar granulomas have also been recently observed in scalene node and liver biopsies in patients with suberosis (Villar, Avila and Telles de Araujo, 1973).

The inhaled particles are usually not identified in biopsies of lung. However, in suberosis particles of cork dust are seen in the granular pneumonocytes in the alveoli, in the histiocytes of the septal infiltrates, and in the granulomas.

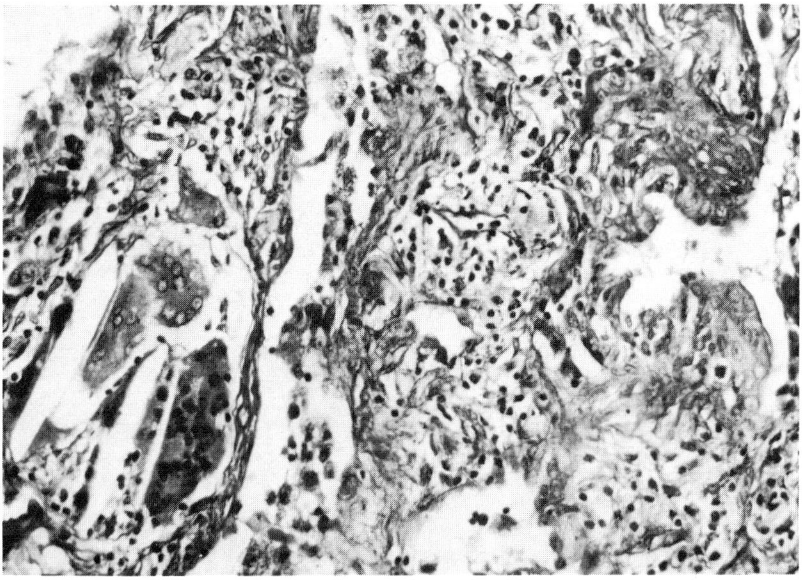

Figure 8.11. Lung biopsy from a patient with extrinsic allergic alveolitis to illustrate non-caseating granuloma and giant cells (by courtesy of Dr. K. Shier).

In maple bark pneumonitis the spores of *Cryptostroma corticale* have been observed. In farmer's lung the presence of antigen in the walls of small bronchi has been detected by immuno-fluorescent techniques (Wenzel, Emanuel and Gray, 1971).

Mechanisms

Allergen inhalation tests provoke a late respiratory response which is associated with fever and polymorphonuclear leucocytosis (Hargreave and Pepys, 1972). Figure 8.12 illustrates the response in a pigeon fancier with extrinsic allergic alveolitis without airways obstruction. The fall in ventilatory capacity which is not reversed by isoprenaline and the fall in CO gas transfer factor reflects the reaction in the peripheral respiratory tissues. In other patients with extrinsic allergic alveolitis and airways obstruction (Figure 8.13) the fall in ventilatory capacity is due to asthma. The respiratory responses in allergen inhalation tests resemble the acute natural presentation of disease.

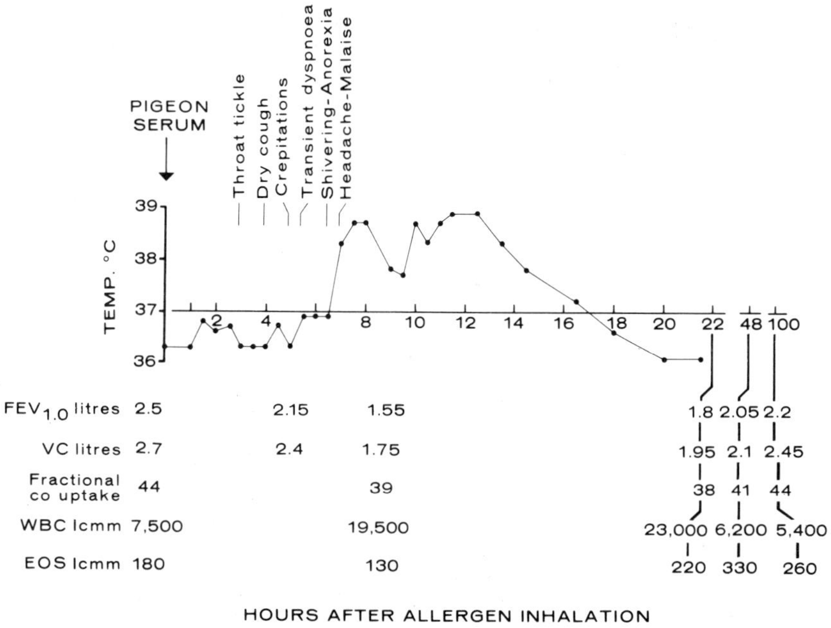

Figure 8.12. Allergen inhalation test with diluted pigeon serum in patient with bird fancier's lung; late pyrexial and peripheral respiratory response.

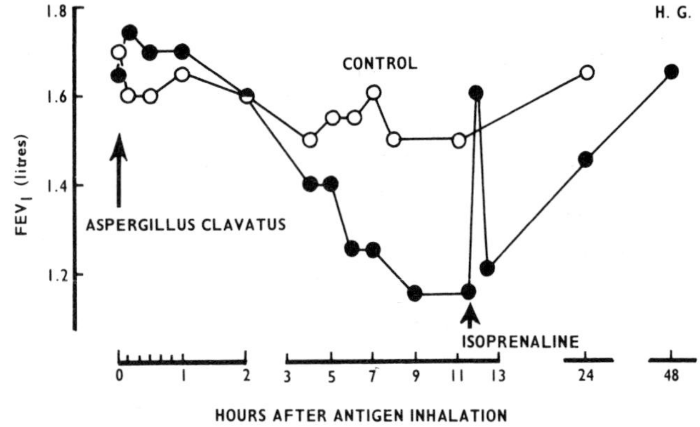

Figure 8.13. Allergen inhalation test with *Aspergillus clavatus* extract in patient with malt worker's lung; late asthmatic response.

Until recently the respiratory responses have been considered to be chiefly type 3 allergic reactions. This view was supported by the time course of the responses provoked by allergen inhalation tests, the occurrence of fever and polymorphonuclear leucocytosis, the usual presence of precipitating IgG or IgM antibodies in the serum, and the skin test responses. Skin tests with suitable extracts may provoke dual skin responses in which there is an early weal and flare followed by a late ill-defined swelling (Figure 8.14) which is maximum at about 6 to 12 hours and resolves over 24 to 48 hours. The early component of the response may not be mediated by IgE antibodies because these usually cannot be demonstrated, and it has been suggested that it could be due to sensitising IgG antibodies of the 'short-term' variety. The histological appearances of the late components show a cellular infiltration which consists of varying numbers of mononuclear cells, neutrophils and eosinophils. Immunofluorescent studies may demonstrate the deposition of complement

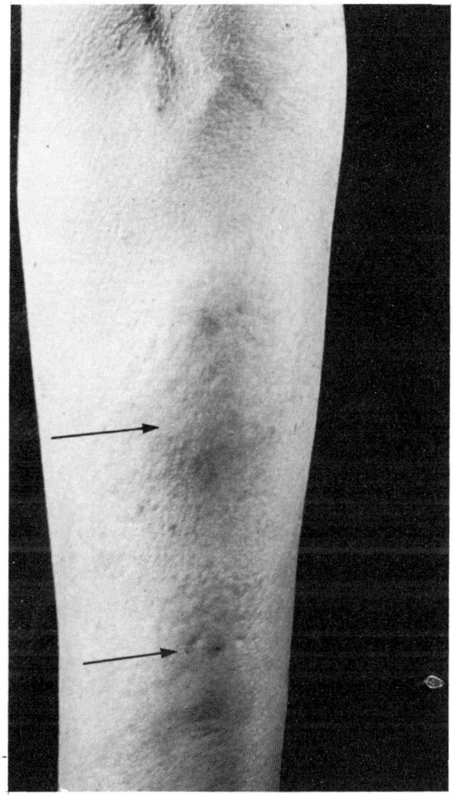

Figure 8.14. Skin tests with budgie serum in patient with bird fancier's lung, showing two late skin responses at 8 hours.

within vessel walls. The latter would support the participation of a type 3 reaction but the histological features are not characteristic of the type 3 allergic reaction seen in animals. Moreover, there is no direct relationship between precipitating antibodies in the serum and the presence of disease. Many persons with large quantities of serum antibody of the IgG and IgM classes have no reaction to the inhalation of the corresponding antigen.

The pathological appearances in the lung are consistent with type 4 hypersensitivity, but the extent to which this mechanism participates in extrinsic allergic alveolitis in man is still unclear. In animals the passive transfer of allergised lymphocytes followed by inhalation challenge with antigen produces an 'alveolitis' which resembles extrinsic allergic alveolitis (Hensley, Fink and Barboriak, 1974). In animal experiments such a response has not been provoked following passive immunisation with serum. In patients with extrinsic allergic alveolitis there is a release of MIF following incubation of lymphocytes with antigen indicating the presence of cellular immunity (Fink, Moore and Barboriak, 1974). By contrast, lymphocytes from exposed persons with precipitins but without disease do not release MIF when they are challenged with antigen. However, skin tests do not show delayed skin responses and the time course of the late skin and respiratory responses is not characteristic of type 4 reactions. On balance, it appears that the pulmonary reactions in extrinsic allergic alveolitis may be due mainly to type 4 hypersensitivity but that type 3 and perhaps even type 1 hypersensitivity may contribute to the disease in some cases.

Diagnosis and investigation

The diagnosis of extrinsic allergic alveolitis should be suspected in any person exposed to airborne allergens which are known to cause the disease if there are febrile episodes or respiratory symptoms, and especially if there

Table 8.4. Some differences in clinical features between the insidious presentation of extrinsic allergic alveolitis and cryptogenic fibrosing alveolitis

Clinical features (selected)	Extrinsic allergic alveolitis	Cryptogenic fibrosing alveolitis
Crepitant rales	+	++ Basal
Clubbing	10 per cent mild	60–70 per cent
Radiograph (early): nodular shadows	Widespread	Lower
Radiograph (late): shrinkage	Upper	Lower
Rheumatoid or antinuclear factors	5 per cent	60 percent

are widespread nodular shadows on the chest radiograph or clinical features of a chronic fibrosing lung disease. Acute episodes are commonly mistaken for pneumonia or bronchitis. The clinical features of the insidious presentation of disease resembles those of cryptogenic fibrosing alveolitis (Table 8.4). Methods of diagnosis include the medical history, serum precipitin tests, skin tests, allergen inhalation tests and lung biopsy.

A careful history of the patient's environment at work, home and in relation to any hobbies is necessary to identify possible sources of allergen exposure. Exposure to large quantities of organic dust should arouse suspicion; however it should be remembered that small amounts of dust, e.g. from budgie, may also induce disease. The relationship of this exposure to symptoms is more likely to be detected if the presentation of symptoms is 'acute' than if it is 'insidious'. In the acute presentation the patient may recognise the association himself. However, in the insidious presentation this is less likely although circumstantial evidence may be detected by the wary physician.

Tests of serum precipitins to antigens considered responsible for disease are useful in diagnosis. A positive precipitin test confirms a level of exposure to antigen of sufficient intensity to potentially cause the disease. Table 8.5 presents the results of surveys of serum precipitin tests with commonly involved antigens in unexposed persons, healthy exposed subjects, and exposed patients with extrinsic allergic alveolitis. Precipitin tests are negative in unexposed persons. They may be positive in healthy exposed subjects. This is more common in the pigeon fanciers where exposure is heavy and less common in persons keeping a budgie in the home where exposure is more limited. Patients with extrinsic allergic alveolitis, except in the case of bagassosis, usually have positive serum precipitin tests to the corresponding allergens. To this extent the precipitin test provides evidence to support the diagnosis. The strength of the precipitin reaction is of no help because it relates to the intensity of exposure and not to the severity of disease.

Allergy skin tests by prick and intracutaneous methods may be useful except in cases of disease due to the thermophilic actinomycetes. Extracts of these organisms cause reactions in unexposed and unaffected people as well as in patients with extrinsic allergic alveolitis.

Table 8.5. Precipitins % against relevant allergen extracts in unexposed subjects and in farmers, bird fanciers and bagasse workers

Extract	Unexposed	Exposed	
		Healthy	EAA
M. faeni	0	18	87–100
Pigeon	0	40	100
Budgerigar	0	5	85
T. vulgaris	0	0	64

Allergy skin tests with extracts of a series of common allergens are usually negative; extrinsic allergic alveolitis usually occurs in non-atopic individuals. However, tests with the particular offending allergen extract may induce small early responses. In one survey of bird fancier's lung skin tests with undiluted bird serum induced early responses in 27 per cent (Hargreave and Pepys, 1972). These responses indicate antibody production and support the diagnosis; however, inhalation challenges do not generally induce early respiratory responses. Intracutaneous tests are useful for the identification of late responses (Figure 8.14), which in one study of bird fancier's lung were observed in 84 per cent (Hargreave and Pepys, 1972). The late skin responses are usually preceded by early skin responses.

Inhalation tests with appropriate antigen extracts may confirm the diagnosis. They are unnecessary when the clinical diagnosis is well supported by a known source of allergen, typical clinical features, and positive precipitin or skin tests. However, they are essential to demonstrate the relevance of a new source of allergen or to confirm a diagnosis when the clinical features are atypical. The allergen inhalation test is safe when done carefully. It should be performed before considering lung biopsy.

Lung biopsy is useful when the patient has features of a chronic fibrosing lung disease and when the aetiology is unknown. The histological features in the early stages of disease differ from those of cryptogenic fibrosing alveolitis, while in the late fibrotic stage there may be no difference (Hinson, 1970). If the histological features resemble those of extrinsic allergic alveolitis renewed search for the allergen should be made.

Management and prognosis

Successful management requires the identification of the allergen and avoidance of exposure. The avoidance of exposure should be complete. For example, if there is a budgie in the house it should be removed, if the humidifier is contaminated it should be changed, or if the hay is mouldy the job location should be changed. In situations like the latter, improved methods may avoid the development of moulding of hay. In patients with diabetes insipidus who have become allergic to their treatment with porcine or bovine posterior pituitary snuff, synthetic lysine vasopressin may be used. Masks are an alternative to the avoidance of exposure only if they can filter the small particles responsible for the disease. If this filtration is not complete the reduced exposure may allow the insidious progression of disease.

Corticosteroids have been shown to inhibit the late skin and respiratory responses provoked by allergen challenge. Their mode of action in these instances is unknown. They should be used in any patient with persisting symptoms to hasten recovery and limit the development of fibrosis. A course of prednisone beginning with 30 mg daily, then reducing by 5 mg every week is usually sufficient. They could also be used to prevent the reaction following unavoidable exposure. However, it is unwise to use them as an alternative to the avoidance of exposure because in this situation the disease may progress insidiously. The effects of treatment should be followed by clinical and radiographic examination and by pulmonary function tests like the vital capacity and CO transfer factor.

Prognosis

The prognosis in terms of the systemic features of disease is universally good. Treatment is followed by the disappearance of febrile episodes, anorexia and malaise, and the recovery of lost weight. However, the prognosis for the recovery of pulmonary function depends upon the amount of fibrosis at the time of diagnosis. In early stages of disease when the chest radiograph is normal or shows only nodular shadows, treatment is followed by clearing of nodular shadows and improvement in lung volumes and CO transfer factor to normal or near-normal values. In the later stages of disease when there are honeycomb shadows and lung shrinkage some symptomatic improvement in cough and effort dyspnoea may occur but a persistence of symptoms can be expected and there is little or no change in the chest radiograph, lung volumes and CO transfer factor.

Cryptogenic Fibrosing Alveolitis

This condition includes cases described under the names of 'diffuse interstitial fibrosis of the lungs', 'Hamman–Rich syndrome', and 'interstitial pneumonia' (Scadding, 1973).

The clinical features are similar to those seen in the insidious presentation of extrinsic allergic alveolitis, but there tend to be some differences which are summarised in Table 8.4. The histological appearances also differ from extrinsic allergic alveolitis. In cryptogenic fibrosing alveolitis (Hinson, 1970; Scadding, 1973) there is an exudation of cells into alveolar spaces and an inflammatory thickening of alveolar walls with a strong tendency to fibrosis. When the former predominates the condition is called 'desquamative' while when the latter predominates it is called 'mural'. In the desquamative pattern large mononuclear cells fill and line the alveolar spaces in a uniform way. These often have the characteristics of granular pneumonocytes. Alveolar wall thickening is less pronounced and alveolar architecture tends to be maintained. In the mural pattern there are fewer cells in alveolar spaces, more alveolar wall thickening with collagenous fibrosis and, generally, distortion of alveolar structure. Granulomas and giant cells are not seen. Most cases show features which are intermediate between desquamative and mural patterns.

Diagnosis is based on the clinical picture and the lung biopsy appearances. Corticosteroids may produce improvement especially in the desquamative type.

Although the cause is unknown the condition is often associated with features considered to be characteristic of immunological disturbances (Turner-Warwick, 1972). These immunological features are as follows.

Cryptogenic fibrosing alveolitis frequently occurs in association with a number of diseases which are characterised by the presence of non-organ specific antibodies. These diseases include rheumatoid arthritis, systemic sclerosis, chronic active hepatitis, Sjogren's syndrome, dermatomyositis and polymyositis.

Non-organ specific antibodies, including rheumatoid factor (RF), anti-nuclear factor (ANF) and non-organ specific complement fixing antibodies, are found in about 60 per cent of cases of cryptogenic fibrosing alveolitis. RF is found in about one-third of cases, while ANF is found in another third. Both RF and ANF are usually found in low titre, except in those patients who also have rheumatoid arthritis. That these antibodies are not just an incidental consequence of the disease is suggested by their lower incidence in patients with other chronic fibrosing lung diseases like extrinsic allergic alveolitis and sarcoidosis.

The pathological processes may develop as a secondary event in lung disease which has been initiated by some external agent. For example, changes very similar to the desquamative type of fibrosing alveolitis have been seen to follow influenza infections, and nitrofurantoin hypersensitivity. However, in most cases of cryptogenic fibrosing alveolitis evidence for the involvement of external agents is lacking.

Alveolitis following Ingested Substances

Ingestion of the weed killer, Paraquat, and of gluten and of a number of drugs like busulphan, nitrofurantoin, PAS and sulphonamides may cause an alveolitis. The mechanisms are not understood and, in at least some instances, may be toxic rather than immunological.

PULMONARY EOSINOPHILIA

The term 'pulmonary eosinophilia', also called 'pulmonary infiltration with eosinophilia (or PIE) syndrome' is used here to indicate the occurrence of pulmonary shadows accompanied by a blood eosinophilia. The pulmonary shadows may or may not be the result of lung infiltration by eosinophils. The condition is often associated with asthma.

Pulmonary eosinophilia may be provoked by a number of fungi which grow in the lung, e.g. *Aspergillus*, *Candida*, *Mucor*, *Helminthosporium*, *Geotrichium*, *Blastomyces* and *Coccidiomyces*. Pulmonary eosinophilia also occurs in a few cases of extrinsic allergic alveolitis. It may be induced by a number of helminthic parasites, and by certain drugs and chemicals. In many cases, however, the cause is unknown and the condition has been referred to as 'cryptogenic pulmonary eosinophilia'.

Allergic Broncho-pulmonary Aspergillosis

The spores of the fungus *Aspergillus* are ubiquitous; they are present in low concentrations in the outside air but may attain high densities in certain environments like barns and breweries. Inhaled spores can become involved in a number of different types of lung disease. In the atopic sensitised subject the spores may provoke extrinsic asthma, or they may grow saprophytically in the airways and induce allergic broncho-pulmonary aspergillosis. In the non-atopic person inhalation of large numbers of spores can lead to extrinsic allergic alveolitis; alternatively, they may grow within a cavity to form a non-invasive fungus-ball (aspergilloma), or they may invade lung. The latter only occurs in patients with deficient immune defence mechanisms, as in patients with leukaemia or those receiving immunosuppressive treatment.

Allergic broncho-pulmonary aspergillosis (McCarthy and Pepys, 1971a) is due to the growth of *Aspergillus fumigatus* within medium-sized bronchi. It generally occurs in patients with a history of extrinsic asthma associated with allergy to other inhaled allergens. The condition is characterised by episodes of pulmonary infiltrations accompanied by blood and sputum eosinophilia. It is the commonest cause of pulmonary eosinophilia in the United Kingdom.

Clinical features

The symptoms include asthmatic symptoms, febrile episodes, expectoration of sputum plugs and pleurisy. The asthma is often severe, as might be expected to result from the continuous allergen exposure. The febrile episodes may occur in association with pleurisy and pulmonary infiltrations or separately, and they may be related to the condition or to separate bacterial infection. The sputum is often purulent and associated with bacterial infection, it is often blood streaked and it often contains plugs. These plugs appear as dirty green, brown or beige cylinders or pellets which are firm and average about 0·5 to 1·5 cm in size. When they are observed at bronchoscopy they may be firmly attached to the bronchial walls and require piece-meal dissection. The pleurisy occurs in association with pulmonary infiltrations.

The radiographic shadows (McCarthy, Simon and Hargreave, 1970) are of consolidation and collapse and tend to involve one or two areas near the hilum most commonly in the upper lobes (Figure 8.15). These shadows may resolve spontaneously or with treatment, but if persistent they may be followed by lung shrinkage and fibrosis. Parallel-line shadows wider than a normal

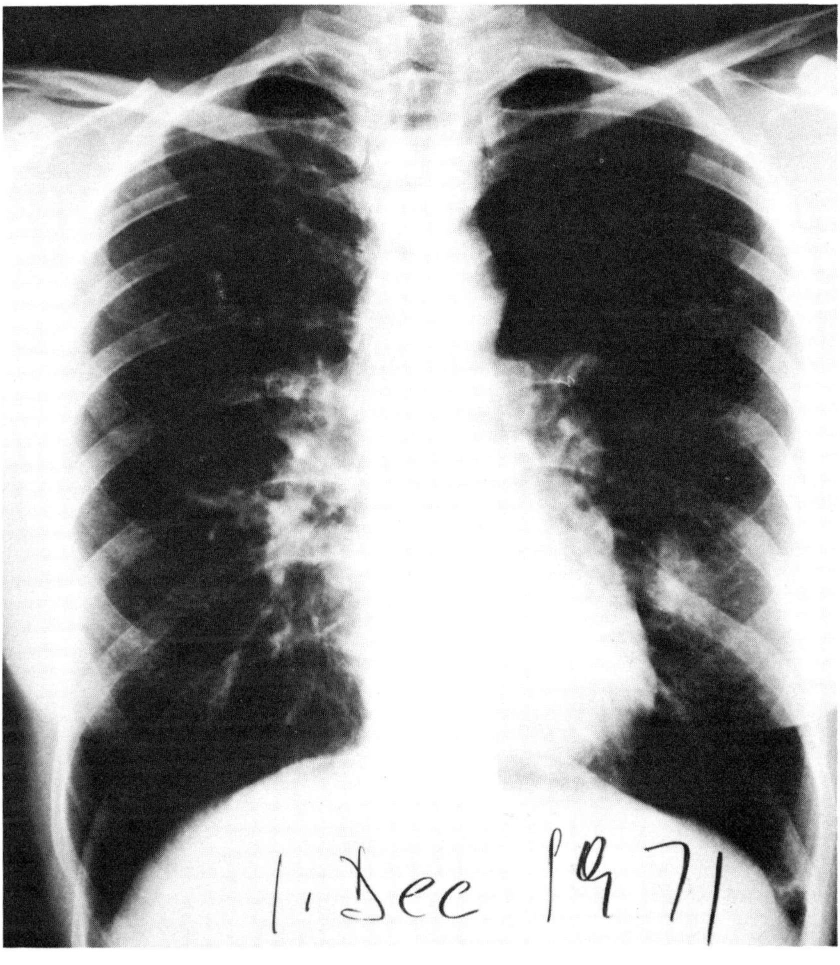

Figure 8.15. Chest radiograph in patient with allergic broncho-pulmonary aspergillosis showing the typical transient shadows.

bronchus may suggest the presence of bronchiectasis. Bronchograms demonstrate a characteristic bronchiectasis, in the region of sputum plugs, affecting proximal bronchi with the distal bronchi normally filled. The distal bronchi, however, may be damaged by secondary infection. Finger clubbing in association with this bronchiectasis is unusual. In a few patients there may be a cavity containing a mobile mass, suggesting an aspergilloma.

The total blood eosinophil counts found in association with the pulmonary infiltrations are elevated in the range of 500 to 2000/mm^3.

Pathology

The sputum plugs are composed chiefly of secretions, and they contain eosinophils and fungal mycelium. Bronchial wall biopsies show changes similar to those observed in asthma. In areas of consolidated lung there may be numerous eosinophils within the alveolar spaces (eosinophil pneumonia), or there may be changes like those observed in extrinsic allergic alveolitis (Chan-Yeung et al, 1971).

Mechanisms

Allergen inhalation tests with extracts of *A. fumigatus* provoke dual (early followed by late) asthmatic responses (McCarthy and Pepys, 1971b). The late responses are stronger and more prolonged than the early responses. They are associated with leucocytosis due to an increase in eosinophils and/or polymorphs and, in about half the cases, with fever. Inhalation tests do not provoke changes in the radiographical appearance of the lung. These radiographical appearances occur in relation to growth of *Aspergillus* and the formation of sputum plugs.

Skin tests with appropriate extracts (McCarthy and Pepys, 1971b) induce dual skin responses, similar in timing and macroscopic appearances to those described in the sections on asthma and extrinsic allergic alveolitis. Biopsies of the late skin responses have shown oedema, and infiltration with scanty polymorphonuclear neutrophils and scanty or moderate numbers of eosinophils. Granular deposits staining for IgG, IgM and IgA, and the beta-1c component of complement may be identified in mononuclear cells, in the perivascular tissues and in the vascular endothelium.

The respiratory features and the changes observed in skin tests with *Aspergillus* extracts have been attributed to types 1 and 3 allergic reactions. There are unusually high serum IgE concentrations and a correspondingly high level of type 1 allergy which is responsible for the early bronchial and skin responses. Late responses have generally been attributed to type 3 reactions. However, as discussed in the section on asthma, there is some evidence that the marked IgE-dependent sensitivity may confer the tendency to late responses. The timing of the late bronchial and skin responses, the occurrence of fever following inhalation challenge, the presence of *Aspergillus* specific precipitating IgG/IgM antibodies in the serum, and the demonstration of the fixation of complement in vascular endothelium in skin biopsies of late responses are all consistent with the possibility of a type 3 mechanism. Type 3 reactions lead to tissue damage, and the occurrence of bronchiectasis and fibrosis in the condition is evidence of a destructive process. Further evidence for the involvement of type 3 allergy has been obtained in passive transfer tests in monkeys. In these, skin and bronchial challenge tests with *Aspergillus* extracts provoked a late skin response and pulmonary infiltrations respectively in one monkey who had received serum from a patient with *Aspergillus* specific reaginic and precipitating antibodies, but not in another monkey who had received serum from a patient with reaginic antibodies only.

Diagnosis and investigation

The diagnosis should be suspected in any patient with pulmonary eosinophilia, and especially those with sputum plugs, pleurisy, transient episodes of consolidation and collapse, bronchiectasis, or radiographical evidence of pulmonary fibrosis. The condition may present with features consistent with pneumonia, tuberculosis, bronchiectasis or bronchial carcinoma. It may complicate cystic fibrosis (Mearns, Longbottom and Batten, 1967), and it may itself be complicated by an aspergilloma (McCarthy and Pepys, 1973a). Confirmation of the diagnosis is provided especially by skin and serological tests, and also by examination of the sputum.

Prick tests with suitable extracts of *A. fumigatus* induce early weal and flare skin responses in virtually all cases, and provide very useful support of the diagnosis. Late skin responses occur following prick tests in up to 25 per cent of cases, and following intracutaneous tests in virtually all patients. Precipitating antibodies can be demonstrated in double diffusion tests in most (92 per cent) cases. The intensity of the precipitin test reaction does not correlate with the severity of the disease, but rather with the intensity of exposure. Aspergillomas provide a particularly intense antigenic stimulus and this is reflected in the multiple lines observed in precipitin tests (McCarthy and Pepys, 1973a).

The sputum should be examined by sectioning and staining for mycelia, as well as by culture. The presence of mycelia in fresh specimens indicates that the organism is growing in the respiratory tract. Culture of the sputum is not a very useful test in diagnosis because cultures are negative in almost half the patients with the disease and they may sometimes be positive in patients with other chronic respiratory disease.

Allergen inhalation tests are not required for routine diagnosis.

Management

The patient should avoid environment with high concentrations of *Aspergillus* spores, e.g. barns, hay and grains.

Hyposensitisation with *Aspergillus* extracts is contraindicated because it is not effective and theoretically it could aggravate the disease by stimulating more IgG and IgM antibodies which contribute to the allergic reactions.

The value of antifungal agents has not been carefully studied. At the moment they are generally regarded as not effective. However, it would seem reasonable to try 5-fluorocytosine which can be taken by mouth.

The asthma should be treated with palliative drugs, taken in the minimum doses necessary to control symptoms. Often it cannot be controlled either by bronchodilators alone or together with disodium cromoglycate, and then corticosteroids are required. Both disodium cromoglycate and corticosteroids have been shown to inhibit the late asthmatic response, and their simultaneous use may reduce the required dose of the latter. The corticosteroids do not seem to enhance further growth of the fungus; in fact their use may contribute to an eradication of the disease, apparently by favouring removal of the fungus by expectoration.

The pulmonary shadows resemble pneumonia and this possibility should be remembered in treatment. They should probably be treated initially with antibiotics and chest physiotherapy, but if there is no response within 5 to 7 days corticosteroids should be added. In this situation prednisone 30 mg daily usually clears the shadows and the drug can be withdrawn rapidly providing that it is not required for treatment of the asthma. Bronchoscopy is not necessary unless collapse is persistent.

Prognosis

The course of the disease is very variable. The asthma is usually troublesome and often requires treatment with prednisone. Consolidation and collapse may occur once or repeatedly. Chest radiographs should be repeated at intervals to insure that further shadows have not recurred and persisted to cause progressive fibrosis.

Pulmonary Eosinophilia Induced by Parasites and Drugs

Pulmonary eosinophilia may be induced by a number of helminthic parasites (Crofton and Douglas, 1969; Liebow and Carrington, 1969) such as *Ascaris lumbricoides*, *Wucheria malayi*, *Dirofilaria immitis*, *Ankylostoma brasiliensis*, *Trichuris trichiura*, *Dispomium hepaticum*, *Taenia saginata* and *Toxacara*. The terms 'Loeffler's syndrome' or 'simple pulmonary eosinophilia' have been used for the condition in which there are wandering pulmonary infiltrations, blood eosinophilia which is usually mild, minimal or no respiratory symptoms and fever, and recovery within one month. 'Tropical eosinophilia' is the condition occurring in the tropics in which there are fever, weight loss, asthma, widespread finely nodular shadows, high blood eosinophilia, and response to treatment with organic arsenicals. It is probably frequently caused by filariasis.

The drugs which are known to cause pulmonary eosinophilia include para-aminosalicylic acid, nitrofurantoin, sulphonamides, penicillin, aspirin, hydrochlorthiazide and hydrallazine (Crofton and Douglas, 1969; Liebow and Carrington, 1969).

The mechanisms underlying the way that parasites and drugs cause these conditions is poorly understood. Skin sensitising and humoral antibodies may be demonstrated against extracts of the parasites.

Cryptogenic Pulmonary Eosinophilia

Pulmonary eosinophilia of unknown cause (McCarthy and Pepys, 1973b; Scadding, 1971b) sometimes complicates asthma but may occur in isolation. In contrast to allergic broncho-pulmonary aspergillosis, it is more common in women, the sputum is usually not prominent, sputum plugs are rare and bacterial infection is uncommon. Total blood eosinophil counts are generally between 2000 and 5000/mm^3. The pulmonary shadows tend to be multiple and peripheral (Figure 8.16), and bronchiectasis, lobar shrinkage and fibrosis are usually not present.

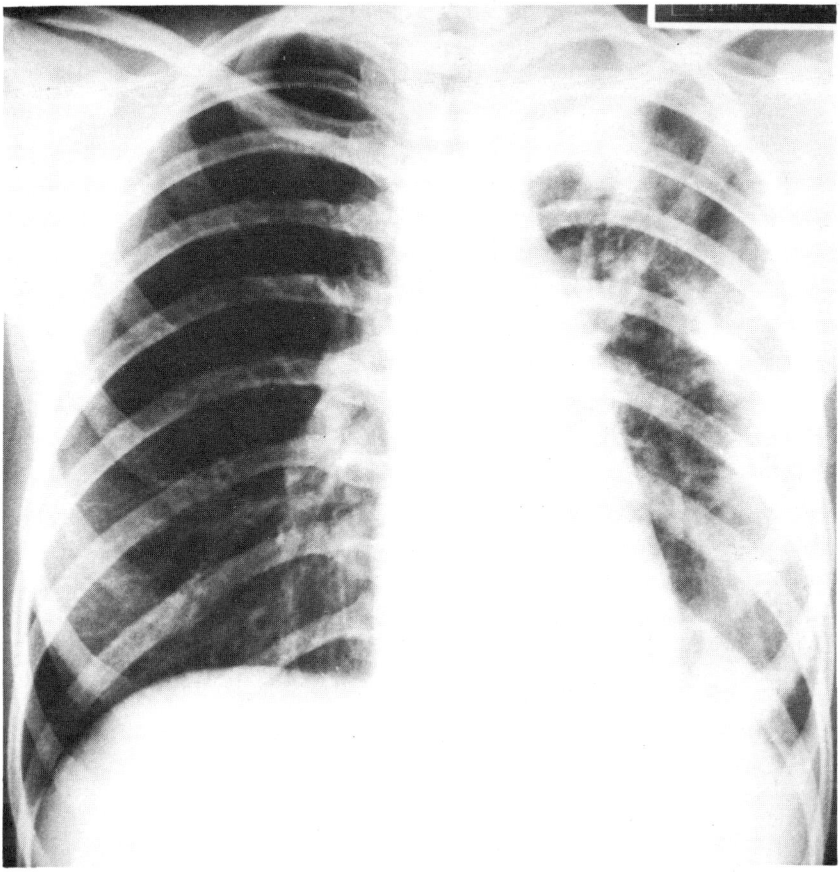

Figure 8.16. Chest radiograph in a patient with intrinsic asthma and cryptogenic pulmonary eosinophilia showing the typical widespread peripheral shadows.

Immunological mechanisms have not been demonstrated. Occasionally pulmonary vasculitis or systemic vasculitis are observed. Non-organ specific autoantibodies are usually not demonstrable.

The condition responds to treatment with corticosteroids.

OCCUPATIONAL LUNG DISEASE

Respiratory diseases provoked by airborne particles in occupational environments include asthma, byssinosis, extrinsic allergic alveolitis and mineral dust pneumoconioses. In many instances, the underlying allergic and non-allergic mechanisms involved are poorly understood.

Asthma

Airborne particles provoking asthma may stimulate the formation of reaginic or other antibodies which can be demonstrated by skin and serological tests.

These particles include fungal spores in agricultural environments such as *Cladosporium fulvum* which may infect tomato plants, *Bacillus subtilis* enzymes in the non-soap detergent industry, wood dusts like Western red cedar, and castor bean. In other instances, antibodies either cannot be demonstrated or have not yet been correlated with the disease. Examples include asthma from exposure to wood dusts, tolylene di-isocyanate in the manufacture of polyurethane products, the fumes of amino-ethyl ethanolamine in certain aluminium fluxes, piperazine dihydrochloride and complex salts of platinum.

Byssinosis

Byssinosis is the disease induced by the dust emitted during the processing of cotton, flax and soft hemp (*Cannibis sativa*) (Schilling, 1972). In cotton manufacture it may occur in workers removing seeds from picked cotton bolls, pressing the cotton into bales, cleaning and combing the fibres in the mixing and card rooms and in the spinning and winding rooms. Flax is used in the manufacture of linens and soft hemp in the making or ropes and twine.

The symptoms consist of chest tightness, dyspnoea, and cough. They initially occur on the first day of work after a weekend or other period away, often with onset near the end of a work-shift and improvement some time after leaving work. The symptoms may be associated with decreases in FEV_1, flow rates on maximum expiratory flow-volume curves and VC, while airways conductance changes little. As the disease progresses, symptoms recur on other days of the week. Finally, usually after many years of exposure, there is persisting and severe effort dyspnoea in association with irreversible airways obstruction which is not improved by giving up the work. At this stage, the illness has the usual features of chronic bronchitis and emphysema.

Antigen-induced respiratory responses appear to be similar in timing to the late asthmatic responses previously discussed. The mechanisms underlying them are not clear; however, both non-specific mechanisms and specific allergic reactions may be involved. The occurrence of non-specific mechanisms is suggested by the provocation of chest tightness and fall in ventilatory capacity by extracts of cotton dust and of the bracts of the cotton plant even in previously unexposed healthy subjects.

The diagnosis is based upon the clinical history, observed changes in ventilatory capacity and lung mechanics following natural exposure.

Extrinsic Allergic Alveolitis

The occupational exposures which induce this condition are listed in Table 8.3.

Mineral Dust Pneumoconioses

Workers exposed to coal dusts develop small pigmented deposits about which there is the development of focal emphysema but little or no fibrosis or hyaline deposit. This is simple pneumoconiosis of coal workers. The chest x-ray examination shows tiny nodulations which may coalesce into larger nodules. At this stage, there are no symptoms and physiologic studies are normal. The immunologic status of the worker is probably a major factor determining whether the occupational exposure will lead to progressive symptomatic lung disease (Turner-Warwick, 1972b). Caplan noted that coal miners with rheumatoid arthritis are especially susceptible to the development of pulmonary nodules. It was subsequently observed that a majority of workers with progressive massive fibrosis or complicated pneumoconiosis but no rheumatoid arthritis also had positive serum tests for rheumatoid factor.

Silicosis is induced by the chronic industrial inhalation of crystalline silica. There is a unique tendency to the production of fibrotic nodules in the lung. The silica has an irritant effect and induces damage to alveolar macrophages. The progressive form of silicosis referred to as conglomerate silicosis may be produced or aggravated by the presence of tuberculosis but in most cases, tuberculosis is probably not present.

Asbestosis may result from the occupational exposure to asbestos in mining and in various industrial applications. The inhaled particles induce a diffuse inflammation and fibroplasia in the peripheral airways leading to restrictive functional abnormalities. Some asbestos induces damage to alveolar macrophages in a manner similar to silica. There is an increased frequency of rheumatoid and antinuclear factors in patients with asbestosis. The greatly increased risk of bronchogenic carcinoma and pleural mesothelioma remains unexplained.

Berylliosis is a diffuse granulomatous lung disease which develops insidiously either in isolation or after acute symptoms relating to the inhalation of beryllium. Stimulation by beryllium sulphate of lymphoblast transformation of peripheral lymphocytes of affected individuals but not control individuals (Deodhar, Barna and VanOrdstrand, 1973) suggest that type 4 hypersensitivity is involved in the disease process.

PULMONARY VASCULITIS

Conditions which are associated with generalised vasculitis such as serum sickness, allergic angiitis and systemic lupus erythematosus can also involve the lung. The so-called allergic granulomatosis of Churg and Strauss is a form of vasculitis which appears to develop as a complication of asthma. Polyarteritis nodosa, while a generalised disease, tends to spare the lung.

Wegener's granulomatosis involves the lower respiratory tract and, less frequently, the upper respiratory tract with necrotising granuloma (Fauci and Wolff, 1973). The disease is associated with glomerulonephritis and less frequently with widespread disseminated vasculitis. It may, however, be limited to the upper respiratory tract. The most common glomerular lesion is one of focal glomerulonephritis. A coarse granular deposition of IgG and beta 1c in the glomeruli may be demonstrated. Virtually any system of the body may be involved in the disease. Wegener's granulomatosis has previously been considered to have a uniformly bad prognosis. The prognosis is now greatly improved, perhaps due to diagnosis of milder cases but certainly, in addition, due to the treatment regimens now employed. Adrenal corticosteroids and particularly cytotoxic agents such as cyclophosphamide used in sufficient suppressive dosage may produce prolonged remissions which ultimately may be maintained after medical treatment is discontinued.

GOODPASTURE'S SYNDROME

Goodpasture's syndrome is characterised by glomerulonephritis and haemorrhagic pneumonia with recurring hemoptysis, typically in young males. The glomerulonephritis is often rapidly progressive. There are linear deposits of IgG and beta 1c on the glomerular and alveolar basement membranes. The relevance of these immunological reactants in the disease has been convincingly demonstrated. Immunoglobulins eluted from affected kidneys have been shown to bind to glomerular basement membrane and to fix complement in vitro and to produce severe glomerulonephritis when infused into monkeys.

The prognosis is poor but prolonged survival may occur. Adrenal corticosteroids and cytotoxic drugs may control the disease. In some instances, the pulmonary disease may be persistent despite this medical treatment but may subside following bilateral nephrectomy, followed by chronic haemodialysis.

References

Bazaral, M., Orgel, A. & Hamburger, R. N. (1971) IgE levels in normal infants and mothers and an inheritance hypothesis. *Journal of Immunology*, **107,** 794–801.

Bryant, D. H., Burns, M. W. & Lazarus, L. (1973) New type of allergic asthma due to IgG 'reaginic' antibody. *British Medical Journal*, **iv,** 589–592.

Chan-Yeung, Moira, Chase, W. H., Trapp, W. & Grzybowski, S. (1971) Allergic bronchopulmonary aspergillosis. *Chest*, **59,** 33–39.

Ciba Foundation Guest Symposium (1959) Terminology, definitions and classification of chronic pulmonary emphysema and related conditions. *Thorax*, **14,** 286–299.

Clark, T. J. H. (1972) Effect of beclomethasone dipropionate delivered by aerosol in patients with asthma. *Lancet*, **i,** 1361–1364.

Coca, A. F. & Cooke, R. A. (1923) On the classification of the phenomena of hypersensitiveness. *Journal of Immunology*, **8,** 163–182.

Crofton, J. & Douglas, A. (1969) *Respiratory Diseases.* Oxford and Edinburgh: Blackwell Scientific Publications, pp. 425–434.

Davis, D. J. (1972). NIAID initiatives in allergy research. *Journal of Allergy and Clinical Immunology*, **49,** 323–328.

Deodhar, S. D., Barna, B & VanOrdstrand, H. S. (1973). A study of the immunologic aspects of berylliosis. *Chest*, **63,** 309–313.

Dolovich, J., Hargreave, F. E., Chalmers, R., Shier, K. J., Gauldie, J. & Bienenstock, J. (1973) Late cutaneous allergic responses in isolated IgE-dependent reactions. *Journal of Allergy and Clinical Immunology*, **52,** 38–46.

Dunnill, M. S. (1971) The pathology of asthma. In *Identification of Asthma* (Eds.) Porter, R. & Birch, J., pp. 35–46. Ciba Foundation Study Group No. 38. Edinburgh and London: Churchill Livingstone.

Fauci, A. S. & Wolff, S. M. (1973) Wegener's granulomatosis: studies in 18 patients and a review of the literature. *Medicine*, **52,** 535–561.

Fink, J. N., Moore, V. L. & Barboriak, J. J. (1974) Cell-mediated and humoral responses in pigeon breeders' disease. *Journal of Allergy and Clinical Immunology*, **53,** 85 (abs.).

Green, G. M. (1970) In defense of the lung. *American Review of Respiratory Disease*, **102,** 691–703.

Hargreave, F. E., Dolovich, J., Robertson, D. G. & Kerigan, A. T. (1974) The late asthmatic responses. *Canadian Medical Association Journal*, **110,** 415–424.

Hargreave, F. E. & Pepys, J. (1972) Allergic respiratory reactions in bird fanciers provoked by allergen inhalation provocation tests. *Journal of Allergy and Clinical Immunology*, **50,** 157–173.

Hensley, J. T., Fink, J. N. & Barboriak, J. J. (1974) Hypersensitivity pneumonitis in the monkey. *Archives of Pathology*, **97,** 33–38.

Hinson, K. F. W. (1970) Diffuse pulmonary fibrosis. *Human Pathology*, **1,** 275–288.

Hubscher, T. & Eisen, A. H. (1973) An eosinophil derived inhibitor (EDI) of histamine release. *Journal of Allergy and Clinical Immunology*, **51,** 83–84. (abs.).

Hyde, H. A. (1972) Atmospheric pollen grains and spores in relation to allergy I. *Clinical Allergy*, **2,** 153–179.

Leskowitz, S., Salvaggio, J. E. & Schwartz, H. J. (1972) An hypothesis for the development of atopic allergy in man. *Clinical Allergy*, **2,** 237–246.

Liebow, A. A. & Carrington, C. B. (1969) The eosinophilic pneumonias. *Medicine*, **48,** 251–285.

Lowell, F. C. (1967) Clinical aspects of eosinophilia in atopic disease. *Journal of the American Medical Association*, **202,** 875–878.

Marsh, D. G., Bias, W. D., Hsu, S. H. & Goodfriend, L. (1973) Association of HL–A7 cross-reacting group with a specific reaginic antibody response in allergic man. *Science*, **179,** 691–693.

McCarthy, D. S. & Pepys, J. (1971a) Allergic broncho-pulmonary aspergillosis. Clinical immunology; (1) Clinical features. *Clinical Allergy*, **1,** 261–286.

McCarthy, D. S. & Pepys, J. (1971b) Allergic broncho-pulmonary aspergillosis. Clinical immunology; (2) Skin, nasal and bronchial tests. *Clinical Allergy*, **1,** 415–432.

McCarthy, D. S. & Pepys, J. (1973a) Pulmonary aspergilloma. *Clinical Immunology*, **3,** 57–70.

McCarthy, D. S. & Pepys, J. (1973b) Cryptogenic pulmonary eosinophilias. *Clinical Allergy*, **3,** 339–351.

McCarthy, D. S., Simon, G. & Hargreave, F. E. (1970) The radiological appearances in allergic broncho-pulmonary aspergillosis. *Clinical Radiology*, **21,** 366–375.

Mearns, M., Longbottom, J. & Batten, J. (1967) Precipitating antibodies to Aspergillus fumigatus in cystic fibrosis. *Lancet*, **i,** 538–539.

Middleton, E. (1972) Autonomic imbalance in asthma with special reference to beta adrenergic blockade. In *Advances in Internal Medicine* (Ed.) Stollerman, G. H., volume 18, pp. 177–197. Memphis: Year Book Medical Publishers.

Muir, D. C. F. (1972) Airborne allergens. In *Clinical Aspects of Inhaled Particles.* (Ed.) Muir, D. C. F., pp. 54–69. London: William Heinemann Medical Books.

Parker, C. W. & Snider, D. E. (1973) Prostoglandins and asthma. *Annals of Internal Medicine*, **78,** 963–965.

Pepys, J. (1959) *Hypersensitivity Diseases of the Lungs due to Fungi and Organic Dusts.* Switzerland: Karger.

Phills, J. A., Pearlmutter, L. & Liakopoulou, A. (1972) Employment of the rat mast cell technique to separate immunologic from nonimmunologic types of allergic reactions to aspirin. *Journal of Allergy and Clinical Immunology*, **49,** 97 (abs.).

Rackemann, F. M. (1940) Intrinsic asthma. *Journal of Allergy*, **11,** 147–162.

Reed, C. E. (1974) Abnormal autonomic mechanisms in asthma. *Journal of Allergy and Clinical Immunology*, **53,** 34–41.

Robertson, D. G., Kerigan, A. T., Hargreave, F. E., Chalmers, R. & Dolovich, J. (1974) Late asthmatic responses induced by ragweed pollen allergen. *Journal of Allergy and Clinical Immunology*, **54,** 244–254.

Scadding, J. G. (1971a) The definition of asthma: general introduction. In *Identification of Asthma.* (Eds.) Porter, R. & Birch, J., pp. 13–34. Ciba Foundation Study Group No. 38. Edinburgh and London: Churchill Livingstone.

Scadding, J. G. (1971b) Eosinophilic infiltrations of the lungs in asthmatics. *Proceedings of the Royal Society of Medicine*, **64,** 381–392.

Scadding, J. G. (1973) Diffuse pulmonary alveolar fibrosis. *Therapeutische Umschau/Revue Therapeutique*, **30,** 191–198.

Schilling, R. S. F. (1972) Byssinosis. In *Clinical Aspects of Inhaled Particles.* (Ed.) Muir, D. C. F., pp. 70–84. London: William Heinemann Medical Books.

Speizer, F. E., Doll, R. & Heaf, P. (1968) Observations on recent increase in mortality from asthma. *British Medical Journal*, **i,** 335–339.

Tada, T. & Ishizaka, K. (1970) Distribution of γ E-forming cells in lymphoid tissues of the human and monkey. *Journal of Immunology*, **104,** 377–387.

Taylor, B., Norman, A. P., Orgel, H. A., Stokes, C. R., Turner, M. W. & Soothill, J. F. (1973) Transient IgA deficiency and pathogenesis of infantile atopy. *Lancet*, **ii,** 111–113.

Taylor, G. & Shivalkar, P. R. (1971) 'Arthus-type' reactivity in the nasal airways and skin in pollen sensitive subjects. *Clinical Allergy*, **1,** 407–414.

Tomasi, T. B. & Bienenstock, J. (1968) Secretory immunoglobins. In *Advances in Immunology*. (Ed.) Dixon, F. J. & Kunkel, H. G., volume 9, pp. 1–96. New York: Academic Press.

Turner-Warwick, M. (1972a) Cryptogenic fibrosing alveolitis. *British Journal of Hospital Medicine*, **7,** 697–704.

Turner-Warwick, M. (1972b) Immunology of the respiratory tract. *British Journal of Hospital Medicine*, **8,** 19–25.

Villar, T. G., Avila Ramiro & Telles de Araujo, A. (1973) Pulmonary granulomatoses due to inhaled particles: personal experience and some immunological considerations. *Clinical Allergy*, **3,** 217–223.

Wenzel, F., Emanuel, D. & Gray, R. (1971) Immunofluorescent studies of the lung in patients with farmer's lung. *Journal of Allergy*, **47,** 102–103 (abs.).

9. Allergic Disease of the Upper Respiratory Tract

GEOFFREY TAYLOR

Allergic disease of the upper respiratory tract is usually termed allergic rhinitis. It also commonly involves the paranasal sinuses and the conjunctivae. The condition may be defined as an acute, recurrent, non-specific, inflammatory disease of the nasal airways due to acquired reactivity to an exogenous antigen (allergen). In this definition the term 'acute inflammatory' is used in the broadest sense. The condition is very common, but the precise incidence is impossible to determine. Not only is the outward conformation of the nose highly individual, but also the day to day behaviour of the nasal airways is subject to considerable personal variation. How often need one sneeze to be abnormal? What are the normal limits of nasal mucus secretion? The interpretation of normality versus abnormality, which determines whether an individual seeks medical advice, depends on his previous experience both of himself and of his fellows. Some individuals will complain of abnormal nasal function with symptoms which others would accept as normal. Others will not complain even if nasal discharge and obstruction are present all the time. Such considerations clearly prevent an accurate estimate of incidence, and may well account for the apparently higher incidence of allergic upper respiratory tract disease in more affluent populations who will seek medical aid with less obvious disease.

Although not a serious disease, allergic rhinitis can produce considerable discomfort, occasionally of sufficient degree to cause a relatively unstable adult sufferer to contemplate suicide. It is often ignored or misdiagnosed, particularly in children, who are considered to have 'catarrh' or recurrent colds. It is important that a correct diagnosis be made because treatment is effective and also because as one marker of the atopic state the occurrence of allergic rhinitis carries implications for the future of the sufferer.

CLINICAL PRESENTATION

Patients classically suffer from the triad of nasal irritation with sneezing, nasal discharge and nasal obstruction although the emphasis on each of these symptoms may vary. Patients may be grouped into those with mainly sneezing and nasal discharge, and those in whom obstruction is the major problem. The incidence of 'blockers' tends to increase with age, being relatively less common in childhood than in older patients. The type of reaction observed may change over the years in an individual patient, and again, an individual may have predominantly sneezing and rhinorrhoea on exposure to one allergen and yet nasal obstruction to another. It is possible that different mechanisms are involved in causing the two types of reaction, and also that the two types carry a different prognosis and call for differences in therapy.

Symptoms may occur under very specific circumstances, such as handling a pet animal, or may only occur during certain months of the year—seasonal allergic rhinitis—or may occur throughout the whole year—perennial rhinitis. The symptoms of allergic rhinitis are commonly associated with evidence of allergic reactivity at other sites. Allergic blepharo-conjunctivitis is common, particularly in patients with seasonal rhinitis, and infantile eczema is often present in children in whom onset of allergic rhinitis is early. The association between allergic rhinitis and asthma is too familiar to be stressed further, but less obvious evidence of lower respiratory tract hypersensitivity is even more common. The occurrence of a dry irritating cough in association with allergic rhinitis commonly precedes overt asthma as does mild exercise-induced asthma.

NATURAL HISTORY

There is considerable individual variation in the course of the disease. The age of onset varies from the extremes of a few months of age to over 60 years, although the latter is very uncommon. Many patients begin to have symptoms before puberty, and there is a further large group who do not start to be troubled until the late 'teens' or early twenties. Spontaneous 'cures' are relatively common and a history of past allergic rhinitis will often be elicited in an older patient presenting for the first time with asthma. The rhinitis may predate the asthma by several decades. Remission of allergic rhinitis, particularly around the age of twenty, will sometimes be followed by a recurrence in later life. Often patients will continue to have symptoms without great change over many years.

The pattern of nasal sensitivity may also change with time; sensitivity to one allergen waning and another sensitivity becoming clinically more important. Not only may this changing pattern be observed in childhood when it might be assumed that immunological experience of environmental allergens is being gained, but may also be seen in adults. In the latter case acquisition of further sensitivities may be associated with obvious change in environment or may appear to be spontaneous.

As already mentioned, some patients when first seen will already have associated asthma and others often will develop asthma at a later date. Often an inverse relationship is seen in which as the allergic rhinitis has improved lower respiratory tract symptoms have become more prominent. It is not possible at the moment to define which individuals will undergo spontaneous cure, which will continue with allergic rhinitis, and which will develop clinically obvious asthma. In general, sensitisation to multiple allergens and a strong family history of allergic disease tend to be associated with continuation of allergic disease of both the upper and lower respiratory tract, and such individuals tend not to recover spontaneously. Too little research effort has so far been devoted to attempts to understand the reasons for the individual variation in the natural history of allergic respiratory tract disease. Such studies are likely to be very profitable.

PATHOGENESIS AND PATHOGENETIC MECHANISMS

Allergic rhinitis is one of the diseases included by Coca and Cooke (1923) as part of the atopic state. As is well recognised, atopy is 'subject to hereditary influence' but whilst there is a familial clustering of asthma, rhinitis and eczema, the mode of inheritance is so far unknown. One reason for the difficulty may be related to the multiplicity of abnormalities found in atopics, each of which may be inherited separately.

It is now well established that the major immunoglobulin class responsible for type 1 (anaphylactic) reactions in man is IgE. Combination of allergen with this immunoglobulin in its mast-cell-bound state results in release of mast cell granules and initiates a complex sequence of events in which a number of vasoactive agents provoke the capillary and smooth muscle changes observed. There is significant correlation between the concentration of circulating IgE and the number of positive weal and flare skin reactions to 'common allergens', the latter being used by some workers as an index of 'atopic status'. It is therefore reasonable to assume that one abnormality of an atopic subject is his greater propensity for producing antibody in the IgE class. This is, however, not the sole abnormality.

There is a growing evidence that atopic subjects have a diminished ability to mount a secretory IgA (SIgA) response. This has been observed in adults by Salvaggio et al (1973) who compared the SIgA response in nasal mucus following nasal instillation of tetanus toxoid in normals and atopics. It has also been demonstrated that nasal mucus from both atopic and non-atopic individuals contains SIgA directed against environmental allergens and is capable of blocking allergen-induced histamine release from sensitised leucocytes (Turk, Lichtenstein and Norman, 1970). These workers did not show any consistent difference between the two groups; however, a major problem in interpretation is the lack of a 'reference point' against which to quantitate any activity present in nasal mucus.

Taylor et al (1973) have investigated serum IgA levels in the children of atopic parents and have observed a delayed maturation of IgA production in those infants who subsequently developed clinical allergic disease as compared with those who did not. From the opposite viewpoint, selective IgA deficiency is not rare, and such subjects have an increased incidence of allergic disease (Kaufman and Hobbs, 1970; Schwartz and Buckley, 1971).

If the atopic does tend to have an impaired SIgA response to mucosally applied environmental allergens then several problems can be resolved. An individual with allergic rhinitis very often develops neither symptomatic nor objective changes on nasal challenge until a particular critical dose of allergen is applied. This phenomenon may be frequently observed in grass pollen sensitive individuals naturally challenged during the summer months. Some respond only when the pollen concentration is very high and have a 'short season', whilst others respond to low concentrations and have symptoms over the whole of the summer. It is difficult to explain this phenomenon solely on the IgE-mast cell model. Binding of allergen to SIgA in nasal mucus with passage through the mucous membrane only when the mucus is fully saturated could account for the 'threshold' effect. Again, those individuals with no detectable nasal sensitivity yet undoubted mast cell sensitivity as shown by positive skin tests could be explained on the basis of a specific mucosal block to allergen entry due to restoration (or full maturation) of an impaired local SIgA response. The author has suggested (Taylor and Shivalkar, 1972; Taylor, 1973) that local nasal desensitisation may operate by this mechanism, and hence be analogous to a 'spontaneous' cure.

Evidence to implicate other immunological abnormalities in atopic individuals is presented by Taylor (1973). Comparing the amount of complement fixing (CF) antibody against a grass pollen antigen in normal and pollen sensitive subjects a significant difference was observed. The atopics produced far less than non-atopics and there was an inverse relationship between an objective assessment of nasal sensitivity and the amount of CF antibody detected. This observation suggests a difference in antigen handling in atopics and non-atopics, but it is not possible to be sure whether this is a primary difference or is due to modification brought about by an IgE-mast cell reaction at the portal of entry. Thus, in summary, the atopic appears to produce greater quantities of IgE and smaller amounts of SIgA and complement-fixing IgG. It is unlikely that all these differences stem from the expression of a single gene and it is likely that an individual inherits some or all of these various abnormalities independently. This would account for the difficulties in understanding the inheritance of atopic disease and also for the great variation in disease presentation and course in different individuals.

NERVOUS CONTROL OF THE NASAL AIRWAYS

As discussed in Chapter 8 (p. 244) the lower airways are under the control of the autonomic nervous system. This control may operate by influencing the tone of the smooth muscle of the airways and also in the context of allergic airways disease by influencing the output of mediators. Similar principles apply in the upper airways; however, there are added complications. The nasal mucous membrane, particularly over the tubinates, behaves as an erectile tissue. Mucosal thickness is largely dependent on the amount of blood contained in the venous sinuses. This may be varied at the level of the afferent arterioles, at arterio-venous anastamoses and directly on the thick-walled, muscular, venous sinuses. In the abnormal situation of rhinitis, mucosal thickness will also be influenced by the amount of exudation from capillaries into the interstitial tissue. Stimulation of the alpha adrenoreceptors results in decreased mucosal thickness with decrease in nasal airways resistance. Blockage of the alpha receptors results in the reverse effect and is seen as a complication of the treatment of hypertension by alpha-blocking agents. These effects are probably mediated via the afferent arterioles. Beta-stimulants produce engorgement of the mucous membrane with increase in nasal airways resistance and beta-blockade a great reduction in resistance. These latter effects are probably brought about by changes in tone of the muscle of the venous sinuses. The nasal glands are supplied by cholinergic nerve fibres, and there is also some cholinergic innervation of the arterio-venous anastamoses. The effect of cholinergic stimulation is to increase the output of mucus and also to increase nasal mucosal thickness. The nervous controls described are involved in the normal changes in nasal patency and mucus output brought about by variation in the temperature and humidity of inspired air, in diurnal variation and in the alternating changes in the patency of the two sides of the airways which take place frequently. In health these nervous pathways may be involved also in the response of the nasal airways to non-specific irritants.

There is good evidence that the atopic individual has some degree of autonomic imbalance and behaves as though he were partially beta-blockaded (p. 246). In the context of the upper respiratory tract such a situation produces increased nasal patency. As an individual with rhinitis usually has nasal obstruction it might be assumed that the effect of the blockade of beta adreno-receptors operates mainly on the output of mediators rather than directly on the smooth muscle of the blood vessels. As with the lower airways, the nose of an atopic individual responds differently from the normal to the administration of a variety of stimuli. These include more violent responses to temperature and humidity changes, non-specific irritants and histamine. This difference in response is likely a function of autonomic imbalance, but precisely at what level this operates is unclear. It is important to make allowance for the greater nasal response of an atopic individual to non-specific stimuli and not immediately to assume a further specific sensitivity.

INVESTIGATION AND DIAGNOSIS

A detailed history is of paramount importance. One major object is to attempt to determine the likely causative allergens. The association of symptoms with specific locale, certain activities, with variations in climatic conditions and with the seasons of the year may point to particular environmental allergens. What appear on first hearing as highly improbable associations should not be ignored; they may well provide valuable clues. In such circumstances it may prove necessary to investigate the potential allergens in the patient's own environment before the reason for an unusual association is clarified. Experience of the distribution and seasonal incidence of the many potential allergens is necessary for the interpretation of the history of allergic respiratory tract disease.

A family history of allergic disease gives a useful index of prognosis and should include where possible two generations. The pattern of progress of a patient is very often similar to that of an affected relative. The previous medical history, particularly of the patient's response to infective conditions, is also pertinent. An association is recognised between IgA deficiency and allergic disease, and a history of frequent, and particularly severe, respiratory tract infections, particularly in childhood, should direct attention to this possibility. Serum immunoglobulin determinations should be carried out in such patients, but this should not be considered as a routine test in all sufferers.

The relationship of frequent tonsillitis often leading to tonsillectomy and allergic upper respiratory tract disease also deserves mention. The onset of allergic disease shortly after tonsillectomy is relatively common. Whether removal of the tonsillar lymphoid tissue has resulted in increased mucosal permeability to antigen by impairing the local secretory IgA response or that individuals with poor IgA responsiveness ab initio have a greater tendency to develop both allergic disease and to suffer recurrent infections is still problematical. The second possibility seems on current evidence to be more likely.

Clinical examination of patients suffering from allergic rhinitis is often perfunctory. Full clinical examination is desirable and examination of the nasal airways, where possible including the post-nasal space, is essential. The presence of nasal polypi, and in children of foreign bodies, is clearly important and the typical appearance of the turbinates in allergic rhinitis is useful confirmation of the diagnosis. Examination of nasal secretions for the presence of eosinophils is a valuable test. Whilst the presence of eosinophils is considered to be confirmatory of a diagnosis of allergic rhinitis, their absence does not exclude such a diagnosis. Eosinophils may be apparently absent or very scanty in some patients. Peripheral blood eosinophilia is common, particularly in patients with multiple sensitivities and with associated allergic disease in sites other than the upper respiratory tract. In patients with isolated allergic rhinitis the peripheral blood eosinophil count is often within normal limits, and therefore cannot be used to exclude allergic disease in a patient presenting with nasal symptoms.

Skin testing, usually using the 'modified prick technique,' is traditional in the investigation of allergic rhinitis. This method of testing is to be preferred to either scratch or intradermal methods as it results in fewer false positive tests, and is rather easier to read. Commercially available extracts are usually used, although under some circumstances home-made extracts will be needed. These are easily produced, but very difficult to standardise. Currently much effort is being devoted to better methods of standardisation of allergen extracts using in vitro IgE binding methods. These are likely to help considerably with skin test and hyposensitisation preparations. Certainly at the moment there is some variation in skin test potency between allergen preparations obtained both from the same and from different manufacturers. This does not usually lead to great difficulties of interpretation.

The clinical history provides a useful guide to the range of skin test allergens to be used. It is preferable to include not only the most likely allergens but also other possibilities as surprises are not uncommon. The skin of the back or of the forearms is usually used for skin testing. The same degree of response is not found over the whole of the skin and whilst the latter is the more convenient site, the skin of the back probably gives more satisfactory results. Responses are read after 15 to 20 minutes as the area or average diameter of the weal and of the flare and should be compared with a negative vehicle control and a positive histamine phosphate control. 'Late' skin responses which appear after about 4 hours and may persist for 12 to 24 hours may also occur following skin testing either by the intradermal or the modified prick testing methods. These are larger and more diffuse than weal and flare responses. Late skin reactions of this type correlate with 'late' nasal reactivity (vide infra).

Whilst a positive weal and flare response provides an index of systemic type 1 (anaphylactic) sensitivity to particular allergens, it is important to appreciate the limitations of this information in relation to respiratory tract sensitivity. The response represents the outcome of the interaction of allergen with IgE sensitised mast cells in the skin. IgE is not produced in the skin but in the mucous membrane-associated lymphoid tissue of the respiratory tract and the intestines, i.e. near to the sites of major allergen entry. As IgE has great binding affinity for mast cells the tendency is for it to bind near to its site of production; that which is found in the circulation and hence is available to bind to skin mast cells representing 'over-spill'. Thus it is possible to find sensitive mucous membranes of the upper and lower respiratory tracts without raised serum IgE levels or positive skin tests. This is particularly common in children and probably represents an early phase of sensitisation—the skin tests usually becoming positive a variable time after mucosal sensitivity has been established.

Competition for IgE binding sites on mast cells between antibodies of different specificities has been demonstrated in experimental animals by Jarrett, Orr and Riley (1971). The poor 'acceptance' of human IgE by the skin of some individuals on P-K testing and the inability to carry out P-K testing in an individual with an IgE myeloma probably represents such competition in human skin. Competition for mast cell IgE binding sites in the skin takes place between IgE molecules of different specificities derived from both the intestines and the respiratory tract. The range of specificities produced in these two regions of major production is likely to be very different and hence local mucosal sensitivity, determined mainly by local production, will be different both quantitatively and often qualitatively from that found in the more competitive situation of the skin. Such factors probably account for the poor *quantitative* correlation between the degree of sensitivity of mucous membrane and skin. A correlation coefficient of only 0·026 was observed by the author when objective quantitative measurement of the skin and nasal sensitivity were studied in pollen sensitive subjects (Taylor, 1973).

The finding of a positive weal and flare reaction to an allergen in the absence of nasal (or bronchial) sensitivity also occurs. This is not uncommonly found in patients who have undergone spontaneous cure of allergic rhinitis. The mechanisms operating are not yet clear but may involve competition for allergen either at the mucosal level by specific secretory IgA or by 'blocking' IgG in the mucous membrane. Alternatively strong competition for mast cell IgE binding sites by antibody of a different specificity produced locally may decrease mucosal sensitivity to another antigen without greatly influencing skin reactivity.

In summary, weal and flare skin responses should be interpreted with circumspection. They provide a useful part of the investigation of the patient with allergic rhinitis but should be viewed alongside the history and the limitations of the information they provide should be appreciated.

Measurement of serum concentrations of IgE though valuable as a research tool is not particularly helpful in the routine diagnosis and management of allergic rhinitis. Levels tend to correlate with atopic status; high levels being associated with multiple positive skin tests. In individual cases of allergic rhinitis the IgE concentration may be within normal limits. Measurement of specific IgE in serum using the radio-allergosorbent test (RAST) (Wide, Bennich and Johansson, 1967) produces results which correlate well with skin sensitivity (Stenius et al, 1971). This would be expected. Significant correlation of the specific IgE content of serum with the clinical manifestations of the disease at target tissue level are not found (Kumar et al, 1971; Stenius, Wide and Seymour, 1972). Thus the information obtained by examining serum for specific IgE antibody adds very little to the information obtained more easily by skin testing. The results have similar limitations to skin testing as far as airways sensitivity is concerned.

Of much greater value in the investigation of allergic rhinitis are nasal challenge tests. These may be either qualitative or quantitative in nature. Qualitative techniques involve applying an extract to the nasal mucosa and observing the reaction by the appearance of nasal mucous membrane, by sneezing, nasal irritation, nasal discharge and obstruction. Quantitative methods involve measuring changes in nasal airflow following challenge.

Allergens may be applied in a number of ways, but it is important to avoid, where possible, entry into the lower respiratory tract. Allergens are usually applied as aqueous extracts, but some workers have used particulate material, e.g. pollen grains, sometimes diluted with inactive carrier particles for ease of handling. An alternative method is to use small filter paper discs impregnated with allergen extracts. These may be dried before use. Aqueous extracts may be applied directly to the nasal mucous membrane as drops from a pipette, using a thin glass rod dipped in an extract and then drained and applied to the inferior turbinates, or as aerosols. The latter method is more reproducible in adults and older children but requires patient cooperation. The aerosol spray is applied through each nostril in turn with the patient in full inspiration. After application he breath-holds for 30 sec before exhaling through the nose. In this way penetration to the lower respiratory tract is minimised and asthmatic reactions have been rare. Using aerosol challenge it is pointless to challenge one side of the nasal airways and to assume that the other side will act as control. Reactions almost inevitably occur bilaterally. Even with carefully applied solutions or particles, reflex changes will occur on the unchallenged side. It is difficult to define the correct concentration of allergen to use, partly because there is no satisfactory method for the standardistaion of allergen extracts, and partly because patients' local sensitivity vary so greatly. The latter is best evaluated before challenge by an assessment of the severity of the patient's rhinitis rather than in relation to his skin tests. It is preferable to err on the side of safety rather than to use a highly concentrated preparation, particularly when using the aerosol spray method. Rather higher concentrations may be used when the allergen is applied directly to the nasal mucous membrane using a pipette or a glass rod.

Quantitative methods involve measuring changes in nasal flow following administration of allergen and are valuable in that they give an objective measure of nasal sensitivity. This is useful in investigating changes taking place in a patient either as a result of therapy or occurring spontaneously. A

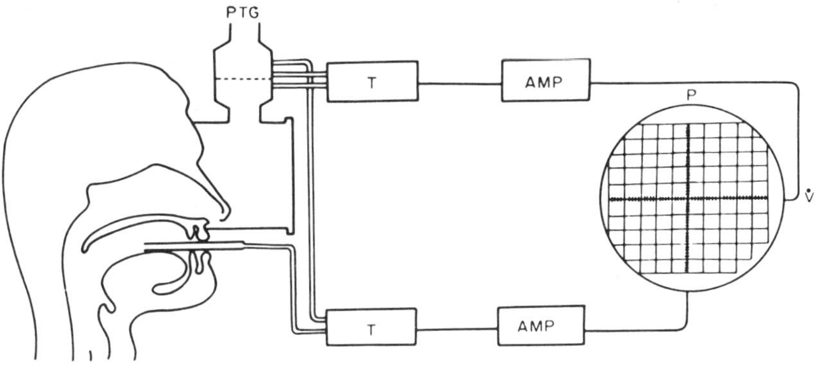

Figure 9.1. To illustrate a suitable apparatus for the measurement of nasal airways resistance. PTG = pneumotachograph; T = pressure transducer; AMP = amplifier. The pneumotachograph is attached to a suitable 'scuba' mask.

variety of methods of rhinometry have been used to measure nasal airways resistance or nasal patency. The principles involved have been reviewed by Ingelstedt, Jonson and Rundcrantz (1969). The most satisfactory methods involve continuously monitoring the flow rate through the nose ($\dot{V}$) and the trans-nasal pressure difference (*P*). A suitable apparatus is illustrated in Figure 9.1 which is described by Taylor and Shivalkar (1971a) and is a modification of the method of Solomon et al (1965). A typical 'loop' as displayed on the oscilloscope is illustrated in Figure 9.2. Only when laminar flow

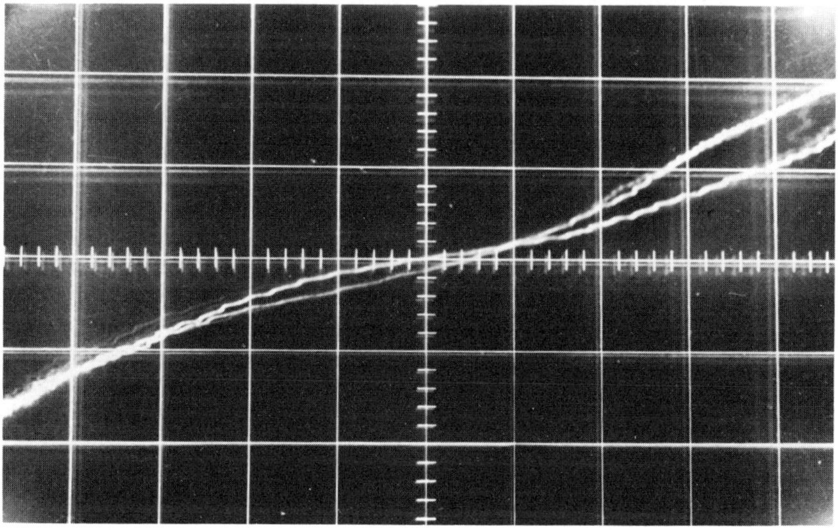

Figure 9.2. The oscilloscope display of one cycle of inspiration and expiration. Nasal airflow is measured on the horizontal axis and trans-nasal pressure difference on the vertical.

is taking place at very low flow rates is a linear relationship found between $\dot{V}$ and P. It follows that resistance measurements must be referred either to an arbitrary flow rate or pressure difference. The author has usually referred measurements of nasal airways resistance (NAR) to a flow rate of 0·4 l/sec. An alternative method using easily available equipment measures a function of the difference between peak expiratory rate through the mouth and through the nasal airways.

The function

$$\frac{\text{PEFR}_{\text{oral}} - \text{PEFR}_{\text{nasal}}}{\text{PEFR}_{\text{oral}}} = \text{'blockage index' (BI)}$$

has a good correlation with nasal airways resistance (Taylor, MacNeil and Freed, 1973).

In objective measurement of nasal sensitivity, dose response curves can be generated by varying the dose of allergen applied. This is very time consuming particularly as there is need to leave several days between challenges. It is however a useful research procedure (Connell, 1968; Taylor and Shivalkar, 1971a). The shape of the dose response curves indicates a 'threshold' effect—below a critical dose of allergen no change in nasal patency occurs, above this dose the response becomes progressively more vigorous. The threshold-dose may be used as an index of sensitivity, or alternatively, the dose which doubles the resting NAR. The two values are numerically very similar.

Three different types of response to nasal challenge may be found. These may be called 'early', 'early + late' and 'late' only. The 'early' response commences within minutes of allergen application and consists of nasal irritation and sneezing, nasal discharge and some nasal obstruction. The symptoms usually subside within 30 min. The 'late' reaction which may follow an early reaction, or occur as the sole response to challenge, commences usually about four to six hours after allergen administration although there may be an even greater delay (Taylor and Shivalkar, 1971b). The changes are essentially those of nasal obstruction with little or no irritation and only slight nasal discharge and this may commonly persist for 24 hours or longer. Systemic manifestations of fever and general malaise are not uncommon and an attack of acute sinusitis may be associated with the late nasal reaction. Figure 9.3 illustrates the course of an 'early + late' nasal reaction. Late nasal reactivity is common in patients with allergic rhinitis—approximately one-third of young adults suffering from simple grass pollen sensitivity exhibit this type of reactivity. Late reactivity is also common in patients sensitive to *Dermatophagoides* and to various moulds and with these allergens may occur without any detectable early component. Because of the possibility of late reactivity following any challenge only one allergen can be investigated on each occasion. An interval of at least 48 hours should elapse between challenges, thus making nasal challenge studies a protracted and very time-consuming investigation.

Late nasal reactivity contributes greatly to the morbidity in allergic rhinitis, particularly perennial rhinitis. Patients with late reactivity tend to have more severe symptoms, particularly of nasal obstruction which may be associated with recurrent sinusitis. It is sometimes possible to infer late reactivity from the clinical history, in which situation a search for late skin reactivity may suggest which allergen is most appropriate for nasal challenge studies. Late reactivity is most commonly found in 'blockers' rather than in 'sneezers'. The response to therapy of individuals with late reactivity is in general less satisfactory than those with pure 'early' reactivity.

Not all patients with nasal discharge and obstruction suffer from allergic rhinitis. Differentiation is required between perennial rhinitis and frequent upper respiratory tract infections and the difficult-to-define entity of non-allergic vasomotor rhinitis. Chronic use of alpha-stimulator nasal drops will

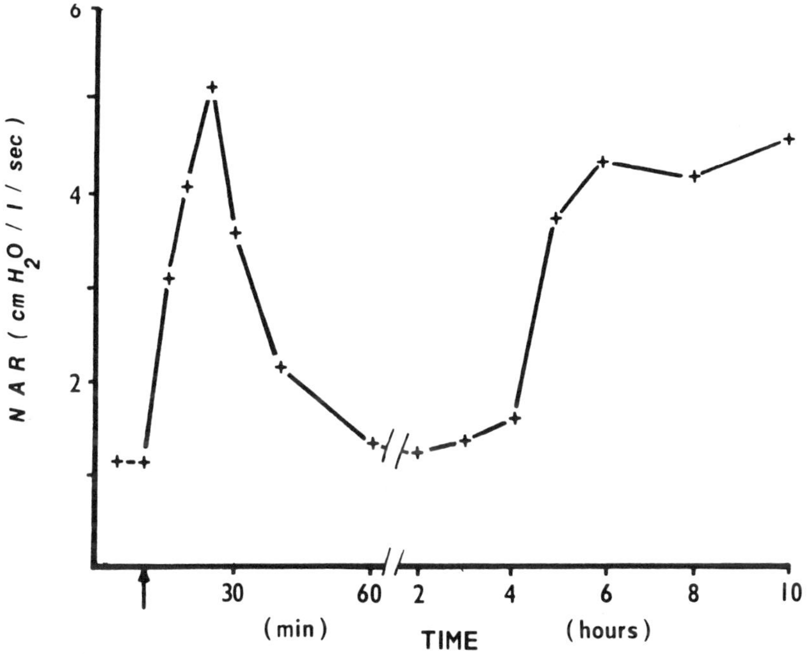

Figure 9.3. Changes in nasal airways resistance following allergen challenge (arrow) in an individual with 'early + late' nasal reactivity.

in itself produce a severe rhinitis and so add further difficulties. From the infective viewpoint the occurrence of similar symptoms at about the same time in other members of the family and the presence of other evidence of infection are often helpful. In both infective rhinitis and 'non-allergic vasomotor rhinitis' protracted nasal itching and sneezing are uncommon and when present suggest allergic rhinitis. The occurrence of associated eye irritation is also strongly suggestive of an allergic aetiology. In a proportion of patients the differentiation between allergic and non-allergic perennial rhinitis can only be partially solved by carrying out an extensive series of nasal challenge tests. This will reveal some to be clearly allergic in nature, particularly ones giving 'late' only nasal reactions, and leave a residue of 'non-proven'. It should be emphasised that absence of positive weal and flare skin tests does not exclude allergic rhinitis.

TREATMENT

Three major approaches are currently used in the treatment of allergic rhinitis. These are: (1) prevent entry of allergen into the patient's respiratory tract; (2) reduce the patient's sensitivity to the allergen (hyposensitisation); and (3) block the acute inflammatory reaction generated by contact with allergen without altering the patient's sensitivity.

Under some circumstances removal of an allergen from a patient's immediate surroundings may be very easily carried out. This applies if the allergen in question is derived from a family pet or a feather pillow. There will often be a delay before the patient improves presumably due to persistence of the allergen after the source has gone. It is therefore unnecessary to seek further possible causes of allergic rhinitis until a period of a month or so has elapsed after removal without evidence of improvement. Problems arise with animal dander sensitivity in environments out of the control of the patient or his parents. This often presents difficulties particularly with children. In the situation of laboratory workers sensitised to experimental animals the reverse approach of removing the individual from animal contact is the best course of action. The intensity of allergen exposure in an animal research facility is often so high that the alternatives of suppression of symptoms or hyposensitisation may not control the problem. House dust allergen sensitivity is very common, and although complete exclusion is impossible, house dust control can be very helpful. Attention is best directed to the bedroom, and involves removal of as much soft furnishing as possible, 'damp-dusting', frequent vacuum cleaning of mattresses and maintenance of a low relative humidity. Efficient air filtration systems are available but are relatively expensive. Their value in the reduction of the symptoms of allergic disease of the respiratory tract has not been fully investigated.

Reduction in patient sensitivity by immunotherapy (hyposensitisation) has been used extensively since first introduced by Noon (1911). Courses prescribed have varied according to the number of injections given, and the type of preparation and amount of allergen included. Results have been evaluated mainly by consideration of subjective reports provided by the patients. There are many problems of interpretation, but no doubt that some reports show definite improvement in a significant proportion of patients treated. More recently changes in objectively measured mucosal sensitivity have been carried out which support the large body of subjective data.

Studies to elucidate the immunological mechanisms involved in hyposensitisation have given conflicting results. In summary, following hyposensitisation there is often the production of allergen-specific IgG antibody which is capable of blocking a P-K test (Loveless, 1940). This can also block release of histamine from sensitised peripheral blood basophils (Lichtenstein et al, 1966). Correlation between such antibody and clinical improvement has varied in different studies but has not in general been very good. Some workers have claimed that there is a reduction in serum reaginic antibody (presumably specific IgE) following hyposensitisation. On the other hand more recent studies have shown that the response is very variable and in many patients hyposensitisation results in an increase in specific IgE. Whilst the increase may be temporary it is difficult to reconcile these data. Decrease in histamine release from peripheral blood leucocytes after hyposensitisation has also been reported by some workers and increased release by others. The situation with respect to IgE production and to changes in target cell sensitisation is very confused and requires further investigation. Decrease in allergen-induced lymphocyte mitogenesis following hyposensitisation has been demonstrated and has led to the suggestion that a state of T-cell tolerance might have been induced to the allergen. This would be expected to reduce production of antibody by lack of T–B cell cooperation. The very variable results obtained when antibody production to allergen has been investigated must leave this hypothesis in doubt. Finally, the possibility that specific SIgA production is induced by hyposensitisation must be considered. This is unlikely as antigens given other than by the mucosal route do not produce good SIgA responses. It is highly desirable that the mechanisms involved should be fully elucidated as this would allow a more critical scientific approach to providing the most satisfactory preparations and courses for therapeutic use.

A variety of allergen preparations have been used for hyposensitisation. In considering their relative merits several factors must be taken into account. These are the proportion of patients who are significantly improved, the incidence of side effects, and patient acceptability related to the number of doses required. The classes of preparations available are soluble extracts, soluble extracts in oil-in-water emulsions, alum precipitated preparations, 'allergoids' (allergen extracts modified by formalin treatment), and allergenic extracts absorbed onto amino acid crystals (e.g. tyrosine). Adequate data are not yet available to evaluate the latter two types of hyposensitisation preparation. The efficiency of the other three methods are very similar, but they differ in the incidence of adverse reactions and in patient acceptability. Soluble extracts require very long courses and have a high adverse reaction rate. Their use has considerably decreased since the introduction of slow release preparations. Water-in-oil emulsions require fewer injections (usually three), but the use of mineral oil, which cannot be metabolised, gives cause for concern; sterile abscesses and dimpled scars at injection sites are not uncommon. Alum precipitated preparations occupying an intermediate position with respect to a number of doses required are probably currently the preparation of choice.

It is most important to limit as far as possible the number of allergens included in a prescribed preparation. Poor results are often due to 'treating the skin tests' rather than the sensitivity really causing trouble to the patient. The author prefers to define by nasal challenge the one allergen causing most trouble and to attempt hyposensitisation against that one alone in the first instance. This approach applies equally to pollen sensitivity. Though skin sensitivity to a wide range of pollens may be present, the nasal airways may react significantly only to a very limited number. Single courses will often produce only partial improvement and three separate courses with intervals between is the usual scheme. The maximum dose of allergen given should if possible increase with each course. In pollen sensitivity the course should be completed ideally just before the pollen season commences. Co-seasonal courses using much smaller doses continuing during the season are far less satisfactory. 'Crash' courses of hyposensitisation in which multiple increasing doses of vaccine are given over a period of a few days have been advocated by some workers. The risk of reactions is such that this procedure needs hospitalisation and constant observation. Good comparative studies are not available to evaluate objectively the results of this type of hyposensitisation.

Reactions to a course of hyposensitisation using alum precipitated preparations are not common but most are of only minor concern. Local redness and swelling in the region of the injection is the commonest adverse reaction. Symptoms of allergic rhinitis may increase shortly after a dose of vaccine (usually within 24 hours), and some patients may also experience mild asthma. Severe reactions are very uncommon using alum precipitated preparations, particularly when compared with soluble preparations, the use of which may provoke systemic anaphylaxis. Though serious reactions do occasionally occur they usually do so after milder reactions to smaller doses have been ignored and the dose nonetheless increased.

Decrease in nasal airway reactivity following repeated doses of aerosols of allergen applied locally has been evaluated by Taylor and Shivalkar (1972). In seasonal allergic rhinitis the results have been good; decrease in sensitivity occurring in most subjects, and in many persisting for a year or more. Eight doses of that dose of allergen which doubles the NAR applied at three-day intervals has been the scheme employed. Preliminary work suggests that a similar result can be obtained in perennial rhinitis. Local nasal desensitisation has improved patients both with 'early' and with 'early + late' nasal responses. It is proposed (Taylor, 1973) that a local SIgA response to the applied allergen may account for the decrease in nasal sensitivity. This approach is still experimental and the results require confirmation.

It is difficult to define which patients are most likely to benefit from hyposensitisation. In general, patients with multiple sensitivity at the mucosal level, reflecting a high 'atopic status' do not greatly improve. It is also a clinical impression that patients with either 'early + late' or 'late only' reactivity are not greatly helped by systemic hyposensitisation. Those having dual reactivity are sometimes converted to the 'late only' type with a tendency to have symptoms of a different character though equally troublesome. Patients with 'early only' reactivity achieve the best results and this applies even if the sensitivity is extreme, providing that only one or two allergens are implicated.

A variety of approaches have been used to block the unpleasant effects of allergic rhinitis. Nasal decongestants, whilst producing temporary relief, are to be condemned. Rebound vasodilatation invariably occurs and the patient then uses the decongestant more and more frequently with a resulting complete dependence on the preparation and eventually serious mucosal damage.

Antihistamines are moderately effective, but all have some sedative effect. In children this may be acceptable, but most adults are unable to take sufficient antihistamine to control severe symptoms without unacceptable drowsiness.

Disodium cromoglycate (DSCG) applied locally to the nasal mucosa blocks the reaction in about 70 per cent of subjects with seasonal rhinitis.

The reason why some subjects respond well and others not at all is not yet known, but those with a 'late' component in their nasal reactivity do not respond as well as 'early only' reactor. The results in perennial rhinitis are not so easy to evaluate, but some patients undoubtedly improve considerably. There appears to be a lag period before nasally applied DSCG produces significant effects particularly in perennial rhinitis. This is of the order of two weeks. In seasonal rhinitis, treatment with DSCG should be started before the rhinitis becomes really troublesome, otherwise again it is ineffective for some days.

Steroids undoubtedly improve rhinitis considerably, but because of their side effects are only rarely indicated for uncomplicated rhinitis. Depot steroids have been used in seasonal rhinitis and two spaced doses will often prevent most of the summer symptoms. It is debatable whether the use of such a preparation in seasonal rhinitis with the likelihood of adrenal suppression is fully justified. I would prefer to limit the use of depot steroids to those situations in which rapid relief of the symptoms of allergic rhinitis is desirable for some clear reason and where antihistamines are unsuitable, e.g. individuals taking important examinations. Steroids applied directly to the nasal mucosa have also been used. This approach carries the theoretical possibility of producing an atrophic mucous membrane and of depressing local immunological reactivity, particularly if used over long periods as would be necessary in perennial rhinitis. Until this problem is resolved, the use of topical steroids in the respiratory tract should be undertaken with caution.

References

Coca, A. F. & Cooke, R. A. (1923) On the classification of the phenomena of hypersensitiveness. *Journal of Immunology*, **8,** 163.

Connell, J. T. (1968) Quantitative intranasal pollen challenge. *Journal of Allergy*, **41,** 123.

Ingelstedt, S., Jonson, B. & Rundcrantz, H. (1969) A clinical method for determination of nasal airway resistance. *Acta Oto-laryngologica*, **68,** 189.

Jarrett, E. E. E., Orr, T. S. C. & Riley, P. (1971) Inhibition of allergic reactions due to competition for mast cell sensitisation by two reagins. *Clinical and Experimental Immunology*, **9,** 585.

Kaufman, H. S. & Hobbs, J. R. (1970) Immunoglobulin deficiencies in an atopic population. *Lancet*, **ii,** 1061.

Kumar, L., Newcomb, R. W., Ishizaka, K., Middleton, E. & Hornbrook, M. M. (1971) IgE levels in sera of children with asthma. *Paediatrics*, **47,** 848.

Lichtenstein, L. M., Norman, P. S., Winkenwerder, W. L. & Osler, A. G. (1966) *In vitro* studies of human ragweed allergy: changes in cellular and humoral activity associated with specific desensitisation. *Journal of Clinical Investigation*, **45,** 1126.

Loveless, M. H. (1940) Immunological studies of pollenosis. I. The presence of two antibodies related to the same pollen antigen in the serum of treated hay fever patients. *Journal of Immunology*, **38,** 25.

Noon, L. (1911) Prophylactic inoculations against hay fever. *Lancet*, **i,** 1572.

Salvaggio, J. E., Waldman, R. H., Fruchtman, M. H., Wigley, F. M. & Johnson, J. E. (1973) Systemic and secretory antibody response of atopic and non-atopic individuals to intranasally administered toxoid. *Clinical Allergy*, **3,** 43.

Schwartz, D. P. & Buckley, R. H. (1971) Serum IgE concentrations and skin reactivity to anti-IgE antibody in IgA deficient patients. *New England Journal of Medicine*, **284,** 513.

Solomon, W. R., McLean, J. A., Cookingham, C., Ahronheim, G. & DeMuth, G. R. (1965) Measurement of nasal airways resistance. *Journal of Allergy*, **36,** 62.

Stenius, B., Wide, L., Seymour, W. M., Holford-Strevens, V. & Pepys, J. (1971) Clinical significance of specific IgE to common allergens. I. Relationship of specific IgE against *Dermatophagoides* spp. and grass pollen to skin tests and history. *Clinical Allergy*, **1,** 37.

Stenius, B., Wide, L. & Seymour, W. M. (1972) Clinical significance of total IgE and of specific IgE to *Dermatophagoides* spp., grass pollen and other common allergens. II. Relationship to clinical manifestations. *Clinical Allergy*, **2,** 303.

Taylor, B., Norman, A. P., Orgel, H. A., Stokes, C. R., Turner, M. W. & Soothill, J. F. (1973) Transient IgA deficiency and pathogenesis of infantile Atopy. *Lancet*, **ii,** 111.

Taylor, G. (1973) The nose as a model for the study of respiratory tract allergic disease. *Annals of the New York Academy of Sciences*, **221,** 117.

Taylor, G., MacNeil, A. R. & Freed, D. L. J. (1973) Assessing the degree of nasal patency by measuring the peak expiratory flow rate through the nose. *Journal of Allergy and Clinical Immunology*, **52,** 193.

Taylor, G. & Shivalkar, P. R. (1971a) Changes in nasal airways resistance on antigenic challenge in allergic rhinitis. *Clinical Allergy*, **1,** 63.

Taylor, G. & Shivalkar, P. R. (1971b) 'Arthus-type' reactivity in the nasal airways and skin in pollen sensitive subjects. *Clinical Allergy*, **1,** 407.

Taylor, G. & Shivalkar, P. R. (1972) Local nasal desensitisation in allergic rhinitis. *Clinical Allergy*, **2,** 125.

Turk, A., Lichtenstein, L. M. & Norman, P. S. (1970) Nasal secretory antibody to inhalant allergens in allergic and non-allergic patients. *Immunology*, 19, 85.

Wide, L., Bennich, H. & Johansson, S. G. O. (1967) Diagnosis of allergy by an in vitro test for allergen antibodies. *Lancet*, **ii,** 1105.

10. Immunology of Skin Diseases

MALCOLM W. GREAVES

At least half of all patients attending an average dermatological outpatient clinic will have a skin disease probably or certainly involving one or more immunological mechanisms. The presence of allergic factors in most types of eczema and urticaria is well known. In addition, the natural history and pathology of other common skin diseases including warts and other virus infections, most fungal and bacterial infections and many cutaneous neoplasms is dependent to some degree on the immunological responses of the patient.

Allergic skin diseases because of their accessibility might at first sight seem to lend themselves to detailed investigation and analysis. This is true for model experimental allergic reactions in skin, but the inherent complexity of skin as an organ and the varied influence of genetic and environmental factors on skin are amongst the reasons why surprisingly little is known of the precise role of immunological mechanisms in many skin diseases. Before considering individual skin diseases it is valuable to consider the main classes of immunological reactions and how they may manifest themselves in human skin.

Immunological reactions

The most practical classification currently available is that of Coombs and Gell (1968) who divide immunological mechanisms into four categories:

Type I: Cells are sensitised passively by antibody produced elsewhere. Reactions of antigen with cell-bound antibody lead to release of pharmacological vasoactive agents. In man the antibody involved has specific characteristics, is termed reaginic antibody and is contained in the IgE fraction of the immunoglobulins. Recent evidence suggests that some types of clinical type 1 hypersensitivity reactions may involve reaginic antibody of IgG class. Immunofluorescent evidence indicates that IgE is preferentially bound to mast cells which are the source of histamine and other pharmacological agents which mediate the observed clinical reaction.

The classical manifestation of type 1 reactions in human skin occurs when specific antigen is pricked into the skin of an allergic subject. Within seconds a weal develops surrounded by a flare. The reaction is accompanied by itching and lasts up to one hour. The Prausnitz–Küstner reaction is essentially the same response. Here a healthy recipient's skin is sensitised locally by intradermal injection of serum from an allergic subject. A wealing reaction develops when the sensitised skin is challenged by an injection of specific antigen. The mediator of the type 1 reaction in human skin is histamine. From a clinical point of view, type 1 reactions are the presenting feature in human skin of acute urticaria.

Type 2: Circulating antibodies react with antigens which are either part of the substance of tissue cells or have become intimately combined with them. Characteristically, complement is involved in this reaction which results in cellular damage. In this reaction, 'antiskin' antibodies react with skin antigen. Usually complement is involved and cytotoxic damage to skin occurs. The importance of this reaction in human cutaneous allergy is uncertain. Evidence of circulating antibodies to skin antigen has been found in some patients with acute generalised eczema. In these patients, the antibody was undetectable during remissions but present during relapses. A weal and flare skin reaction was obtained when the skin of a sensitised patient or healthy skin was challenged by intradermal injections of serum containing the antibody. The antibody was also found to be cytotoxic to epidermal cells in vitro in the presence of complement. The antibodies have only been found in a small minority of patients which argues against their importance in the pathogenesis of acute generalised eczema. Possibly the use of newer more sensitive immunological techniques may reveal their presence in a higher proportion.

Circulating antiskin autoantibodies are present in a majority of patients with the blistering diseases pemphigus and pemphigoid. The relationship of these antibodies to the pathogenesis of the diseased skin is uncertain. These and other immunological aspects of pemphigus and pemphigoid are considered in more detail below.

Type 3: Antibodies and antigens in the blood or tissue fluids react togheter to produce antigen–antibody complexes which accumulate in small blood vessels causing tissue damage and local inflammation through their mechanical and toxic effects on blood vessels. Complement is also involved in this type of reaction. Accumulation of antigen–antibody complexes in cutaneous blood vessels leads to a variety of clinical manifestations in the skin including weals which resemble those seen in cutaneous anaphylactic (type 1) reactions, purpura due to extravasation of blood from damaged skin blood vessels, necrotic papules, more extensive ulceration due to occlusion of skin vessels, and indurated nodules in which involvement of deeper cutaneous vessels has led to a local chronic inflammatory reaction. The pathological lesion common to these clinical changes is the formation of intravascular leucocyte–platelet thrombi. This process is common to a wide variety of diseases which involve the skin including serum sickness, anaphylactoid purpura (Henoch–Schönlein), primary cutaneous vasculitis, collagen vascular diseases (rheumatoid arthritis, polyarteritis, systemic lupus erythematosus, systemic sclerosis) and erythema nodosum.

Type 4: A reaction occurs between sensitised lympyhoctes and specific antigen which is independent of free antibodies or complement. Reactivity can be transferred from a sensitive subject to a normal one by lymphocytes or subcellular fractions of lymphocytes but not by serum. Characteristically, a delayed indurated inflammatory reaction develops following challenge of skin by specific antigen. In man it reaches a maximum at about 48 hours. Histologically, the main feature is perivascular infiltration by mononuclear cells. One classical clinical manifestation of this type of allergy in skin is allergic contact eczema. Another manifestation is the skin homograft reaction. Deeper cutaneous reactions of this type occur in the response of the skin to beryllium and zirconium. Granulomatous reactions to microorganisms including mycobacteria (lupus vulgaris) and some deep fungus infections fall in the same category. Much work has been done on the mechanism of allergic contact eczema. During skin sensitisation antigen combines with epidermal protein, or possibly with lymphocytes passing through the skin. Lymphocytes then transport the epidermal antigen to the corticomedullary zone of local lymph glands. Proliferation of immunoblasts in this zone results in formation of a clone of sensitised lymphocytes. Combination between antigen in the skin and sensitised lymphocytes results in local release of mediators of inflammation.

Urticaria

The cardinal feature of urticaria is the development of disseminated weals. Characteristically, the periorbital skin and lips are especially severely affected. The weals fade within about 12 hours. The distinction between acute and chronic urticaria is ill-defined. Acute urticaria is frequently extensive and runs a short-lived course. Usually the cause is obvious as, for example, following a penicillin or serum injection or in response to ingestion of shell fish or other food to which the patient is known to be allergic. Often there may be a history of other forms of allergy including hay fever or asthma. Chronic urticaria implies occurrence of scattered weals daily or weekly over a period of weeks or months. Very often the cause of chronic urticaria is not at all apparent. The main pathological lesion in the skin is local vasodilation accompanied by increased vascular permeability. A principal mediator in this reaction is histamine released from mast cells in the dermis although possibly other mediators are involved.

Acute urticaria

Acute urticaria is extremely distressing and disabling mainly because of the disfigurement produced by extensive facial wealing and because of the associated pruritus.

Diagnosis. Frequently the offending antigen is easily recognised by the patient or doctor in which case no further diagnostic effort is necessary. There may, however, be some uncertainty or total ignorance of the cause. In such cases challenge of the patient with the suspected antigen by systemic administration is undesirable for obvious reasons and resort should be made to skin testing. Most antigens likely to be involved in urticaria are contained in the standard Bencard diagnostic kit (Bencard Limited, Brentford, Middlesex), and additional antigens can be prepared by the suppliers to order. Initially prick tests should be carried out. A drop of prick test solution is placed on the flexor surface of the forearm and the skin lightly pricked through the solution using force sufficient only to demonstrate the elasticity of the skin. The positive response is indicated by the development, 10 minutes after the pricking into the skin, of a weal at least 5 mm in diameter. All tests should include a control injection in which physiological saline (0·9 per cent NaCl in water) is pricked into the skin. Interpretation of prick tests is often difficult in atopic subjects who frequently give positive reactions to a variety of antigens. If prick testing is negative or equivocal intradermal tests should be carried out. In this procedure 0·05 ml of antigen solution is injected intradermally. In other respects the procedure is the same as for prick testing.

Chronic urticaria

This is a common problem and presents great difficulty both in diagnosis and management. It is particularly common in female adults. In most cases the urticaria runs a course of weeks or months before clearing up spontaneously. Usually no cause is found. Since in a small minority the apparent cause can be identified, investigation of patients with urticaria is worthwhile. Food allergy is a rare cause which can be confirmed by skin tests as described above. Parasitic infestation is a well-established cause of urticaria particularly in those who have lived in tropical climates. The presence of a blood eosinophilia together with identification of parasites or ova in the stools suggests this diagnosis. Occasional patients are infected with *Candida albicans* and treatment with nystatin has resulted in remission of the urticaria. These patients usually have a positive immediate wealing reaction to the skin testing with *Candida* extract. There have also been isolated case reports in which treatment of focal sepsis including chronic urinary or gallbladder infection or dermatophytosis has been followed by apparent cure of chronic urticaria. Chronic urticaria can also be a rare manifestation of internal malignant disease. The relationship of aspirin ingestion to urticaria is of some interest. Undoubtedly aspirin can occasionally cause urticaria through an immunological mechanism. Aspirin may also exacerbate pre-existing urticaria by an apparently non-immunological mechanism, since aspirin has been shown to enhance skin wealing in a non-specific way. Thus the possibility of regular ingestion of one of the multiple proprietary preparations containing aspirin must be excluded in all cases. Chronic urticaria can, of course, be a hypersensitivity reaction to continued ingestion of almost any drug. Although this relationship is usually easy to establish, antibiotics (especially penicillin) may present some difficulty since trace amounts may be present in milk and other dairy products. Skin testing by the methods described above may be helpful in confirming the diagnosis.

Treatment. In the great majority of cases when a cause cannot be established treatment is directed to suppression of wealing until such a time as the urticaria undergoes spontaneous remission. Systemic antihistamines are effective in reducing itching and cause some reduction in the extent and frequency of wealing. Antihistamines should be given to the limit of tolerance, i.e. until drowsiness, dryness of the mouth and other side-effects become intolerable. It is often a good policy to give a strongly sedative antihistamine such as promethazine at night time and a less sedative form such as chlorpheniramine by day.

Patients with acute urticaria involving the mouth may, rarely, suffer airway obstruction. In these cases, intravenous hydrocortisone and adrenaline should be given in addition to an antihistamine. Occasionally tracheostomy may be required.

Other forms of urticaria

Chronic urticaria may occasionally be due to identifiable physical causes. The commonest form of physical urticaria is factitious urticaria in which rubbing or minor trauma to the skin provokes wealing. Pressure urticaria presents as local often painful subcutaneous swellings in response to local pressure. Cholinergic urticaria occurs in association with eccrine sweating usually in response to physical exertion or emotional stimuli. Cold, heat and ultraviolet radiation may occasionally cause urticaria.

Papular urticaria is a common form of relapsing urticaria which occurs particularly frequently in children. Lesions are most prolific on the exposed parts of the skin mainly the face, neck, forearms, hands and legs. Each weal is a response to an insect bite. Fleas, mosquitoes, sandflies and ticks are extremely common causes of papular urticaria. The weal represents a hypersensitivity reaction to either the saliva or mouth parts of the causative insect and this form of urticaria can readily be diagnosed by the grouped distribution of the weals and by the presence on the weals of a central punctum at the point where the insect penetrated the skin. Patients often give the history of contact with an infested pet dog or cat and frequently several members of the same family are affected. Treatment consists of avoiding the source of the offending insect and the use of an insect repellent such as dimethyl phthalate lotion. If the insect repellent lotions are unsuccessful it may be necessary to apply a cream containing DDT. Calamine cream containing 2 per cent DDT and 2 per cent benzylbenzoate is extremely effective.

Angioneurotic oedema

This is sometimes called 'giant' urticaria and is distinguished from urticaria by involvement of the deeper part of the dermis and subcutaneous tissues. The swellings are pale and redness and itching are not prominent. Frequently urticaria and angioneurotic oedema coexist. The causes, investigation and treatment are the same as for urticaria though antihistamines are less effective in angioneurotic oedema than in urticaria.

One special and potentially fatal form of angioneurotic oedema is the hereditary or familial type (HAE). It is due to an inherited deficiency of a plasma inhibitor of the activated first component of complement (C1-esterase inhibitor). Apart from eliciting a family history of angioneurotic oedema, several other points in the history can suggest HAE. There are often episodes of abdominal pain and vomiting which are due to oedema of the intestinal mucosa, the cutaneous lesions are often precipitated by trauma, and the lesions fail to respond to adequate doses of either antihistamines or corticosteroids. The mechanism of the increased vascular permeability is almost certainly due to kinin-like agents derived from the uninhibited action of activated C1 on the complement cascade. Because the C3 and C5 anaphylatoxins operate by causing histamine release, and as the oedema is unresponsive to antihistamines, these are unlikely to be important causes of increased vascular permeability. 'HAE kinins', probably derived from C2, are the most likely agents involved.

The diagnosis can be best confirmed by demonstrating a deficiency of the inhibitor by enzymic methods. If the inhibitor is measured immunochemically two types of HAE can be demonstrated—true deficiency and a type with normal quantities of very inefficient inhibitor. Demonstration of reduced quantities of the early complement components, either directly or by measuring serum complement by the immune-adherence method, is also useful but less reliable than the estimation of the inhibitor. Treatment is by the use of the antifibrinolytic agent epsilon aminocaproic acid which is thought to have an inhibitor-sparing effect. The dosage is the smallest that will control symptoms and varies from 9 to 18 g per day. Fresh frozen plasma has been used successfully to treat acute laryngeal oedema and abdominal colic.

Eczema

Eczema is an inflammatory papulovesicular disorder of the skin characterised histologically by spongiosis (epidermal intercellular oedema). It is the final result of a number of alternative and widely diverse aetiological factors and pathogenetic processes. Although there is no general agreement on the classification of eczema, it is convenient to divide eczema into two types: *exogenous*, which includes allergic contact eczema and non-allergic eczema due to exposure to primary irritants, and *endogenous*, in which genetic and constitutional factors play a major role. Endogenous eczema includes atopic (infantile) eczema, and seborrhoeic eczema. Terms such as discoid eczema, infective eczema, nummular eczema and pityriasis alba should probably not be used other than in a purely descriptive way for they depend for their distinction from other forms of eczema solely on the morphological variations, there being no available evidence that these variations imply any specific aetiology and pathology. The histological appearances of the dermis in eczema with a dense lymphocytic infiltrate suggest an immune mechanism, but there are only two forms of eczema where immunological abnormalities have been unequivocally established—allergic contact eczema and atopic eczema—and these two forms of eczema will be considered in the present account. It is nevertheless probable that application of newer immunological techniques will reveal immune mechanisms in other forms of eczema.

The region of the involved skin and the degree of acuteness or chronicity considerably modify the clinical appearances in eczema. Because of the thickness of the stratum corneum, acute eczema of the palms and the soles is characterised by persistent multilocular blisters (pompholyx) which coalesce to form large bullae. For the same reason deep painful fissures and cracks occur in chronic eczema of the palms and the soles. Blistering, weeping, crusting, redness and oedema are characteristic of acute eczema in any region. In chronic eczema, especially where pruritus leads to constant rubbing, marked epidermal thickening and hyperkeratosis accentuate the normal creases of the skin (lichenification). Secondary infection increases the wetness of the involved skin and produces pustulation, crusting and pain.

Allergic contact eczema

Allergic contact eczema is due to a specific delayed cell-mediated allergic reaction to antigen applied to the surface of the skin in a sensitised subject. This sensitivity can be transferred from a sensitised donor to a normal recipient by the donor's leucocytes or by a cell-free extract of these but not by the donor's serum. Challenge of sensitised skin by antigen applied topically evokes a delayed eczematous response in the challenged skin. Although knowledge of the immunology and pathogenesis of allergic contact eczema remains incomplete, some general conclusions on the mechanism have been reached. Contact sensitisation can be evoked by a variety of agents ranging from complex substances present in plants such as the primula and poison ivy, to simple chemicals or elements including paraphenylenediamine, nickel and chromate. Simple chemicals behave as haptens, by conjugating with proteins, the complex then behaving as an antigen. Lymphocytes circulating through the skin containing antigen become altered in a specific way which enables them to 'recognise' the antigen. These lymphocytes then circulate to the corticomedullary zone of local lymph glands and proliferate there to form a 'clone' of sensitised lymphocytes. Reaction of these with skin containing antigen leads to local release of pharmacological agents which evoke eczematous changes. Thus a locally intact lymphatic system is an essential prerequisite for sensitisation. Fortunately, although man is continuously in contact with a variety of potential contact sensitisers, sensitisation only occurs in a tiny minority. Genetic factors, local concentration of antigen, duration of exposure and local variations in permeability of skin and development of immune tolerance are amongst the more important factors which determine whether or not sensitisation occurs. Susceptibility to sensitisation declines in old age. Sensitisation to more than one allergen at the same time occurs in about 20 per cent of patients with allergic contact eczema. This may be due to a genetic predisposition or because allergic contact eczema lowers the threshold of sensitisation by other agents. A third possibility is cross-sensitivity between chemically closely related antigens as for example with paraphenylenediamine, sulphonamides and benzocaine.

Diagnosis and investigation. The detailed physical signs of allergic contact eczema do not differ significantly from those of other forms of eczema. However, the history, general pattern and distribution of the eruption may suggest contact eczema. For example, a chronic eczematous rash under the watch strap, metal fastenings of underwear, or jewellery suggests sensitivity to nickel. Acute eczema in linear streaks on the backs of the hands and extensor surfaces of the forearms often associated with acute eczema of the face and periorbital oedema should lead to close questioning about the relationship of the eruption to contact with plants such as primula. Occasionally patients present with allergic contact eczema predominantly in light-exposed areas. Clinically and histologically the eczematous skin is indistinguishable from ordinary allergic contact eczema, and passive transfer can be demonstrated using the same methods. Sulphonamides and antibacterial agents present in soaps, halogenated salicylanilides and hexachlorophane may cause photo-allergic contact eczema. The precise mechanism is the subject of some dispute but it seems likely that sensitivity develops to the products of ultraviolet-induced degradation of the parent compound. Although the pattern of contact eczema is often diagnostic, secondary spread may occur to areas totally unrelated to direct contact with the offending agents. For example, nickel or chromate allergy may result in generalised discoid eczema.

Histologically, allergic contact eczema does not differ significantly from other non-allergic types of eczema although using skin window techniques an increased proportion of basophil leucocytes is present in the dermal infiltrate.

The standard method of detecting contact sensitivity is by patch testing. The antigen is applied on a patch of cotton or linen material 1 cm square and occluded on the skin of the back by adhesive tape. The patch is removed at 48 hours. Redness and oedema and vesiculation signify a positive patch test. The basis of the patch test is that a concentration of the suspected antigen is employed which does not normally produce an irritant reaction. It is impossible to use concentrations of antigen which will never produce irritant reactions in normal subjects because this concentration would frequently be insufficient to produce a positive specific response in a sensitised subject. Thus, the concentrations used are inevitably a compromise between these two requirements. It is frequently necessary to do tests of substances in which the appropriate concentration for patch testing is unknown. In these instances the concentration selected usually depends upon the results of patch testing in a small group of control subjects. Obviously false positive and false negative reactions are common in this situation and the significance of results is correspondingly low. The test site should not be evaluated until at least 20 minutes after removal of the patch to allow the erythematous reaction to stripping off the patch test to subside. Positive reactions are conveniently scored as follows: + is weak non-oedematous, non-vesicular reaction; ++ is oedematous or vesicular reaction. Ideally patients with negative results should be seen again 24 hours later (72 hours after application of the patch test), in order to identify occasional delayed positive results. Some dermatologists claim they can distinguish primary irritant from positive allergic reactions on the basis of clinical appearances. This is extremely difficult even after wide experience.

In many instances the general pattern of an eczema may raise the possibility of contact sensitivity but neither the history nor the clinical appearances help in identification of the offending substance. In these cases patch testing with a standard range of antigens is often helpful. The agents included in the battery are those which together are known to account for the majority of cases of contact sensitisation in the region where the patient is domiciled. This method frequently uncovers unsuspected allergies but battery patch testing involves a significant risk of producing sensitisation to agents to which the patient was previously unreactive. The battery of antigens used in the Department of Dermatology, Royal Victoria Infirmary, Newcastle upon Tyne, is given in Table 10.1. Photo-patch testing is carried out in suspected cases of photo-allergic contact eczema. The suspected antigen is applied to the skin and irradiated, then occluded under a patch for 48 hours in the usual way. Most cases of photo-allergic contact eczema are provoked by wavelengths greater than 320 nm and the light source used should produce a continuous spectrum of light from 320 nm to the visible range. Obviously natural sunlight is the best source of radiation in climates where this is available.

Treatment. Acute weeping contact eczema is best treated by a short course of systemic corticosteroids: prednisone should be given in dosage 60 mg a day and gradually reduced to zero once the inflammation has subsided. Systemic antihistamines are given to allay pruritus and pieces of gauze soaked in a weak antiseptic solution such as 1/10 000 potassium permanganate should be applied to the inflamed skin several times daily. In chronic contact eczema the simplest and most effective treatment is obviously withdrawal of the offending antigen. This may be done easily in the case of contact eczema due to cosmetics or topical medications. However, it may be somewhat impractical

Table 10.1. Standard battery of patch test solutions

Antigen	Strength (%w/v)
Potassium dichromate	0·5
Paraphenylenediamine	1·0
Neomycin sulphate	20·0
Cobalt chloride	1·0
Benzocaine	5·0
Nickel sulphate	2·5
Chinoform	5·0
Colophony	20·0
Parabens	3·0
Wool alcohols	30·0
Mercaptobenzthiazole	2·0
Ethylenediamine	1·0
Chlorquinaldol	5·0
Balsam of Peru	25·0
Turpentine	1·0
Formaldehyde	2·0

for economic reasons in some instances of industrial contact eczema. Complete withdrawal of the antigen may also be virtually impossible because of the prevalence of the antigen in the every-day environment as, for example, in patients with rubber or nickel allergy. In the latter two instances, recourse must be made to suppression by topical corticosteroid medications. Hyposensitisation has been attempted in some patients but with little success except in the occasional case of antibiotic sensitivity. Causes of failure of eczema to clear up despite apparently successful withdrawal of the offending agent include unrecognised sensitisation to one or more other antigens (including antigens which cross-react with the already identified agent), increased susceptibility to primary irritants due to impairment of barrier-function of the stratum corneum and overtreatment by topical medications. The role of ingestion of antigens in the exacerbation of allergic contact eczema due to nickel, chromate and cobalt is uncertain. These agents find their way into food from metal cooking utensils.

Atopic eczema

Atopic eczema is a form of constitutional eczema with a characteristic distribution associated with increased incidence of asthma, hay fever and urticaria and other allergic manifestations. Total serum IgE immunoglobulin concentration is often raised.

A family history is present in about 70 per cent of cases, and about 3 per cent of infants have some evidence of atopic eczema during the first few months of life. Although atopic eczema can develop soon after birth, or as late as in middle age, the most frequent age of onset lies between two and six months. Characteristically the face, hands, feet, backs of the knees and antecubital fossae are affected but spread often occurs to the trunk and extensor surfaces of the limbs. All degrees of eczema occur ranging from the acute vesicular and weeping eruptions, to chronic and lichenified eczema sometimes called Besnier's prurigo. Pruritus is invariable. There is an increased incidence of ichthyosis vulgaris (an hereditary extensive dry scaliness of skin) in patients with atopic eczema. Occasionally atopic eczema is associated with ocular abnormalities including cataracts and keratoconus. There is a marked tendency for spontaneous improvement to occur during childhood and adolescence.

Histologically, atopic eczema is normally indistinguishable from other types of eczema although the dermal inflammatory infiltrate may contain an increased proportion of eosinophils. There may also be a blood eosinophilia.

Diagnosis and investigation. A raised serum IgE concentration lends considerable support to the diagnosis of atopic eczema but it may be within normal limits, particularly in patients with limited skin involvement. Serum IgE is usually measured by radioimmunoassay. The presence of reaginic antibody can be detected by prick testing with a wide range of food and inhalant antigens. Patients with atopic eczema frequently have multiple positive weal and flare reactions to these antigens, often without a corresponding history of clinical hypersensitivity. Withdrawal of antigens causing positive prick tests does not influence the course of the eruption. Skin testing should be carried out cautiously in patients when there is associated asthma.

The cutaneous vasculature in atopic eczema readily vasoconstricts in response to certain physical and pharmacological stimuli. Light stroking of the skin produces a transient local blanching (white dermographism) and blanching occurs one to five minutes after intradermal injection of 10 μg acetylcholine. However, these tests are not specific to atopic eczema and occur in other inflammatory skin disorders. Bronchoconstrictor drugs including histamine and acetylcholine when inhaled produce enhanced bronchoconstriction in subjects with atopic eczema, but these tests involve significant risk. Recent evidence raises a possibility that defective beta-adrenergic receptors may be important components of the atopic syndrome. An imbalance between alpha (excitatory) and beta (inhibitory) adrenergic responses in smooth muscle of blood vessels and bronchi results in abnormal pharmacological responses. Beta-adrenergic receptors are probably identical with the cell membrane enzyme adenylcyclase which catalyses the conversion of ATP to cyclic AMP; attempts to identify qualitative and quantitative abnormalities of adenylcyclase, cyclic AMP and phosphodiesterase (which degrades cyclic AMP) in atopic subjects are at present in progress. This theory receives some support from biochemical and pharmacological studies of sweat glands in atopic individuals.

The significance of reaginic antibodies and raised IgE concentrations in atopic eczema is uncertain. Histologically, involved skin resembles delayed (type 4) hypersensitivity which makes a direct role for IgE unlikely, but the possibility that antigen–IgE antibody reactions in skin may play a synergistic role with other immunological and pharmacological mechanisms remains to be excluded.

Treatment. Both humid, hot climates and cold dryness exacerbate atopic eczema and should be avoided if possible. Unless there is a direct risk of infection by smallpox, vaccination is inadvisable because of the risk of developing eczema vaccinatum. The dominant symptom in atopic eczema is pruritus, and this is aggravated by woollen clothes and by warmth. Thus, light cotton or linen clothes should be worn and bed clothes should be light. Addition of emulsifying ointment to the bath water prevents excessive drying of the skin after bathing. Systemic antihistamines are often effective in the management of itching and are tolerated extremely well by children even in adult dosage. An antihistamine which combines both antipruritic and sedative effects, such as promethazine, can be given each night. By day an antihistamine with less potent soporific actions (e.g. chlorpheniramine) can be given. Systemic corticosteroids have little or no place in the management of atopic eczema because, although initially effective, they frequently lose their effect and a flare-up may follow their withdrawal. Furthermore, side-effects are a serious risk, especially impairment of growth in children. Topical corticosteroids are used widely and are undoubtedly effective but the advent of the more potent fluorinated steroids has led to an increased incidence of steroid atrophy of the skin and even cushingoid side-effects due to percutaneous absorption through the eczematous skin. They should be used with extreme caution, especially in children (whose surface area relative to mass is great). One per cent hydrocortisone ointment is safe since it produces no local or systemic steroid side-effects, and can be used liberally. Coal tar paste is also highly effective for chronic lichenified eczema and can be used with complete safety. A sudden acute exacerbation of previously well-controlled atopic eczema should raise the possibility of bacterial or virus infection; the latter may be the result of herpes simplex infection or vaccination either in the patient himself or someone with whom he has been in close contact. Eczema vaccinatum and eczema herpeticum are serious complications which necessitate hospital admission and vigorous antiviral therapy.

Autoimmune Connective Tissue Diseases

Under this loose heading are grouped a variety of systemic disorders which have in common multisystem involvement, widespread abnormalities of connective tissue, fibrinoid changes in blood vessels and a high incidence of organ and non-organ specific autoantibodies. In the present account, three of these disorders will be considered: lupus erythematosus, systemic sclerosis and dermatomyositis. The non-cutaneous features of these diseases are described in detail elsewhere (Chapter 4) and only the skin manifestations and immunological features will be considered here. The occurrence of patients with connective tissue diseases whose clinical signs and laboratory investigations do not enable satisfactory pigeon-holing into one or other of these designations is widely recognised and there is no doubt that many intermediate forms exist.

Lupus erythematosus

There are two main types of lupus erythematosus: systemic lupus erythematosus, and chronic discoid lupus erythematosus. Present evidence strongly supports the view that these two types are variants of the same disorder. Skin manifestations of both types of lupus erythematosus may coexist and patients with discoid lupus erythematosus occasionally develop systemic lupus erythematosus. Immunopathological abnormalities in involved skin of both forms of lupus erythematosus are also similar.

Chronic discoid lupus erythematosus

The eruption of chronic discoid lupus erythematosus is destructive and leads to scarring. It most commonly occurs on the exposed parts of the skin, particularly on the cheeks, bridge of the nose, forehead, ears and the backs of the hands. The main clinical features are circumscribed areas of atrophy, telangiectasia, follicular plugging, scaling and hypopigmentation. About half the patients have haematological and serological abnormalities including a raised ESR, leucopenia, antinuclear factor and hypergammaglobulinaemia, although the precise relationship of this group to systemic lupus erythematosus is debatable and depends on the controversial problem of the definition of systemic lupus erythematosus. The onset of lesions may be triggered by exposure to sunlight and by ingestion of drugs including sulphonamides and griseofulvin. Histologically, there is atrophy of the epidermis, plugging of follicles with keratin, liquefaction degeneration of the basal layer, oedema and hyalinisation of connective tissue in the dermis. There is also a dermal perivascular and periappendigeal inflammatory infiltrate.

Diagnosis and investigation. About 60 per cent of patients with chronic discoid lupus erythematosus have an abnormal reaction to 300 nm ultraviolet rays (UVR), and in about half of these the resulting inflammatory reaction has the features of discoid lupus erythematosus. Direct immunofluorescent tests for bound immunoglobulins are positive in the involved skin of 90 per cent of patients with discoid lupus erythematosus but are usually negative in uninvolved skin. The fluorescence is granular in character and is located at the dermo-epidermal junction alongside the basement membrane (Figure 10.1d). IgG is demonstrable more frequently than IgA or IgM and complement is demonstrable in most lesions. The globulin deposits probably form part of the antigen–antibody complexes. The specificity of basement membrane fluorescence is low since similar basement membrane fluorescence is also seen in a number of other conditions including rosacea, morphoea, porphyria and lichen planus. Several serological abnormalities are found in chronic discoid lupus erythematosus. Antinuclear antibodies are present in about 30 per cent of patients although lupus erythematosus cells are demonstrable in only 1 to 2 per cent. Rheumatoid factor is present in 17 per cent. Occasionally Coombs' test and the Wassermann reaction are positive and there is also increased incidence of gastric parietal cell and thyroid autoantibodies. The presence in the serum of anti-native DNA antibodies suggests the development of systemic lupus erythematosus.

Management and treatment. About 5 per cent of patients with discoid lupus erythematosus develop evidence of systemic lupus erythematosus. It is therefore important to carry out a full clinical, haematological and serological examination at the first examination, as a baseline for subsequent evaluations. Patients should be warned about the risk of light-provoked exacerbation and should use a preparation such as titanium dioxide or 5 per cent para-aminobenzoic acid in 70 per cent alcohol as sun screen. Topical corticosteroid creams usually control the lesions but are rarely curative. For extensive cases and ones in which topical steroids are ineffective, oral antimalarial treatment can be helpful. Hydroxychloroquine (Plaquenil) 400 mg daily should be given. It is important to obtain an ophthalmological assessment at the beginning and at intervals during chloroquine treatment because of the risk of corneal and retinal changes due to this drug.

Systemic lupus erythematosus

Although skin lesions occur in about 80 per cent of cases the skin abnormalities of systemic lupus erythematosus are extremely variable and frequently non-specific. In contrast to chronic discoid lupus erythematosus, destructive skin lesions leading to atrophy and scarring are unusual except in cases where chronic discoid lupus erythematosus coexists with systemic lupus erythematosus. The classical 'butterfly' rash on the nose, cheeks and forehead consists of erythema with or without oedema and scaling. This rash is frequently light-provoked and frequently also occurs in other light-exposed areas. Blisters may be present. Alternatively the rash may be more extensive and diffuse resembling eczema. On the hands reticular telangiectasia is common and may be associated with Raynaud's phenomenon. The nailfold capillaries are often prominent and may be accompanied by nailfold and nailbed haemorrhages. Gangrene of the fingertips is a common sequel of Raynaud's phenomenon in these patients. Other skin manifestations include erythema multiforme, livedo reticularis, and purpura which may be due to capillaritis or thrombocytopenia or both. Diffuse alopecia is common and mucous membrane lesions, usually of the mouth, occur in about 15 per cent of cases. Histologically, the appearances are less characteristic than in chronic discoid lupus erythematosus. Hyperkeratosis, follicular plugging and liquefaction degeneration of the basal layer of the epidermis may be seen and dermal oedema is frequent, in association with a diffuse inflammatory infiltrate. Often, however, the changes do not amount to more than those of a non-specific inflammatory reaction of the skin. In nearly all patients the direct immunofluorescent technique reveals the presence of globulin in the basement membrane zone, but unlike discoid lupus erythematosus these changes can be demonstrated in clinically normal skin as well as in the lesions themselves in 60 per cent of patients. Complement can also be demonstrated in these sites by the same method. Lupus erythematosus cells, anti-nuclear and anti-native DNA antibodies are often demonstrable. The general pathology, diagnosis and management of systemic lupus erythematosus are considered fully elsewhere.

Systemic sclerosis

The three most important skin manifestations of systemic sclerosis are Raynaud's phenomenon, scleroderma and small vessel vasculitis. About 90 per cent of patients with systemic sclerosis develop Raynaud's phenomenon and this is frequently the presenting symptom. It is nearly always bilateral and is associated with telangiectasia of the hands, abnormal fingernail-fold capillaries and nailfold haemorrhages, and eventually by infarcts and scarring of the fingertips. Digital calcinosis may develop in longstanding cases. Scleroderma (literally hardening of the skin) begins peripherally and proceeds centrally. The facial appearance of systemic sclerosis is characteristic. The nose becomes beaked, radial furrows develop around the lips which become thin, the forehead loses its normal creases and this confers a spuriously youthful appearance. Facial telangiectasia is common. The facial skin feels immobile on palpation and it is difficult to evert the lower eyelids. Similar changes affect the hands (sclerodactyly), wrists, forearms, feet and ankles; the mobility of the involved limbs becomes markedly impaired. Evidence of arteritis of the skin vasculature is frequently present in the form of livedo reticularis or small areas of skin infarction. Generalised melanin pigmentation is also a frequent finding. Histologically, the basic change in sclerodermatous skin is replacement of subcutaneous fat by abnormal connective tissue. The collagen appears homogeneous and histological evidence of vasculitis is often present. Atrophy of sweat glands and other skin appendages is also a frequent feature. Involvement of internal organs occurs to some extent in nearly all patients. This subject is considered more fully elsewhere.

Diagnosis. This is made mainly on clinical grounds. There is ample evidence of associated immunological abnormalities in systemic sclerosis. Direct immunofluorescent studies have shown evidence of globulin deposits and complement at the dermo-epidermal junction in telangiectatic sclerodermatous skin but not in sclerodermatous skin without telangiectasia. Serological abnormalities include antinuclear factor in 80 per cent and rheumatoid factor in about 30 per cent. Cold agglutinins are present in about 25 per cent of cases and LE cells are present in about 8 per cent.

Treatment. Treatment of systemic sclerosis is unsatisfactory. Little or nothing can be done to arrest the fibrosis of the skin and other tissues. Systemic corticosteroids are ineffective and the value of immunosuppressive therapy is unproven. Frequently the dominant symptom in systemic sclerosis is Raynaud's phenomenon or other manifestation of cold sensitivity. Patients should be kept as warm as possible and ideally should live in centrally heated accommodation. Intermittent infusions of low molecular weight dextran given over 48 hours at intervals of three to four weeks on three or four occasions cause significant improvement in peripheral blood flow and considerable symptomatic improvement. Vasodilator drugs are occasionally beneficial.

Dermatomyositis

In dermatomyositis erythematous changes in skin are associated with myopathy and there is an increased incidence of internal malignant disease in adult cases.

The rash of dermatomyositis is characteristic. A purple-red telangiectactic eruption involves the eyelids, cheeks and forehead, and oedema is often so prominent as to provoke a diagnosis of acute contact dermatitis of the face. Similar changes are seen on the backs of the hands, especially the knuckles where the rash has a linear configuration. The nailfold capillaries are often abnormally prominant. When lesions remit there is often residual atrophy with pigmentation and telangiectasia giving a poikilodermatous appearance. Occasionally the rash may look eczematous. Raynaud's phenomenon occurs in about 10 per cent and, although livedo reticularis is fairly common, in general small vessel arteritis is less prominent than in other autoimmune connective tissue diseases. Calcinosis of the involved skin may occur, particularly in childhood cases. Myositis usually presents as an aching and weakness of the pelvic and shoulder girdle muscles causing difficulty in getting up from a supine position, climbing stairs or raising the arms above the head. Occasionally the pharyngeal muscles may be affected causing dysphagia. The histological changes of the skin may resemble those of acute lupus erythematosus with dermal oedema and inflammatory perivascular infiltrate. In poikilodermatous cases there is additional liquefaction degeneration of the basal layer, epidermal atrophy and hyperkeratosis. Mucin is often present in the dermis in involved skin in dermatomyositis.

The relation of the disease to malignant tumours in adults suggests that dermatomyositis may be due to an immunological reaction to tumour antigens. In support of this concept the condition may improve when the tumour is removed and there are reports which await confirmation of complement-fixing antibodies to autologous tumour tissue and positive skin reactions to aqueous tumour extracts. Convincing immunofluorescent evidence of the immune nature of the disease is as yet unavailable.

Diagnosis. The antinuclear factor and rheumatoid factor are usually absent in the serum, and LE cells are rarely found in the blood. Diagnosis is usually confirmed by muscle biopsy, determination of the serum glutamic oxaloacetic transaminase, and estimation of 24-hour urinary creatine. The serum creatine phosphokinase may be raised. The presence of scattered deposits of calcium in muscles is also strongly suggestive of dermatomyositis.

Treatment. Treatment consists of systemic corticosteroid therapy. The occasional patients who fail to show some degree of remission on this treatment or who develop incapacitating steroid side-effects may respond well to chemical immunosuppressive treatment by azathioprine or cyclophosphamide.

Allergic Vasculitis

The clinical appearances of allergic cutaneous vasculitis are pleomorphic and depend in part on the size of the involved vessels and on regional differences in the anatomy of the blood supply in the skin. Characteristically, lesions range from crops of urticated papules, vesicles and pustules to purpura, necrotic papules and larger areas of skin necrosis due to infarction. Vasculitis lesions have a predilection for the legs, presumably because for gravitational reasons the cutaneous circulation in the legs is often more precarious than elsewhere. Local minor trauma and lower skin temperatures are additional localising factors. Vasculitic lesions are often associated with livedo reticularis—a reticulate pattern of dull-red erythema on the trunk and limbs indicative of sluggish blood flow through the superficial cutaneous blood vessels. Continuous livedo reticularis often occurs in healthy skin but broken livedo indicates pathological stasis of blood in the involved skin. Vasculitis is one cause of this. Cutaneous vasculitis may be associated with systemic disease including arthritis, nephritis and intestinal complications.

There is no satisfactory classification of cutaneous vasculitis, and dermatological textbooks contain under this heading accounts of a confused array of rather similar disorders. However, from a histopathological point of view, the changes in most of these share a resemblance to the Arthus (type 3) reaction. Vessels show endothelial thickening and fibrinoid necrosis of the vessel walls with perivascular haemorrhage. In early lesions the involved vessels show migration of polymorphonuclear leucocytes through the walls leading to a cuff of neutrophils around the vessels. Eosinophils are also often prominent. In older lesions mononuclear infiltrates may predominate. Resemblance of the vasculitis to the Arthus reaction has led to investigation of the possibility that cutaneous vasculitis is due to deposition of antigen–antibody complexes in the skin blood vessels. There is now good evidence that cutaneous vasculitis is frequently allergic in origin. A number of animal models of allergic vasculitis have been described. In human lesions immunofluorescent studies have demonstrated the presence of globulin and complement. In some patients it has been possible to identify bacterial antigens in the lesions including streptococcal, staphylococcal and *Mycobacterium tuberculosis* antigen. In these lesions the antigen and globulins were almost certainly bound in the form of complexes because double staining with rhodamine and fluorescein showed discrete globulin deposits superimposed on a more diffuse intracellular bacterial antigen. Serum of patients with cutaneous vasculitis frequently contains circulating immune complexes and these may be cold precipitable as cryoglobulins. These circulating mixed cryoglobulins are of the same immunoglobulin classes as those globulins present in the skin lesions. Although the importance of immunological mechanisms in cutaneous vasculitis is becoming widely recognised, not all cases of vasculitis have an allergic basis. Vasculitis with a similar clinical presentation may be the result of degenerative changes in vessel walls as in diabetes mellitus, or due to an increased blood viscosity as in hyperglobulinaemia or polycythaemia.

Diagnosis. The presence of cutaneous vasculitis is usually easily established on the basis of the clinical appearances and histological evidence of Arthus-like reactions, but it is difficult to confirm that the vasculitis is allergic. Immunofluorescent evidence of immune complexes and complement in the lesions is not absolute proof since these could have been deposited secondarily in pre-existing non-allergic vasculitis lesions. Thus it can be argued that a recent streptococcal respiratory infection in a patient with vasculitis may result in deposition of streptococcal antigen–antibody complexes in vasculitic lesions as a secondary 'trapping' effect. Skin testing by bacterial antigens has been advocated but the significance of results is too uncertain for its use to be recommended except on an experimental basis. The ESR, serum globulins and blood eosinophil count may be raised or normal and are of little or no diagnostic help.

Treatment. No specific treatment is available. Since bacterial antigen has been implicated in some cases it is reasonable to identify and treat any chronic infection. Systemic corticosteroid therapy is usually ineffective. There is good evidence that in some cases of vasculitis the fibrinolytic activity of the blood is lowered and these patients may benefit from therapy with fibrinolytic agents. Phenformin 50 mg twice daily and ethyloestrenol (Orabolin) 2 mg twice daily have been used together with success in some patients. There is no evidence that this treatment is ever beneficial in patients with vasculitis who have normal blood fibrinolytic activity.

Henoch-Schönlein purpura

This form of allergic vasculitis occurs predominantly in children and is frequently associated with arthritis, nephritis and gastrointestinal complications. The role of streptococcal infections in Henoch–Schönlein purpura is uncertain. Results from recent controlled studies do not support the earlier reports of an increased incidence of haemolytic streptococci in the respiratory tracts of patients.

Abdominal symptoms in the form of diarrhoea, colic and vomiting occur in about 50 per cent of children, and evidence of renal involvement in 25 to 50 per cent. Although attacks of Henoch–Schönlein purpura last about three to six weeks, relapses occur in almost half the patients. Although the role of streptococcal infection is unproven, penicillin should be given to patients with evidence of streptococcal infection. Systemic corticosteroids probably do not influence the course of the disease but are sometimes justifiable on the grounds of systemic relief. Patients should be carefully investigated for evidence of renal involvement at the beginning and at frequent intervals during attacks of Henoch–Schönlein purpura. A final assessment should be made three months after the attack has subsided.

Erythema nodosum

This form of vasculitis presents as a dull-red nodular eruption on the extensor surfaces of the legs and forearms. The nodules are tender and often show bruising but they do not ulcerate and clear up in about one to two months without scarring. Fever and joint pains frequently accompany the eruption. More important aetiological factors are shown in Table 10.2.

Table 10.2. Causes of erythema nodosum

Infections:	Streptococcal infections
	Tuberculosis
	Virus infections
	Leprosy
Sarcoidosis	
Drugs:	Sulphonamides
	Contraceptive pill
Enteropathies:	Ulcerative colitis
	Crohn's disease
Malignant disease:	Reticulosis

Diagnosis. The ESR is usually high. Evidence of streptococcal infection should be sought by taking throat swabs and determining the blood ASO titre. The Mantoux reaction is positive in patients with tuberculosis but may be negative in sarcoidosis. The Kveim test is positive in sarcoidosis. Radiological examination of the chest may show evidence of sarcoidosis or tuberculosis.

Treatment. In the presence of painful erythema nodosum arthralgia and pyrexia, the patient should be kept in bed. Aspirin is effective in relieving both pain and fever. Systemic corticosteroids are of little or no value. The patient should be allowed up when the pain and fever have subsided. The most important aspect of the management of erythema nodosum is the investigation of the underlying cause.

Bullous Diseases

It is only comparatively recently that the classification of chronic blistering diseases has been established on a rational basis. Blistering eruptions are classified as intra- or sub-epidermal depending on whether the blister originates above or below the basal layer. Pemphigus, eczema, and many virus infections cause intraepidermal blistering. Subepidermal blistering occurs in dermatitis herpetiformis, pemphigoid, and erythema multiforme. The discovery that some chronic bullous diseases are associated with immunological abnormalities is a recent development, and has important implications in terms of the pathogenesis, diagnosis and treatment of these conditions.

Pemphigus vulgaris

This extremely severe and progressive blistering eruption occurs predominantly in middle or old age. The essential pathological change in the epidermis is loss of intercellular bridges between adjacent epidermal cells—a process called acantholysis. Acantholytic cells are round in shape. Their presence in a skin biopsy or in blister fluid is highly suggestive of the diagnosis of pemphigus. Since the blister in pemphigus characteristically does not heal and spreads in untreated cases, the involved areas may become very extensive indeed. That normal-looking skin between the areas of blistering is really abnormal can often be demonstrated by the ease with which the apparently normal epidermis can be dislodged with the finger (Nikolsky sign). The majority of patients develop painful oral erosions. Without treatment the average duration of survival from the onset is 14 months.

Diagnosis. The clinical diagnosis is confirmed by demonstration of acantholysis in skin biopsies. Acantholytic cells can also be identified in centrifuged deposits of blister fluid or in stained smears from a blister base.

Almost all patients with active pemphigus have antiepidermal antibodies both in the serum and in the epidermis. These antibodies, which are in the IgG or less often the IgM fraction, react with antigen in the intercellular zone between adjacent epidermal cells. They can readily be detected by immunofluorescent techniques either in the skin itself (direct immunofluorescent test) or by the indirect method using the patient's serum. The direct test is positive both in involved and clinically uninvolved skin in pemphigus vulgaris. Skin biopsy material is treated with fluorescein-conjugated rabbit antihuman gamma globulin. Fluorescent microscopy reveals intercellular fluorescence in the epidermis (Figure 10.1a). The presence of complement concommitantly bound with globulin can also be demonstrated. In the indirect test, serum from patients with active pemphigus is reacted with squamous epithelial substrate (usually guinea pig oesophagus). The serum antiepidermal antibody is taken up by the epidermal antigen in the substrate and is then detected by the same technique as with the direct test. The serum antibodies cannot react with non-squamous epithelial substrates and are not species specific. Their titre correlates with the activity of the disease and is held by some to be of prognostic value. The presence of these antibodies in the serum is specific for pemphigus with the exception that the serum of patients with burned skin shows apparently identical auto-antibodies.

The role of these antibodies in the pathogenesis of pemphigus is uncertain. Circumstantial evidence supports a pathogenic role since:

1. They react with antigen located at the exact site of the histological damage in involved skin.
2. Their titre varies with the disease activity.
3. They fix complement.

However, the critical test of their role would be successful passive transfer of pemphigus using the patient's serum but this has yet to be convincingly demonstrated. At the moment the existing evidence is equally compatible with the hypothesis that the antibodies are a result of epidermal damage rather than the cause. It is, however, of interest that there is an increased incidence of antinuclear factor as well as of some other autoantibodies in the serum of patients with pemphigus vulgaris. The presence of antinuclear factor may also produce apparent false-positive results in the indirect immunofluorescent test of pemphigus antibodies.

Treatment. Blister tops should be removed and weak antiseptic soaks applied (soaks of saline or 1/10 000 potassium permanganate are suitable). Systemic antibiotics should also be given as secondary infection is almost invariable. The use of systemic corticosteroids has lowered the mortality in pemphigus vulgaris from almost 100 per cent to around 30 to 40 per cent. In the average-sized patient at least 120 mg of prednisone should be given daily until no new blisters appear, after which the dose can be gradually reduced. Topical corticosteroids are usually unhelpful in pemphigus vulgaris although they are sometimes of value in the management of oral pemphigus. However, present evidence indicates that spontaneous remissions are excessively rare in pemphigus vulgaris so that patients have to continue with prednisone maintenance treatment for an indefinite period. Very often these elderly patients have to take quite high maintenance doses of prednisone of the order of 10 to 20 mg daily or more, so that the incidence of morbidity and mortality from treatment in this disease is high. Because of the occurrence in pemphigus of antiepidermal antibodies, attempts have been made in several centres to use immunosuppressive drugs in an attempt to replace corticosteroid treatment or at least to reduce the minimum necessary dose of corticosteroid necessary to control the blisters. Methotrexate, cyclophosphamide and azathioprine have been used in several studies, and the concensus of opinion is that administration of one of these drugs usually enables lowering of corticosteroid dosage or total withdrawal of corticosteroid treatment. Methotrexate has the disadvantage that it readily produces cirrhosis of the liver. Reports of the effectiveness of cyclophosphamide, though very encouraging, are mainly limited to accounts of isolated cases. On present evidence azathioprine is probably the best available choice, a steroid-sparing effect being demonstrable in the majority of cases. Since control by azathioprine is slow (at least four weeks), initial rapid control should be achieved by large daily doses of prednisone as outlined above. At the same time azathioprine treatment should be started using a dose 2·5 mg per kilogram body weight per day. During the first month prednisone dosage can be diminished gradually depending on the activity of the skin. Maintenance treatment is then continued with the same dosage of azathioprine and the minimum necessary daily dosage of prednisone. It is important to carry out a full haematological, renal and liver function evaluation before and at weekly or fortnightly intervals during treatment. Obviously pre-existing renal and liver diseases are a contraindication to azathioprine therapy. Leucopenia which is a frequent complication during azathioprine treatment should be dealt with by stopping the azathioprine for one to two weeks or reducing the dose, depending upon the degree of leucopenia.

Bullous pemphigoid

Like pemphigus, pemphigoid is a chronic blistering eruption of the latter half of life which is associated with the presence of antiskin autoantibodies and which responds to treatment with high dosage of corticosteroids. It was not clearly distinguished from pemphigus as a separate clinical entity until the 1950s. However, it differs from pemphigus in several very important ways. The bullae are subepidermal in origin, there are no acantholytic cells, and the Nikolsky sign is negative. Blisters arise on a background of inflamed oedematous skin and are associated with a variable degree of itching. The inflammatory changes frequently precede the onset of blistering. The blisters are thick-roofed and often haemorrhagic, and individual blisters heal whilst new ones are appearing elsewhere. About one-third of cases have oral mucosal erosions. The disease runs a chronic course with alternate relapses and remissions but the mortality is about 30 per cent.

Diagnosis. The clinical diagnosis is confirmed by histological evidence that the blisters are arising subepidermally. About 80 per cent of patients with pemphigoid have circulating antiepidermal antibodies which react with the basement membrane zone of the epidermis. These antibodies, which fix complement, are usually found in the IgG immunoglobulin fraction although occasionally IgM antibodies have been identified. Antibodies are demonstrable in serum by the indirect immunofluorescent test, a positive result being the presence of a band of fluorescence in the basement membrane zone. The direct immunofluorescent test is also positive in involved skin and skin immediately adjacent to the involved skin. A continuous band of fluorescence is seen in the basement membrane zone. (Figure 10.1b). Similar immunofluorescent staining is seen in the skin in patients with systemic lupus erythematous but in this disease the band of fluorescence has a granular appear-

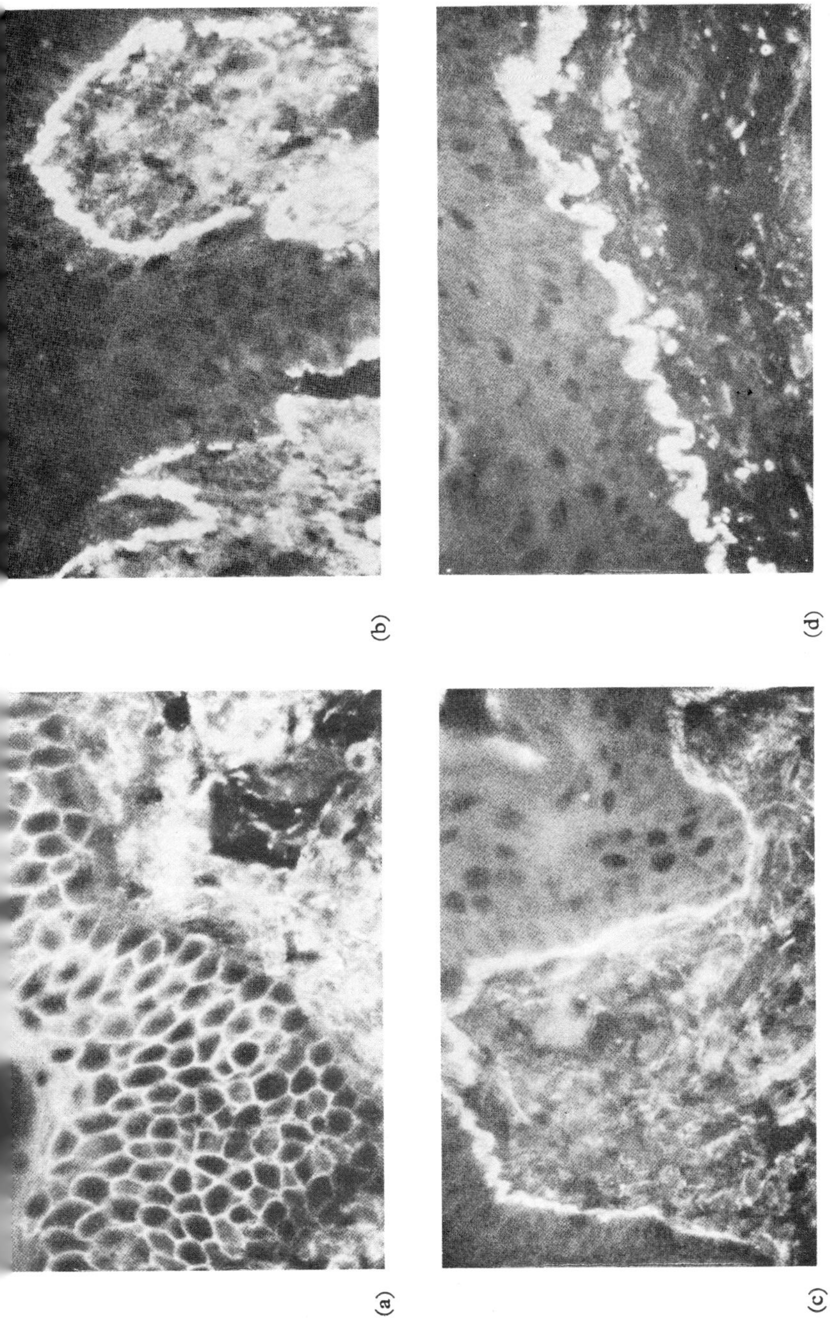

(a) (b) (c) (d)

Figure 10.1. Direct immunofluorescent test in bullous diseases and lupus erythematosus. (a) Fluorescence in the intercellular zones of the epidermis in uninvolved skin in pemphigus vulgaris. (b) Basement membrane zone fluorescence in involved skin in bullous pemphigoid. (c) Basement membrane fluorescence due to deposits of IgA in uninvolved skin in dermatitis herpetiformis. (d) Granular basement membrane fluorescence in uninvolved skin in systemic lupus erythematosus.

ance (Figure 10.1d). As in pemphigus, the importance of the antibodies in the pathogenesis of pemphigoid is unknown. The antibodies are not found in all cases and the titre of serum antibodies does not correlate well with the activity of the blistering eruption in the skin.

Treatment. Bullae should be opened and the roofs removed, and soaks (potassium permanganate 1/10 000, or saline) should be applied to the underlying erosions twice or three times daily. Secondary infection should be treated by systemic antibiotics. The only sure way to achieve rapid control of the eruption is to give large daily doses of corticosteroids systemically. At least 120 mg of prednisone should be given daily in the average-sized adult. After the blistering has been brought under control (i.e. no new blisters are appearing) the daily dosage can be gradually reduced. Although in occasional cases it is possible to reduce prednisone dosage to zero soon after the acute illness, in most cases maintenance treatment with prednisone is necessary, often with high doses. However, one-third of patients with pemphigoid go into sustained remission within five years of the original attack. In the remaining two-thirds, azathioprine is an effective alternative to prednisone in suppression of pemphigoid and it is of especial value in patients who in the long term require substantial daily doses of prednisone to achieve suppression. The dosage precautions and principles of administration of azathioprine are identical with those for the treatment of pemphigus and are discussed in the preceding section on pemphigus. Because of the significant incidence of spontaneous remission in pemphigoid, periodic attempts should be made to withdraw treatment altogether. Evidence that there is an increased incidence of carcinoma in patients with pemphigoid is inconclusive. Nevertheless, this possibility should be borne in mind.

Dermatitis herpetiformis

This chronic blistering eruption is most common in young or middle-aged adults and is characterised by recurrent groups of vesicles mainly on the extensor surfaces, arising on a background of inflamed skin. Pruritus is an almost invariable feature and is often intense. As in pemphigoid, the blisters of dermatitis herpetiformis arise subepidermally, usually developing at the tip of the dermal papillae. Eosinophils are often prolific at the site of vesiculation. Mucosal lesions are rare. There is no acantholysis and the Nikolsky sign is negative. About 70 per cent of patients have a gluten-sensitive enteropathy which is essentially similar to the enteropathy of coeliac disease. The relationship of the enteropathy to the skin in dermatitis herpetiformis is disputed.

Diagnosis. Histologically, the presence of papillary tip microabscesses with numerous eosinophils is characteristic. These can be seen to evolve into subepidermal vesicles in other parts of the section. Similar clinical and histological appearances are often seen in pemphigoid and this may present considerable diagnostic difficulty. This difficulty can be resolved by giving diaminodiphenyl sulphone (dapsone) 100 mg daily by mouth which causes remission of dermatitis herpetiformis within 48 hours but has little or no effect on pemphigoid. Pemphigoid and dermatitis herpetiformis differ immunologically. The presence of basement membrane globulin deposits can be demonstrated in both conditions by immunofluorescence but in dermatitis herpetiformis the fluorescence is due to IgA globulin (Figure 10.1c) unlike pemphigoid where the immunoglobulin is predominantly IgG. Furthermore, no serum antiskin antibodies have been identified in dermatitis herpetiformis although circulating antireticulin antibodies have been demonstrated in a minority of patients. Their significance is uncertain. The possibility that delayed cell-mediated hypersensitivity may be important in the intestinal changes of dermatitis herpetiformis is suggested by the presence of a heavy infiltration of lymphocytes in the small bowel mucosa.

Treatment. Dapsone in a dosage of 100 mg daily is effective in almost all cases, although much higher doses are required in the occasional patient. This subgroup probably includes rapid acetylators of dapsone. Because of the variability of the disease at different times, patients can often learn to adjust their dosage depending on the activity of the skin at the time. This is of some value because side-effects including central cyanosis due to methaemoglobinaemia are extremely common with the dosage of dapsone usually given in dermatitis herpetiformis.

Erythema multiforme

Erythema multiforme is a highly distinctive acute eruption in which bullae are a common but by no means invariable feature. Erythema multiforme is considered here because in its bullous form it is occasionally confused with pemphigoid and because it has a number of features which suggest that it has an immunological basis. Patients characteristically give a history of abrupt onset of an extensive symmetrical eruption involving the palms and the soles as well as other areas. Individual lesions range from pink papules and macules with a purple centre ('iris' or 'target' lesions) through oedematous red vesicular plaques to extensive haemorrhagic bullae. The mucous membranes are often involved. In the rare Stevens–Johnson syndrome bullous erythema multiforme is associated with severe oral conjunctival and genital ulceration, pneumonitis and high fever. Nephritis is an occasional complication of erythema multiforme and may be precipitated by a number of factors including virus infections (especially herpes simplex), *Mycoplasma* infection, streptococcal infection especially streptococcal pharyngitis, drug reactions, internal malignant disease, radiotherapy, and collagen diseases including lupus erythematosus and polyarteritis nodosa. Evidence that erythema multiforme involves allergic mechanisms is only circumstantial and is based on the histological appearances of vasculitis in the epidermis, the frequent history of a recent infection and the multifocal nature of the disease.

Diagnosis. This is clinically based and depends on the symmetrical distribution of the rash, the target lesions and bullae, together with the histological appearances of vasculitis.

Treatment. No treatment is necessary for mild forms of erythema multiforme. Systemic corticosteroids produce symptomatic relief in acute erythema multiforme and in the Stevens–Johnson syndrome, especially where there is severe oral ulceration. There is, however, no evidence that systemic corticosteroids can cure the disease or reduce the morbidity or mortality. Oral ulceration often causes severe discomfort and disability and should be treated by frequent mouthwashes and a topical corticosteroid such as triamcinalone 0·1 per cent in Orabase.

Review References

Beck, P., Wills, D., Davies, G. T., Lachmann, P. J. & Sussman, M. (1973) A family study of hereditary angioneurotic oedema. *Quarterly Journal of Medicine*, **42,** 317–339.

Beutner, E. H., Jordan, R. E. & Chorzelski, T. P. (1968) The immunopathology of pemphigus and bullous pemphigoid. *Journal of Investigative Dermatology*, **61,** 63.

Coombs, R. R. A. & Gell, P. G. H. (1968) Classification of allergic reactions responsible for clinical hypersensitivity and disease. In *Clinical Aspects of Immunology*, eds. Gell, P. G. H. & Coombs, R. R. A., p. 575. Oxford: Blackwell.

Cream, J. J., Gumpell, J. M. & Peachey, R. D. G. (1970) Schönlein–Henoch purpura in the adult. *Quarterly Journal of Medicine*, **39,** 461.

Turk, J. L. (1971) The cytologic basis of immune responses. In *Advances in the Biology of Skin*, Vol. XI, eds. Montagna, W. & Billingham, R. E., p. 45. New York: Appleton-Century-Crofts.

11. Drug Hypersensitivity

J. F. ACKROYD

Untoward reactions to drug therapy have become increasingly common as more and more pharmacologically active drugs have become available. One of the commonest problems confronting the physician nowadays, when faced with a patient who has developed a new symptom, is that of deciding whether this is due to the drugs he has been taking, and if so, what the underlying mechanism may be. It is the purpose of this chapter to indicate how this problem can be approached. Since this book is concerned with clinical immunology the main emphasis will be on immunological mechanisms, although the mechanism by which many allergic drug reactions are caused is very incompletely understood. In fact it must be stated at the outset that, in many cases, even the most careful investigation fails to reveal a mechanism or even to establish beyond doubt that the supposed reaction was due to the drug and was not either an unusual manifestation of the disease being treated or due to coincidental disease. Homologous serum jaundice provides an interesting example of the latter, for that disease, now known to be due to viral infection, was for long thought to be due to arsenobenzol compounds and other drugs given by injection.

Another fact which makes the diagnosis of allergic drug hypersensitivity so difficult and which will become apparent in the course of this chapter is that, with few exceptions, the presence of a drug-dependent antibody in the serum of a patient who has developed a reaction apparently due to that drug does *not* prove that the reaction was in fact due to the drug. It often means only that the patient has developed a perfectly harmless antibody to the drug. Penicillin provides an interesting example of this. Penicillin can cause the production of an antibody that agglutinates penicillin-coated red cells and, if a sufficiently sensitive technique is used, this antibody can be demonstrated in all patients who have been treated with this drug (Levine et al, 1966a). This type of antibody does not, however, reduce the bactericidal activity of penicillin and is not, except on very rare occasions, associated with haemolytic anaemia.

The following classification may be found helpful in the initial assessment of a suspected drug reaction:

Overdosage: The symptoms are due to excessive intake or to a failure to metabolise and detoxicate or to excrete the drug.

Intolerance: The symptoms are those of overdosage, but they occur in the presence of normal blood and tissue levels of the drug.

Idiosyncrasy: The symptoms are unlike those of overdosage. They are not immunologically determined.

Side-effects: These are the undesirable, but unavoidable, pharmacological reactions to the drug.

Secondary effects: These are indirect but not inevitable consequences of the primary action of a drug, e.g. fungal infections in patients being treated with antibiotics.

Hypersensitivity: As in idiosyncracy, these reactions are qualitatively unlike those of normal drug action, or of overdosage. They do, however, have an immunological mechanism.

This classification makes it clear that the major difficulties will be likely to arise in the differentiation of idiosyncracy and hypersensitivity. A few examples will show how closely idiosyncracy can mimic hypersensitivity. Primaquine, and certain other drugs, will cause haemolytic anaemia in patients whose red cells are deficient in the enzyme glucose-6-phosphate dehydrogenase. Patients who acetylate isonicotinic acid hydrazide rapidly rarely develop peripheral neuritis, whereas those who acetylate the drug slowly do so much more commonly. This difference in acetylation is genetically determined. Heterozygous carriers of a gene which causes deficiency of the enzyme-reduced nicotinamide adenine dinucleotide diaphorase develop methaemoglobinaemia and cyanosis after taking certain drugs such as chloroquine, primaquine and diaminodiphenylsulfone. Some patients metabolise phenacetin abnormally by a metabolic pathway that results in the production of metabolites which cause haemolytic anaemia and methaemoglobinaemia, even if only normal therapeutic doses of the drug are taken. This abnormality appears to be familial (Shahidi, 1967). Patients with certain unstable haemoglobins (Hb Zurich, Hb H, Hb Torino and Hb Shepherds Bush) experience an exacerbation of haemolysis, often with the development of frank haemolytic anaemia, when treated with sulphonamides (Dickerman, Holtzman and Zinkham, 1973). Finally, it should be remembered that the symptoms of acute intermittent porphyria are precipitated by certain drugs, notably barbiturates.

The complexity of the situation is exemplified by a consideration of reactions to the drug phenacetin. This drug can cause haemolytic anaemia in at least three ways. First, it may stimulate the formation of an anti-red cell antibody active only in the presence of the drug (MacGibbon et al, 1960). Second, phenacetin may cause haemolytic anaemia in patients deficient in the enzyme glucose-6-phosphate dehydrogenase (G-6-PD). Dern, Beutler and Alving (1955) showed that this drug would cause haemolysis of G-6-PD deficient cells in vivo and although Houston and Barlow (1959) did not measure the level of the enzyme in the patient's red cells, their case of haemolytic anaemia produced by phenacetin was clearly one of G-6-PD deficiency. Third, as already stated, phenacetin may cause haemolytic anaemia as a result of an abnormality in the metabolism of the drug, resulting in the formation of excessive amounts of compounds that cause red cell lysis (Shahidi, 1967). The first mechanism is clearly one of hypersensitivity; the two latter are idiosyncratic.

The differentiation of idiosyncracy from hypersensitivity is by no means always possible, and it may well be that increasing knowledge will show that many drug reactions now thought probably to be due to immune mechanisms are due to enzymatic or other abnormalities in the patient.

Factors Predisposing to the Development of Drug Hypersensitivity

Hypersensitivity to drugs can develop at any age and in either sex. Although the few limited studies that have been made have shown minor predispositions to the development of certain reactions in one or other sex, or at a particular age, no consistent pattern has emerged and certainly such findings are of no help in the diagnosis of the individual patient.

Genetic factors may be involved. This is certainly true for contact sensitivity in the guinea pig and Walker, Smith and Maibach (1967) have reported that the children of parents who are readily sensitised by dermal contact with para-nitrosodimethylaniline are more readily sensitised by this allergen than are the children of parents who are not so readily sensitised. Patients with atopic hypersensitivity which is thought, in part, to have a genetic basis, have been shown to have a greater than normal tendency to develop skin-sensitising antibodies to penicillin (Levine et al, 1966b). Finally, Sheba and Shani (1969) have made the fascinating observation that chloramphenicol aplastic anaemia is extremely rare in Israel, although the drug is widely used in that country in which, with a population of only two million, 15 tons of this drug were consumed within five years. The reason for this low incidence of aplastic anaemia is unknown, but a genetic basis would seem probable. Further support for the concept that chloramphenicol aplastic anaemia may have a genetic basis comes from a report by Nagao and Mauer (1969) that this condition has been observed in identical twins.

Disease

The frequency of reactions to many antibiotics and other chemotherapeutic agents has raised the question whether infections could predispose to the development of drug hypersensitivity. There is some evidence that this may be true for one or two infections. The most striking example is the extremely high incidence of exanthematic rashes due to ampicillin in patients with infectious mononucleosis. The nature of exanthematic rashes is considered below. Another possible example has been reported by Watkinson and Hillis (1947) who observed a high incidence of photosensitisation to sulphonamides in recently vaccinated subjects. This curious relationship has never been confirmed and is unexplained. Apart from these isolated reports it can be said that no disease is known to predispose to the development of drug hypersensitivity. The early impression that there is an abnormally high incidence of hypersensitivity reaction to drugs in patients with systemic lupus erythematosus has not been confirmed. These patients are subjected to a great deal of drug therapy in the course of their long illnesses, and it is doubtful whether any increased incidence of drug reactions that they may develop is more than a reflection of increased exposure with a consequent increase in opportunity for sensitisation.

In hypogammaglobulinaemia, contact sensitivity, which is cell mediated, can be readily induced, but other forms of drug reaction are very rare. In sarcoidosis, in which, as is well known, delayed hypersensitivity to tuberculin is depressed, there is also a reduced susceptibility to contact dermatitis.

The drug

Some drugs rarely cause reactions whereas others do so commonly, but attempts to correlate chemical structure and sensitising capacity have, so far, been unsuccessful. In general it is thought that drugs or their metabolic breakdown products act as haptens and must combine covalently with a carrier macromolecule—usually a protein—before they become immunogenic. Eisen (1959), working with halogenated dinitrobenzene compounds, has demonstrated a direct correlation between the rate of reactivity with protein and potency for producing anaphylactic sensitivity. However, it must be accepted that some of the drugs which cause allergic reactions are not known to react directly with plasma macromolecules, or to have metabolic breakdown products which are capable of doing this.

Although on theoretical grounds reactions to a drug metabolite rather than to the drug itself might be expected to occur commonly, such reactions have very rarely been reported. Eisner and Shahidi (1972) have recently reported a case of immunologically determined thrombocytopenic purpura due, not to paracetamol (*N*-acetyl-*p*-aminophenol) which the patient was taking, but to a major metabolite, *N*-acetyl-*p*-aminophenol sulphate. A further case of thrombocytopenic purpura apparently due to a drug metabolite has been reported by Eisner and Kasper (1972). The patient developed thrombocytopenic purpura whilst taking para-aminosalicylic acid but tests using this drug failed to demonstrate a drug-dependent antibody. The tests were however positive when the patient's serum was mixed with the platelet-rich plasma of a donor who was taking this drug.

An important possibility with any allergic drug reaction is that the patient may have become sensitised to an impurity in the pharmaceutical preparation. This has been shown to be of particular importance in connection with the penicillins. Knudsen, Dewdney and Trafford (1970) found that purification of ampicillin approximately halved the incidence of rashes due to this drug.

Cross-sensitisation

A patient who has developed allergic symptoms in response to one compound sometimes develops similar symptoms in response to related compounds. This phenomenon, known as cross-sensitisation, can be of great clinical importance. Failure to appreciate the immunochemical relationship between two different drugs may lead to the substitution of a cross-reacting drug for one causing a severe drug reaction. If this is done, the reaction will clearly be perpetuated and may even be intensified with a possible fatal outcome. A few examples of drugs which can cross-react in this way may be given. Cross-reactivity occurs between all the penicillins and between penicillin and cephalosporin derivatives.

Cross-reactions between phenothiazines are common. Neomycin may cross-sensitise to streptomycin. A patient sensitised by the topical application of the local anaesthetic benzocaine may develop allergic reactions if exposed to paraphenylenediamine in a hair dye, and a patient who has become sensitised to sulphonamides may also show sensitisation to procaine (see Baer, 1954; Hjorth and Fregert, 1972). The possibility of cross-sensitisation must be considered whenever a reaction thought to be due to a drug persists when the drug is withdrawn: it may be due to a cross-reacting drug the patient is still receiving or to the substitution of a cross-reacting drug for the one withdrawn. It may also be due to a cross-reacting chemical in an unsuspected form. Penicillin in milk products is a good example of this and is believed by Levine (1966) to be the reason for the persistence of some cases of urticaria due to the penicillins.

Route of administration and the vehicle

Contact dermatitis occurs in man only after repeated exposure of the skin to the drug. Apart from this very common form of dermatitis, the route of administration is of little importance in determining the type of hypersensitivity reaction the patient develops. Nonetheless, it does seem to be clearly established that the anaphylactic type of reaction occurs much less commonly after oral than after parenteral drug administration.

Penicillin, when given in oil and beeswax, causes a higher percentage of reactions than does this drug given in aqueous solution. The oil and beeswax probably acts as an adjuvant.

Sensitisation to the vehicle in which the drug is administered has been reported in cows which developed anaphylactic shock or generalised oedema when injected with penicillin. The reaction was not, however, due to the penicillin, but to the vehicle—carboxymethycellulose (Leemann, De Weck and Schneider, 1969). This substance is not known to cause sensitisation in man.

Dosage

The risk of sensitisation rises as the dose and the period of administration are increased. In some sensitised patients the reaction may be provoked by very small doses of the drug. An extreme example of this is the fatal case of anaphylactic shock reported by Dogliotti (1968) which followed a scratch test performed through a drop of a dilute solution of penicillin containing only 40 000 units/ml. If no further drug is given the antibody titre will fall. This may occur so slowly that a reaction can be provoked by a single small dose after an interval of several years. On the other hand, it may fall quite rapidly and it may not be possible to demonstrate the antibody by in vitro tests for more than a few days after the reaction occurred. Ultimately the antibody concentration may fall to a level at which even a therapeutic dose given on a single occasion may fail to cause a reaction. Further administration of the drug will, however, stimulate antibody formation so that eventually the drug will again cause the reaction. On rare occasions, however, this may not occur until after several days of drug administration.

Clinical Patterns

Allergic reactions to drugs rarely develop after less than a week of continuous treatment in patients who have not taken the drug before. On the other hand, the patient may have taken the drug for years before developing a reaction to it. Once the patient has become sensitised, the reaction sometimes develops rapidly, sometimes within minutes or even seconds. Symptoms of hypersensitivity may not occur during the first course of a drug but may occur in response to the first dose of a second or subsequent course. In such cases it appears that sensitisation occurred after the last dose of the previous course. Some types of drug reaction do not usually develop until after treatment has stopped; the serum sickness type of reaction caused by penicillin is an example. If the drug forms a depot from which it is only slowly released the reaction may not occur until weeks or even months after treatment has been discontinued, because sensitisation has only then occurred. An example of this is a patient who developed thrombocytopenic purpura six months after his last injection of a gold salt. This responded to treatment with dimercaprol (BAL), but relapsed when treatment was discontinued (Hazlett and Yendt, 1958). As already stated, a patient who has developed signs of hypersensitivity and who has not taken the drug again for a long period may have experienced such a fall in antibody titre that he does not develop symptoms again in response to the first re-exposure to the drug and will not, in fact, develop symptoms until further treatment with the drug has resulted in a sufficient rise in the level of the antibody.

A very large number of conditions have been thought to be due to drug hypersensitivity, although the evidence has often been tenuous in the extreme. In the following section only a relatively small number of reactions are considered. These have been chosen either because there was strong evidence that they were immunologically determined, or because it was felt that a physician seeing such a case might have a reasonable suspicion that it was so determined and might therefore wish to have a brief statement of the evidence. The selection has clearly been arbitrary and some conditions have undoubtedly been included which further knowledge will show not to be examples of drug hypersensitivity.

Although the different reactions are described separately, it must be realised that more than one type of reaction is commonly seen simultaneously in the same patient. Systemic and cutaneous reactions coexist more commonly than published case reports would suggest because such reports are often concerned only with one type of reaction, and a second and less conspicuous reaction may not be mentioned. The drugs listed below have been chosen only as examples of familiar drugs thought to have caused the reactions described. For detailed lists, the periodical reviews of the world literature edited by Meyler (1957, 1958, 1960, 1963, 1966), Meyler and Herxheimer (1968, 1972) and Meyler and Peck (1962, 1964, 1968, 1972) should be consulted. The *Toxicity Bibliography* (1968 et seq.) will be found an invaluable source of references.

Cutaneous reactions

Some excellent colour plates of cutaneous reactions to drugs will be found in an article by Baer and Harris (1967).

Pruritus

This is a feature of many drug eruptions. Rarely, it is the only symptom of drug hypersensitivity.

Urticaria

Since penicillin became so widely used, this has become the commonest drug reaction; aspirin is also a well-recognised cause. Urticaria frequently occurs alone, but it is also a distressing component of the serum sickness type of reaction. Urticaria usually subsides rapidly when treatment is stopped and, when due to penicillin, it may disappear even if treatment is continued. Urticaria due to penicillin, however, particularly when it is part of the serum sickness type of reaction, sometimes persists for weeks or months.

Exanthematic eruptions

These are common and may closely simulate an infectious exanthem. If treatment is continued they may, on rare occasions, progress to exfoliative dermatitis. The penicillins—particularly ampicillin—barbiturates, phenazone and related drugs, and sulphonamides are common causes. Exanthematic eruptions are extremely common in cases of infectious mononucleosis treated with ampicillin.

Exfoliative dermatitis

This is rare and often fatal. The widespread cutaneous dilatation with exudation and exfoliation cause severe loss of heat, fluid and protein. Heavy metals, barbiturates and sulphonamides are known causes.

Bullae

When occurring alone these are classically associated with iodides and bromides. Bullae are features of erythema multiforme and fixed eruptions.

Erythema multiforme

Dull-red maculopapules are the characteristic lesions, and they may show central bullae. Fever, joint and abdominal pain may occur. Sulphonamides, barbiturates, phenazone and related compounds are amongst many drugs that have been implicated. Phenobarbitone has caused a severe variant resembling the Stevens–Johnson syndrome, with involvement of ocular, genital and oral mucous membranes.

Lichenoid eruptions

Shiny, purplish, often polygonal papules which may very closely resemble lichen planus can be caused by many different drugs including gold salts, thiazides, mepracrine and chloroquine. This type of reaction also occurs commonly after contact with developer used in the processing of colour films, the responsible chemicals being substituted paraphenylenediamines.

Fixed eruptions

The characteristic lesion in this condition is an oedematous plaque which may become bullous. These lesions may be single or multiple and recur in the same site or sites each time the drug is taken, although additional lesions may occur on each readministration of the drug. Buccal or genital mucous membrane lesions may accompany the skin lesions, or may occur alone. The patient is sometimes febrile. Causative drugs include phenolphthalein, phenazone and related drugs, barbiturates and sulphonamides.

Contact dermatitis

This is a form of delayed hypersensitivity to substances applied topically to the skin. In the acute stages, papules and vesicles—sometimes bullae—are seen on an erythematous and oedematous background. Rupture of the vesicles or bullae leads to exudation. In the chronic stages there is crusting and scaling with little vesiculation. Pruritus is a feature at all stages.

Contact with an extraordinary variety of substances can produce this type of reaction. Amongst drugs, the following are a few examples. Contact dermatitis to neomycin, streptomycin and penicillin are occupational hazards of nurses, doctors and pharmacists handling these drugs. Local anaesthetics such as benzocaine and procaine are strong sensitisers. Contact dermatitis to adhesive tapes is frequently seen as is sensitisation to ointment bases, particularly lanoline. An exhaustive list is given by Fregert and Hjorth (1972).

The patient may have been exposed to the sensitising agent for weeks, months or years before developing contact dermatitis and, in general, only very few of those exposed become sensitised, although with very potent sensitising agents used experimentally, such as dinitrochlorobenzene, almost every individual exposed rapidly becomes sensitised. The genetic factor in sensitisation has been discussed above. Once sensitisation is established it tends to persist for years.

The diagnosis of contact dermatitis can most easily be confirmed by patch testing. This and other forms of investigation are discussed in detail elsewhere (see Chapter 10).

Drug-induced eczematous reactions

When sensitisation of the skin has been caused by the topical application of a compound, the same compound, or an immunochemically related one, administered systemically, may cause a widespread eczematous reaction, the appearance of these lesions being virtually identical with those of contact dermatitis. A fascinating study of the cross-reactions which may give rise to this type of skin lesion is given by Fisher (1966). A few examples must suffice. A patient who has been sensitised to quinine in, for instance, hair tonic may subsequently develop generalised eczema in response to quinine taken by mouth in cold cures or tonic water. Patients sensitised to balsam of Peru in cosmetics may develop this type of eczema from taking the flavouring agent cinnamon by mouth, and patients sensitised to hydrazine hydrobromide through industrial exposure may develop eczema as a result of taking isoniazid or hydrallazine by mouth.

The relationship of this type of eczema to contact dermatitis is obviously very close and Sulzberger has called this condition 'contact-type' dermatitis. As might be expected, patch testing with the causative drug is often positive.

Photosensitisation

Phototoxic reactions are not allergic. The drug increases the degree of sunburn caused by a given dose of ultraviolet light. Demethylchlortetracycline causes this type of reaction.

Photoallergic reactions. These occur in a very small proportion of those taking the drug. Initially the patient shows no abnormal sensitivity to light, but whilst still taking the drug he develops an abnormal reaction to light: eczematous, urticarial, papular, bullous or lichenoid. The reaction tends to recur with every re-exposure to light and may be observed even months after the drug has been withdrawn. The fact that only very few of those taking the drug develop this type of reaction, and the existence of a symptom-free period, both suggest an allergic mechanism. For further details, the review of Kirshbaum and Beerman (1964) should be consulted. Causative drugs are thought to include sulphonamides, thiazides, sulphonylurea compounds (e.g. tolbutamide), and chlorpromazine and related compounds.

Non-thrombocytopenic purpura

This condition was fairly commonly seen when the hypnotic carbromal (bromodiethylacetylurea) was widely used, but has become uncommon since other hypnotics became more popular. The purpura due to carbromal is associated with a scaling, itching dermatitis. In longstanding cases the fresh haemorrhages are seen in a skin stained with numerous punctate haemosiderin deposits, the sites of previous petechiae. The legs are predominantly affected. Healing is rapid once the drug is withdrawn, but complete resolution takes up to a month. The causative mechanism is unknown. Patch testing is often positive. Two facts suggest an immunological mechanism. First, the basophil degranulation test is sometimes positive. Second, carbromal is chemically closely related to Sedormid (allylisopropylacetylurea) which is known to cause thrombocytopenic purpura by an immunological mechanism.

Non-thrombocytopenic purpura unaccompanied by other lesions in the skin or elsewhere is uncommon. Thiazides are a well authenticated cause (Levin, 1974). Iodides, gold salts, sulphonamides, barbiturates and quinine are also thought to be causes. A well investigated case due to tartrazine, a dye used in the pharmaceutical industry and for colouring butter and margarine, has been reported by Criep (1971). The mechanisms causing non-thrombocytopenic purpura are unknown.

Systemic reactions

Fever

This is a very common manifestation of drug hypersensitivity. It can accompany almost any type of drug hypersensitivity reaction. Occasionally it occurs alone.

Reaction resembling anaphylactic shock

This alarming reaction occurs within minutes of the administration of the drug. The patient becomes pale and extremely apprehensive. He has central chest pain and increasing difficulty in breathing. The skin becomes ashen grey and unconsciousness and death may ensue within minutes. If the patient does not die, erythema and urticaria may be noted and these are important in distinguishing this from other causes of collapse. The patient often also complains of severe upper abdominal pain. The dyspnoea mentioned above is due to a combination of bronchospasm and bronchial oedema. With adequate treatment (subcutaneous adrenaline, intravenous antihistamines, intravenous pressor agents and perhaps intravenous hydrocortisone) the majority of patients recover. Penicillin, local anaesthetics, sera and pollen extracts are the commonest causes.

Bronchial asthma

Bronchospasm occurs as part of the anaphylactic shock-like syndrome. Apart from this, asthma due to drug hypersensitivity, although it occasionally occurs alone, is more frequently associated with urticaria. Aspirin appears to be much the commonest cause although many other drugs have been implicated. When due to aspirin the patient frequently has nasal polypi (Samter and Beers, 1968). Patients who develop asthma in response to aspirin frequently develop asthma in response to other analgesics; notably indomethacin, paracetamol, mefenamic acid, dextropropoxyphene and pentazocine. They may also develop asthma after taking the yellow dye tartrazine.

The serum sickness type of reaction

The essential features of this type of reaction are fever, joint pains and urticaria. Whereas urticaria, when it occurs alone, usually develops during treatment, the serum sickness type of reaction usually develops a few days (3 to 21) after treatment has stopped. This type of reaction usually subsides spontaneously, but it may persist for weeks or months (see below). It can be due to a wide variety of drugs but penicillin is by far the commonest cause.

Vasculitis

The interrelationship of the different forms of vasculitis, and particularly the relationship of polyarteritis nodosa to those forms of vasculitis involving only the small vessels, is obscure. In the following discussion all forms of vasculitis will be considered together. However, because of its very distinctive clinical picture, anaphylactoid (Henoch–Schönlein) purpura will be considered separately, although it is almost certainly closely related to other forms of vasculitis affecting the small vessels.

It is widely believed that vasculitis (including polyarteritis nodosa) may be caused by drug hypersensitivity. There is certainly often a history of drug administration before the vasculitis was diagnosed although it is often not certain that the drug was not given for symptoms of early manifestations of the vasculitis itself.

There is no doubt that vasculitis can be produced experimentally by methods involving immunological mechanisms. This was first shown by Rich and Gregory in 1943. These workers injected rabbits intravenously with large doses of heterologous serum and found that the animals developed vascular lesions histologically resembling those of polyarteritis in man. This suggests that vasculitis may be due to a mechanism similar to that which causes serum sickness; that is, that vasculitis may be mediated by immune complexes in the vessel walls. However, for reasons discussed below, immune complex formation by drugs is probably rare and it is not known whether drugs can cause vasculitis or, assuming that they can, whether they can do so by such a mechanism.

It has been claimed that vasculitis may develop in cases of the serum sickness type of reaction to drugs (fever, joint pains, urticaria, etc) if treatment has been continued. Such a history is, however, rarely obtained in cases of vasculitis and it is clearly possible that, in the rare cases with such a history, the fever and joint pains were early manifestations of the vasculitis itself.

The most convincing evidence for an association of drug hypersensitivity with vasculitis, although it provides no indication of the mechanisms involved, is the occasional case in which readministration of the drug on more than one occasion has been associated with exacerbation or even recurrence of the vasculitis. Very striking examples of this type have been reported by McCormick (1950) and by Björnberg and Gisslén (1965).

Anaphylactoid purpura (Henoch–Schönlein syndrome)

This syndrome is rarely attributable to any cause. Occasionally foods have been implicated (see Ackroyd, 1953). As with other forms of vasculitis, the best evidence for drug hypersensitivity as a cause comes from the rare cases in which recurrence of the disease has resulted on more than one occasion from readministration of the drug. A case which appears to satisfy these criteria has been reported as being due to chlorothiazide (Reid, Stevenson and Orr, 1969). The case reported by Symmers (1958) was probably one of anaphylactoid purpura due to aspirin. The case described by Creger and Houseworth (1954) as one of the Henoch–Schönlein syndrome due to quinine was clearly due to this drug but it is open to question whether it was really an example of the Henoch–Schönlein syndrome. Cases apparently due to azo dyes have been reported by Michaëlsson, Pettersson and Juhlin (1974). Some of these patients also reacted with purpura to aspirin by mouth. Michaëlsson and his colleagues (1974) describe an interesting extension of the patch test in connection with these cases due to azo dyes and claim that an ester of nicotinic acid (Trafuril) applied to the skin in an ointment makes the skin locally more reactive so that lesions may develop in the skin in the treated area in response to orally administered allergens even when they do not develop in other areas of the patient's skin. Drug hypersensitivity is probably a very rare cause of anaphylactoid purpura. The mechanism is unknown and what has been written above about the pathogenesis of other forms of vasculitis applies equally to the Henoch–Schönlein syndrome.

Syndrome resembling systemic lupus erythematosus

In 1953 it became clear that treatment of hypertension with the drug hydrallazine could be associated in some patients with the development of a syndrome resembling systemic lupus erythematosus. In the fully developed condition the patient might have fever, skin rashes, arthritis and enlargement of the liver, spleen and lymph nodes. In addition, the lupus erythematosus cell phenomenon could be demonstrated in a small proportion of the more severely affected of these patients. Some elements of this syndrome were seen in 7 to 10 per cent of patients who had taken large doses of hydrallazine for several months. Withdrawal of the drug usually resulted in rapid clinical improvement, although in a few patients some elements of the syndrome persisted. Since the discovery that this syndrome could be caused by hydrallazine, it has been found that it can also be caused by a number of chemically unrelated drugs, the most important of which are: procainamide, isonicotinic acid hydrazide, and a number of anticonvulsant drugs including troxidone and primidone. Penicillamine and practolol have recently been described as causes. Procainamide is probably the most active drug in producing this syndrome. Dubois and his colleagues (1968) reported that 15 of 22 patients being treated with this drug developed antinuclear antibodies.

Antibodies to the causative drug have been demonstrated in sera of cases due to hydrallazine and procainamide using as indicator the agglutination of red cells coated with the drug. As already emphasised, the demonstration of an antibody to a drug does not prove that the symptoms the patient has developed whilst taking the drug were caused by that drug, and Russell and Ziff (1968) found that although antibodies to procainamide could be demonstrated in this way with sera from some patients with the lupus-like syndrome due to this drug, these antibodies were widespread and could be demonstrated in the sera of 30 per cent of normal subjects. It is clear, therefore, that anti-drug antibodies have not been shown to cause drug-induced lupus-like syndromes.

The possibility that drug-induced lupus-like syndromes may be associated with pharmacogenetic abnormalities has been considered by several workers. The relatives of patients with lupus-like syndromes due to anticonvulsants and to procainamide have been shown to have a high incidence of abnormalities which might be found in idiopathic systemic lupus. Similar abnormalities were also found in the previous histories of patients who had ultimately developed a lupus-like syndrome due to hydrallazine. Furthermore, it has been reported that the development of antinuclear factors in patients being treated with hydrallazine is related to the total dose of the drug and to the rate of acetylation. Acetylation rates are genetically determined and these findings therefore suggest a pharmacogenetic basis for the hydrallazine-induced lupus syndrome. It seems unlikely, however, that, as Alarcón–Segovia and his colleagues have suggested, drug-induced lupus-like syndromes develop in patients with a 'lupus diathesis' (Alarcón–Segovia et al, 1965). Over two-thirds of one group of patients being treated with procainamide developed antinuclear antibodies as compared with 11 per cent of patients being treated with quinidine. An even higher percentage of patients taking isoniazid developed antibodies to a soluble nucleoprotein which had been altered by reaction with isoniazid, whereas only 6 per cent of normal controls had this antibody, and then only in low titre. It is clearly highly improbable that over two-thirds of these populations of patients, had a 'lupus diathesis'.

One possibility, for which there is some evidence, is that a large proportion of patients metabolise these drugs in a way which produces a metabolite which reacts with nucleoprotein, making it auto-immunogenic. Two observations can be cited in support of such a view. The first observation was made in tuberculous patients being treated with isoniazid: in such patients it was found that antibodies to a soluble nucleoprotein which had reacted in vitro with isoniazid were more common than were antibodies to the soluble nucleoprotein itself. The second observation was that the photoproduct of deoxyribonucleic acid (DNA) with procainamide was considerably more immunogenic in rabbits than was DNA itself (Blomgren and Vaughan, 1968). However, the same group of workers in a later paper (Blomgren, Condemi and Vaughan, 1972) reported that coupling procainamide to DNA did not increase the immunogenicity of the DNA itself in rabbits. They therefore considered that combination of DNA with the drug would not explain the appearance of antibodies to DNA in the procainamide-induced lupus syndrome.

Liver damage

Many drugs cause jaundice and liver damage by mechanisms which are almost certainly not immunological. The following are important examples. Carbon tetrachloride invariably causes widespread hepatic necrosis if given in sufficient quantity. Paracetamol can also produce fatal hepatic necrosis when taken in large doses with suicidal intent. Tetracycline given intravenously in large doses late in pregnancy has caused gross fatty changes in the liver. This is thought to be due to the action of tetracycline in interfering with protein synthesis. Apart from conditions such as these in which the drug exerts a direct toxic effect on the liver, jaundice resulting from drug therapy can be classified as follows:

Cholestatic jaundice due to drugs. Type I. In this type of cholestatic jaundice the drug, if given for long enough in sufficient quantity, always causes intrahepatic obstruction. The main causes of this type of liver involvement are a number of C-17 alpha-alkyl substituted testosterones including methyltestosterone, methandienone (Dianabol) and constituents of some oral contraceptives. The mechanisms of this type of liver involvement are obscure. They are probably biochemical and almost certainly not immunological.

Cholestatic jaundice due to drugs. Type II. This type of cholestatic jaundice develops only in a small proportion of those taking the causative drug. In addition to intrahepatic cholestasis some degree of hepatocellular damage is always present. The jaundice may be associated with fever, skin rashes and eosinophilia. Withdrawal of the drug is almost invariably followed by complete recovery, although on rare occasions the jaundice has persisted for up to three years before recovery has ensued. In these cases, the condition may closely resemble primary biliary cirrhosis. Sometimes the jaundice has cleared even if treatment has been continued. The drugs most frequently involved are the phenothiazines (chlorpromazine and related compounds). Chlorpropamide and phenylbutazone are occasional causes. The subject has been reviewed by Hollister (1957) and by Sherlock (1968, 1972). The causative mechanism is unknown. Serological studies have given conflicting results, some workers having reported the presence of antimitochondrial antibodies in a considerable proportion of cases, whereas others have failed to find them. Although jaundice has usually appeared during the second, third or fourth weeks of treatment, readministration of the drug after recovery has often caused jaundice in under two days. This finding and the occurrence in some cases of skin rashes and eosinophilia suggests drug hypersensitivity as the most probable cause.

Jaundice resulting from hepatocellular damage due to drugs. This type of liver damage can be caused by many different drugs, although only very few of those taking any of these drugs are affected. Unlike cholestatic jaundice due to drugs, the mortality is high. Some progress to a macronodular cirrhosis but about 20 per cent die in the acute stages with liver failure. Jaundice recurs if the drug is readministered after recovery. The drugs most commonly implicated are the hydrazine monoamine oxidase inhibitors, including iproniazid (Marsilid) and phenelzine (Nardil) to name only two of many. Isonicotinic acid hydrazide has also been involved, although only very rarely. It has been reported that this drug causes a rise in serum transaminases in about 10 per cent of those taking it. Apparently these enzymes can return to normal even if treatment is continued. Rifampicin, which is not a hydrazine derivative, has been reported to cause a similar transient rise in serum transaminases. Drugs which are not hydrazine derivatives and which are known causes of hepatocellular damage include sulphonamides, cinchophen, methyldopa, para-aminosalicyclic acid, diphenylhydantoin and halothane. The aperient oxyphenisatin is also a cause (Reynolds et al, 1970; Reynolds, Peters and Yamada, 1971).

Cases due to para-aminosalicylic acid often have a major cholestatic element and may be associated with fever, rashes, arthralgia, lymph gland enlargement, eosinophilia and a white cell picture in the peripheral blood resembling infectious mononucleosis. Recurrence of this syndrome may occur rapidly if even only a small dose of the drug is given after recovery, which suggests that the syndrome may be due to hypersensitivity to para-aminosalicylic acid. Lymphocyte transformation in the presence of this drug has been reported in a single case.

The anaesthetic agent halothane is a very rare cause of hepatocellular jaundice. The evidence for a causal relationship is reviewed by Sherlock (1971, 1972). The condition occurs more frequently after multiple halothane anaesthetics than after a single exposure. This increase in susceptibility following repeated exposure is compatible with a hypersensitivity mechanism. Serological studies have given conflicting results. Both the lymphocyte transformation test in the presence of halothane and attempts to demonstrate antimitochondrial antibodies have given positive results in the hands of some workers, but others have failed to confirm these findings. One group of workers claims to have demonstrated inhibition of macrophage migration by the drug in each of two cases (Williams et al, 1972).

The subject of hepatocellular jaundice due to drugs has been reviewed by Sherlock (1968, 1972) and by Sherlock and Ajdukiewicz (1972). It seems clear that although there is some evidence to suggest an immunological mechanism, no immunological test has proved of any value in diagnosis or in elucidating the pathogenesis of this type of drug reaction.

Nephropathy

Many drugs can cause renal damage. The mechanism is often not immunological. Thus, sulphonamides can cause an obstructive nephropathy if crystals of the drug are deposited within the renal tubules. Accumulation of oxalate crystals in the tubules and interstitium of the kidney appears to be a major factor causing the renal failure associated with methoxyfluorane anaesthesia. Some drugs such as bacitracin, capreomycin and amphotericin have a direct toxic effect on the kidney which is presumably due to biochemical and not to immunological mechanisms. Many other drugs, although not generally nephrotoxic, occasionally cause renal damage probably as a result of immunologically determined drug hypersensitivity.

The following renal conditions have been ascribed to drug hypersensitivity:

1. Acute glomerulonephritis.
2. Polyarteritis.
3. Tubular degeneration and necrosis.
4. Membranous nephritis.
5. Interstitial nephritis. In this condition the interstitium is oedematous and is infiltrated with lymphocytes and plasma cells and sometimes eosinophils. The term interstitial nephritis is often used to describe the combination of interstitial infiltration with inflammatory cells together with tubular degeneration. As either can occur alone it seems preferable to classify the two conditions separately and to reserve the term interstitial nephritis for kidneys showing interstitial inflammatory infiltration but no significant tubular or glomerular lesions by light microscopy. The combined lesion is sometimes referred to as tubulo-interstitial nephritis.

No convincing evidence has ever been produced to prove that the first two types of renal lesion mentioned above can be due to drug hypersensitivity (see Baldwin et al, 1968; Ackroyd, 1974), and the following discussion will therefore be restricted to interstitial nephritis, tubular degeneration and necrosis, and to membranous nephritis. Apart from a brief reference to interstitial nephritis occurring as an isolated condition, the renal lesions will be classified according to the causative drug or drugs.

Interstitial nephritis occurring in the absence of tubular or glomerular damage visible by light microscopy has been reported in cases of nephropathy due to sulphathiazole, to colistinmethanesulphonate (Colomycin) and to troxidone (Tridione). It is not clear why this condition should be associated with renal failure. The most likely explanation would seem to be that the rise in interstitial pressure caused by the oedema and inflammatory infiltration is sufficient to cause a gross reduction in glomerular filtration.

Analgesic nephropathy. It has been known for 20 years that the prolonged and excessive consumption of analgesics is often associated with renal failure. Histologically, the kidneys in advanced cases show interstitial fibrosis with round cell infiltration, tubular degeneration, and necrosis of the papillae. Although the condition is commonly referred to as chronic interstitial nephritis it is now generally considered that the primary lesion is papillary necrosis and that the interstitial fibrosis and tubular degeneration are secondary to this.

The relationship of this type of chronic interstitial inflammation to the infiltration with lymphocytes, plasma cells and sometimes eosinophils which can occur much more acutely in some types of drug-induced nephropathy, and which has been referred to above as interstitial nephritis is not certain.

The mechanism by which this type of renal lesion is caused is unknown. The fibrosis and round cell infiltration of the interstitium and the fact that not all those taking large doses of analgesics are affected have been construed as implying an immunological mechanism.

Phenindione is an occasional cause of oliguric renal failure which is often preceded by fever and a rash. The kidneys usually show tubular degeneration and necrosis, and gross interstitial oedema and cellular infiltration with lymphocytes, plasma cells and eosinophils. The glomeruli have shown little change by light microscopy. Tubular degeneration can occur without the interstitial infiltration. The association of the renal lesion with fever and a rash and the infiltration of the interstitium with inflammatory cells strongly suggest an immunological mechanism.

Sulphonamides are occasional causes of renal failure with tubular degeneration and necrosis, and interstitial inflammatory cell infiltration. The interstitial infiltration may occur in the absence of tubular or glomerular damage visible by light microscopy.

The penicillins are important causes of interstitial nephritis and tubular damage. There is often a coexistent fever with a rash and eosinophilia. Baldwin and his colleagues (1968) have reported seven cases with azotaemia and fever; four developed a rash. Detailed immunological studies were performed on one of these cases. When the nephropathy developed, the patient was being treated with 24 g of methicillin a day for osteomyelitis. His serum contained IgG and IgM benzylpenicilloyl-specific antibodies. Skin testing showed an immediate-type reaction to penicilloyl-polylysine but no reaction to the methicillin homologue. Delayed-type skin tests were, however, negative with benzylpenicillin but positive with methicillin. Frozen sections of a renal biopsy were treated with fluorescein-conjugated rabbit antibody to the major haptenic antigenic determinant of methicillin—the dimethoxyphenylpenicilloyl (DPO) group. This caused fluorescent staining of the glomerular basement membrane and, to a lesser extent, of the tubular basement membrane. There was also some staining of the tubular epithelium and the interstitium. The staining was specific for the DPO group and therefore clearly demonstrated the presence of DPO groups in the kidney. IgG was demonstrated in the same distribution by fluorescence microscopy, but complement could not be shown. These findings suggested that the DPO groups were present as immune complexes, which Baldwin et al (1968) then tried to prove by exposing unstained sections to excess of the hapten, washing and then staining with fluorescein-conjugated anti-DPO antiserum. They did this in the hope that if the DPO was present as immune complexes, these would dissociate in excess hapten as complexes sometimes do. No diminution in fluorescent staining could, however, be demonstrated. This result, although it provides no evidence that the DPO was present as immune complexes does not disprove the existence of such complexes. Baldwin and his colleagues (1968) concluded that the renal lesion was not due to immune complexes because, if it was, glomerular lesions should have been visible. It must, however, be pointed out that, in the absence of electron microscopic studies, minimal lesions could not be excluded. Baldwin et al (1968) suggested that since the patient had a delayed-type skin reaction to methicillin, and since the cellular infiltration of the interstitium was suggestive of delayed hypersensitivity, it might well be that this type of nephropathy is a manifestation of delayed hypersensitivity.

Oxazolidinediones. The drug troxidone, and related compounds used in the treatment of petit mal, can cause a nephrotic syndrome. Very few studies have been made of the renal histology. The usual lesion is a membranous nephritis, although apparently interstitial nephritis can occur with only slight changes in the glomeruli and tubules visible by light microscopy (see above).

Penicillamine. Both the DL and the L forms have been associated with the development of a nephrotic syndrome. The histological picture appears to be characteristic of membranous nephritis. Deposits of IgG and complement have been demonstrated in a granular pattern on the glomerular basement membrane, and electron microscopy has shown subepithelial deposits with fusion of the foot processes, particularly in the region of these deposits. Lachmann (1968) attempted to show that the deposits of IgG and complement were immune complexes, the antigen being the drug, presumably combined with a macromolecule. Using a technique similar to that of Baldwin and his colleagues (1968) in methicillin nephropathy (see above), Lachmann (1968) tried to dissociate the complexes with excess of hapten (penicillamine). This procedure did not, however, abolish the immunoglobulin staining. Although, therefore, it seems likely that penicillamine nephropathy is an example of immune complex nephritis, the antigen being a penicillamine–macromolecular complex, this has not been established beyond doubt.

Mercury compounds. Inorganic mercury compounds, principally in ointments, or organic mercurial compounds as diuretics are occasional causes of nephropathy. In some cases the lesion is principally in the tubules, whereas in others the main lesion is a membranous nephritis. Either type may be associated with a nephrotic syndrome, although when the main lesion is in the tubules the clinical picture may be one of oliguric renal failure. In the cases with predominantly tubular damage the interstitial tissue has sometimes, but not always, shown diffuse infiltration with lymphocytes and plasma cells. The glomeruli have appeared normal by light microscopy.

Very few studies have been made of membranous nephritis due to mercury. Subepithelial deposits in the glomeruli have been demonstrated by electron microscopy in two cases.

Gold salts can also cause a nephrotic syndrome. The histological picture is that of membranous nephritis. Electron microscopy has shown subepithelial deposits in the glomeruli and the foot processes have been fused, particularly in the region of these deposits. Gold particles have been shown by electron microscopy in glomerular epithelial and mesangial cells and in tubular cells, but such particles have not been demonstrated in the subepithelial deposits. Katz and Little (1973) in a recent detailed study of a single case have confirmed these electron microscopic appearances and have reported in addition granular staining in the glomeruli with fluorescent anti IgG, anti IgM and anti β_1C. Like other workers, they were unable to demonstrate gold particles in the subepithelial deposits although such particles were present in the mesangial cells and in the proximal tubules.

The subepithelial deposits seen in the kidneys in membranous nephritis due to gold, mercury and penicillamine closely resemble those seen in systemic lupus erythematosus which have been shown almost beyond doubt to be antigen–antibody complexes. It would seem probable, therefore, that the deposits seen in membranous nephritis due to drugs are also immune complexes. The nature of these deposits is discussed more fully below.

Phenacetin. Except by the dangerous procedure of drug readministration, in none of the drug-induced diseases of the kidney described above would it be possible in any individual case to prove that the condition was due to the suspected drug. Even less would it be possible to prove that an immunological process was involved. This is true, however good the circumstantial evidence. In the case of acute tubular necrosis and interstitial nephritis due to phenacetin described below (MacGibbon et al, 1960), the evidence on both counts almost achieved the level of proof.

CASE HISTORY: This patient developed haemolytic anaemia due to a phenacetin-dependent antibody. There was jaundice and she had severe oliguria. She had had two previous attacks of jaundice in the second of which there was also oliguria. A renal biopsy performed during the latter attack showed interstitial nephritis and tubular necrosis. All three attacks followed the taking of analgesic tablets containing aspirin and phenacetin and either caffeine or codeine or both.

As neither aspirin nor caffeine nor codeine is known to cause renal damage when taken occasionally in normal doses as in this case, and as the haemolytic anaemia was clearly due to phenacetin and was immunologically determined, it seems virtually certain that the renal lesion was due to an immunological reaction to phenacetin. There remains, however, a remote possibility that the tubular necrosis and interstitial nephritis could have been secondary to the haemolysis. Intravascular haemolysis with haemoglobinuria can be associated with this type of renal lesion, but this seems an unlikely cause in this particular case because the haemolysis was not very severe. This case is quoted in detail partly because of its intrinsic interest, and partly because it emphasises some of the difficulties of establishing a diagnosis of drug hypersensitivity even in a case as apparently clear-cut as this.

Pleuropneumonic reaction to nitrofurantoin

This interesting condition is characterised by attacks of fever, cough, dyspnoea and cyanosis. The symptoms may be severe enough to suggest myocardial infarction or pulmonary embolism. Eosinophilia is common. The chest x-ray may not show any change or there may be diffuse mottling sometimes accompanied by pleural effusion. Rapid recovery follows withdrawal of the drug. The duration of treatment before symptoms appear tends to get shorter with each attack. The causative mechanism is obscure. The progressive shortening of the incubation period and the eosinophilia suggest an allergic process. However, Israel and colleagues (1973) concluded that the condition was not due to immune complexes as they were unable to demonstrate immunoglobulin or complement in the lung lesions. The subject of the pleuropneumonic reaction to nitrofurantoin has been reviewed by Murray

(1968). Disodium cromoglycate, a drug which is inhaled into the lungs as a powder in the prophylactic treatment of allergic asthma has recently been reported as having caused a similar condition (Löbel, Machtey and Eldror, 1972).

Many other drugs including particularly busulphan and bleomycin are known causes of lung disease. An extensive review is given by Rosenow (1972).

Fibrosis associated with methysergide therapy

Retroperitoneal fibrosis develops in a small proportion of those taking methysergide. Partial or complete remissions have nearly always occurred if the drug has been withdrawn, and recurrence has been observed on readministration. Histologically, this extraordinary drug reaction is indistinguishable from spontaneously occurring retroperitoneal fibrosis, showing areas of infiltration with lymphocytes and plasma cells. Germinal centres may be seen. In fact, the appearances are reminiscent of many autoimmune diseases. Methysergide is also believed to cause pleuropulmonary and endocardial fibrosis. The subject of fibrosis associated with methysergide has been reviewed by Graham (1968). The mechanisms causing this type of reaction are unknown. The histological appearances strongly suggest an immunological process.

Lymph node enlargement simulating malignant lymphoma

This condition has been caused most frequently by hydantoin derivatives (e.g. phenytoin) and oxazolidine derivatives (e.g. troxidone). Phenylbutazone is also a cause. These three drugs are all based on a five-membered heterocyclic nitrogen-containing ring system. The reaction is characterised by the development of fever and enlargement of one or more groups of lymph nodes. Occasionally the liver and spleen are enlarged. There may be a rash. Histologically the lymph nodes sometimes closely resemble malignant lymphoma and may even be mistaken for it. The patient usually recovers rapidly when the drug is withdrawn (but see below). Immunological investigations have, in general, failed to throw much light on this subject. In one case, possibly due to phenytoin, the drug caused degranulation of rabbit basophils in the presence of the patient's serum. In another, which was almost certainly due to phenytoin, the drug caused lymphocyte transformation. In a case due to phenylbutazone, patch testing with the drug gave rise to an extraordinarily extensive reaction which involved the whole of the arm proximal to the area to which the patch was applied and extended on to the patient's face. In this case there was a progressive shortening of the incubation period with each readministration of the drug. All these findings make it clear that a mechanism of drug hypersensitivity cannot be excluded as a cause of this syndrome.

Although, in the vast majority of cases, the condition recovers when the drug is withdrawn, in a few cases the lymph nodes show the appearances, and run the clinical course, of true malignant lymphoma or Hodgkin's disease. In such cases it is clearly impossible to say whether these were malignant ab initio or whether drug-induced lymph node enlargement may sometimes be premalignant and therefore that some of these cases may be examples of drug-induced malignant disease. The possibility is suggested by the occasional case which has initially regressed on withdrawal of the drug, but which has ultimately developed frankly malignant change (Gams, Neal and Conrad, 1968). The relationship of hydantoin therapy to malignant lymphoma is discussed in a *Lancet* Editorial (1971).

Immunological deficiency and immunological stimulation

The importance of immunosuppression in organ transplantation has led to increasing interest in the effects of drugs on the immune response. Apart from drugs such as steroid hormones and azathioprine (Imuran) which are given for their immunosuppressive activities, some drugs, given for completely different purposes, have been found to have quite unexpected effects on the immunological apparatus.

It has recently been found that patients being treated with hydantoin derivatives sometimes develop various types of immunological deficiency (Sorrell et al, 1971; Grob and Herold, 1972). Complement levels are reduced in about half the patients being treated with these drugs and serum levels of immunoglobulins—particularly IgA—are sometimes reduced. Humoral immunity as measured by antibody responses to defined antigens is strikingly diminished in some patients, and in some there has been evidence of diminished cellular immunity as shown by skin testing. There is apparently no correlation between lymph node enlargement caused by hydantoin derivatives and immunological deficiency (Grob and Herold, 1972).

Another drug which appears to be able to cause immunological deficiency is diazoxide which is used in the treatment both of hypertension and of hypoglycaemia. Diazoxide therapy for persistent hypoglycaemia was associated with a significant reduction in serum IgG in five of seven children (Baker and Miller, 1967). An indication of the possible mode of action of this drug is provided by the observation that diazoxide inhibits the mitotic response of lymphocytes to phytohaemagglutinin.

Unlike the drugs just mentioned, the anthelminthic levamisole can apparently act as an immunological stimulant. It has been reported that this drug can restore reactivity to tuberculin in a considerable proportion of anergic patients with negative Mantoux reactions. This drug has also been found to increase skin reactivity to dinitrochlorobenzene (Brugmans et al, 1973). Furthermore, it appears to be able to cause a rise in the total haemolytic complement titre of some patients (Verhaegen et al, 1973). The mechanisms by which these effects are produced are not understood. The actions of this drug are, at present, under intensive investigation. The action of an ester of nicotinic acid (Trafuril) applied to the skin, in increasing skin reactivity to drugs in cases of drug hypersensitivity has already been mentioned (see above).

Blood dyscrasias

Thrombocytopenic purpura, haemolytic anaemia and agranulocytosis can all be manifestations of drug hypersensitivity and in many cases have been shown to be due to drug-dependent antibodies. With regard to aplastic anaemia, there is suggestive evidence but no proof that this can be due to drug hypersensitivity. These conditions are all clinically indistinguishable from cases not due to drugs. Unless the causative drug forms a depot from which it is slowly released, cases of thrombocytopenic purpura, haemolytic anaemia or agranulocytosis usually recover rapidly when the drug is withdrawn, but aplastic anaemia persists long after treatment has stopped although occasionally recovery may ultimately occur.

Thrombocytopenic purpura. An immunological basis has been demonstrated in cases due to many different drugs, the most commonly used being quinidine, quinine, chlorothiazide, antazoline and stibophen in that order. It has been claimed that thiazides given to the mother antepartum can cause thrombocytopenic purpura in her newly born child, even though the mother developed neither thrombocytopenia nor purpura (Rodriguez, Leikin and Hiller, 1964). The thrombocytopenia and other haematological changes in the infants were apparently due to depressed marrow function. The relationship to thiazide therapy was not proved and an immunological mechanism was not established. Sedormid, which was by far the commonest cause has been withdrawn from the market and cases are now no longer seen. Exhaustive lists of causatic drugs are given by Karpatkin (1971), Böttiger and Westerholm (1972a) and by McVie (1973).

As mentioned above, two cases of thrombocytopenic purpura due to an immunological reaction to a drug metabolite have been reported. One was due to a metabolite of paracetamol (Eisner and Shahidi, 1972); the other, a metabolite of para-aminosalicylic acid (Eisner and Kasper, 1972).

Haemolytic anaemia has been shown by immunological methods to have been caused by hypersensitivity to a large number of different drugs, including penicillin, phenacetin, para-aminosalicylic acid, quinine, quinidine, salicylazosulphapyridine, stibophen and chlorpropamide. The haemolytic anaemia caused by alpha-methyldopa and by mefenamic acid has also been shown to have an immunological basis. The subject has been recently reviewed by Worlledge (1973a, b) and by Böttiger and Westerholm (1973a).

Agranulocytosis. The drugs which have most commonly caused agranulocytosis are amidopyrine, the sulphonamides, the antithyroid drugs, particularly thiourea and thiouracil, the rauwolfia alkaloid ajmalin, phenylbutazone, and the coagulation-inhibiting drug phenylindanedione. Detailed lists are given by Palva and Mustala (1970), Böttiger and Westerholm (1973b) and by Hartl (1973). An immunological mechanism can be demonstrated only infrequently. The agranulocytosis caused by the phenothiazines (chlorpromazine and related compounds) is rarely due to an immunological mechanism (see below).

Aplastic anaemia. By far the commonest cause is chloramphenicol. Other important causes are the sulphonamides, the hydantoins, phenylbutazone, gold salts and the arsenobenzole compounds. For comprehensive lists see Böttiger and Westerholm (1972b), Williams, Lynch and Cartwright (1973) and Nieweg (1973). Some cases in which an initial course of chloramphenicol has been well tolerated have developed pancytopenia when given a relatively small quantity in a subsequent course. Huguley, Erslev and Bergsagel (1961) have reported a case of marrow depression thought to be due to chloramphenicol from which the patient recovered. He was subsequently given a further very brief course of the drug and almost immediately developed signs of marrow depression. Findings such as these strongly suggest the possibility that aplastic anaemia due to chloramphenicol may be a manifestation of drug hypersensitivity. However, as already mentioned, chloramphenicol appears to be a very rare cause of aplastic anaemia in Israel although a large amount of this drug is consumed in that country (Sheba and Shani, 1969). This, and the fact that chloramphenicol aplastic anaemia has occurred in identical twins (Nagao and Mauer, 1969) raise the possibility that the aplasia may be due to a pharmacogenetic mechanism.

It has been found that temporary reversible marrow depression is not uncommon in patients given large doses of chloramphenicol. This may well be due to a disturbance of bone marrow metabolism, for it has been shown that chloramphenicol has a strongly inhibitory effect on bone marrow mitochondrial protein synthesis (see Yunis, 1973). The importance of this observation in the pathogenesis of chloramphenicol aplastic anaemia is uncertain. The fact that the chemically related antibiotic thiamphenicol does not apparently cause aplastic anaemia although it causes as much reversible bone marrow depression as does chloramphenicol, suggests that reversible bone marrow depression is not important in the pathogenesis of chloramphenicol-induced aplastic anaemia (see review by Yunis, 1974).

Immunological Mechanisms

Initiation of an immune response by simple chemicals

In general, small molecular weight chemicals (haptens) can induce an antibody response only if they or their metabolites form a stable, covalent union with a carrier macromolecule, usually a protein, thus producing a complete antigen. There is some evidence that electrostatic bonding may occasionally be adequate. Haptens reversibly bound to protein are not immunogenic, but haptens can block the interaction of the hapten–macromolecular antigen with antibody by combining reversibly with the antigen combining site on the antibody. This phenomenon, which is known as hapten inhibition, has been utilised by de Weck and Girard (1972) to inhibit allergic reactions to penicillin in man (see below).

De Weck (1971a) has pointed out that even if a drug does form a covalent union with a protein, the unconjugated drug will often be present in sufficient concentration to block the interaction of the conjugate with antibody by a process of hapten inhibition. This probably explains the rarity of allergic drug reactions in relation to the total number of patients exposed. It probably also explains why skin tests with drugs are so often negative.

Although irreversible binding of the drug to a macromolecule appears to be a prerequisite for immunogenicity, it must be stated that some drugs which cause allergic reactions cannot be shown to form or to have metabolites which form anything other than the loosest union with any bodily constituent. The hypnotic sedormid which caused allergic thrombocytopenic purpura (see below) was a good example. Such drugs do not cause hapten inhibition. The mechanisms by which they cause allergic reactions are incompletely understood.

Mechanisms underlying different manifestations of drug hypersensitivity

In the following paragraphs, conditions which have been discussed above are referred to only if immunological studies have thrown some light on their pathogenesis or if, as in the case of fixed eruptions, they have been extensively investigated only to produce results that cannot yet be interpreted.

In current practice, the immediate reactions including reactions resembling anaphylactic shock, late urticarial reactions, the serum sickness type of reaction, and exanthematic eruptions are most commonly due to the penicillins and they have been studied mainly in connection with this group of drugs. For this reason the following account refers almost exclusively to penicillin allergy. The subject of penicillin allergy has recently been reviewed by Stewart (1973).

The causative haptens and antibodies

The penicillin haptenic groups. The major determinant is the penicilloyl group which is the determinant in perhaps 95 per cent of the benzylpenicillin that reacts irreversibly with protein (Levine, 1966). There are thought to be at least two minor determinants, the nature of which is not certain. One may be the benzylpenamaldic acid mixed disulphide group (Levine, 1966). The term 'minor' is used purely in a quantitative sense. Both major and minor determinants are almost certainly important in causing hypersensitivity reactions.

IgG and IgM antibodies. These are measured by observing the titre of serum antibody causing agglutination of penicillin-coated red cells.

IgE antibodies. These are responsible for immediate-type reactions. They are almost certainly the same as the skin-sensitising antibodies described below.

Skin-sensitising antibodies. These cause the development of a weal and flare reaction following scratch or prick testing or intradermal injection. This type of investigation has on very rare occasions been fatal when penicillin itself has been used. It is preferable therefore to use penicilloyl-polylysine which is the major determinant mentioned above, coupled to a polypeptide chain. This is considerably safer than benzylpenicillin itself, but it should be used with care as it has occasionally caused generalised reactions.

Unfortunately the correlation between immediate-type reactions to penicillin and a positive skin test with penicilloyl-polylysine has not always been close (see Idsøe et al, 1968). In particular, false-positive reactions are common and it has frequently been shown that patients with a positive skin test may not develop any untoward reactions when given a therapeutic course of the drug (see Brown, Price and Moore, 1964). False-negative reactions, that is negative skin tests in patients who subsequently develop adverse reactions to penicillin, are uncommon although they do occur (Brown et al, 1964; Perlman, 1965). It is clear, therefore, that in the individual case, valid conclusions cannot be drawn from the results of skin testing with penicilloyl-polylysine.

According to some workers considerably better results are obtained if an attempt is made to do skin testing not only with the major penicilloyl determinant, but also with the minor determinants, using for this purpose either benzyl penicillin or the 'minor determinant mixture' devised by Voss, Redmond and Levine (1966). This contains potassium benzylpenicillin, sodium benzylpenicilloate and benzylpenilloic acid. Adkinson and his colleagues (1971), using both penicilloyl-polylysine and a slightly different 'minor determinant mixture' as skin testing reagents and, as a precautionary measure, performing scratch tests before proceeding to intradermal testing, have reported highly satisfactory results in predicting which patients can safely be given penicillin. They have recommended the procedure for routine ward use. However, it should be noted that the mixture contains benzylpenicillin and at least one death has been reported which was due to scratch testing with this reagent (Dogliotti, 1968). Furthermore, because of the large number of false-positive results which occur from testing with penicilloyl-polylysine, many patients will be denied penicillin who are not sensitive to it except by the intradermal route. In conclusion, it appears that the routine use of skin testing is not a satisfactory procedure. Clinically more useful information will probably be obtained if the patient is always asked if he has experienced a reaction to the drug in the past (see Perlman, 1965). A positive answer to this question should, except on very rare occasions, be regarded as an absolute contraindication to the use of the drug.

Very recently Juhlin and Wide (1972) have investigated the level of penicilloyl-specific IgE antibodies in the patient's serum as a means of detecting hypersensitivity to penicillin. Although 15 patients who had developed immediate-type reactions less than a month previously gave positive results, two patients who had developed shock-like reactions to procaine penicillin during the past month gave negative results, as did 12 patients whose reactions to penicillin had occurred over seven months previously. This type of test needs further investigation.

Immediate reactions: *reactions resembling anaphylactic shock, bronchial asthma, urticaria*

The anaphylactic shock-like syndrome is almost certainly mediated by IgE skin-sensitising antibodies. The significance of skin test results and the value of assaying IgE antipenicilloyl antibodies have already been discussed. Bronchial asthma, which is commonly associated with urticaria is, as stated above, most commonly due to aspirin. Very little is known of the mechanism of its causation. Yurchak, Wicher and Arbesman (1970) investigated a series of aspirin-sensitive patients most of whom had perennial asthma and in whom aspirin caused acute attacks of asthma. Nearly all the patients in whom aspirin caused asthma had nasal polypi. Skin testing these patients intradermally with a variety of aspiryl-protein conjugates, and tests for lymphocyte transformation using such conjugates as antigens gave entirely negative results, as did tests for haemagglutinating antibodies reacting with red cells coated with aspiryl-protein conjugates. Using fluorescent antibody techniques, these workers then attempted to demonstrate complement and antibodies reactive with aspiryl-protein conjugates in polypi from these patients; again with negative results. Yurchak, Wicher and Arbesman (1970) therefore concluded that it was possible that this form of aspirin sensitivity is not immunologically mediated. Halpern, Ky and Amache (1967), however, observed lymphocyte transformation in all their cases with either asthma or urticaria or both, due to aspirin, unless the patients had been on intensive or prolonged cortical steroid therapy. Moreover, de Weck (1971b) observed positive skin tests with aspiryl polylysine—a conjugate also used by Yurchak, Wicher and

Arbesman (1970)—in three cases of aspirin-induced urticaria. It seems virtually certain that both asthma and urticaria occurring as immediate drug-induced reactions can be caused by skin-sensitising IgE antibodies, but it is not certain whether this applies to cases due to aspirin.

Late urticarial reactions

The urticaria begins between two hours and two days after starting penicillin therapy. It is associated with skin-sensitising and IgG antibodies of penicilloyl specificity. The IgG antibody titre rises within a few days, and when this happens the urticaria disappears although the skin test remains positive (Levine, 1966). This can happen even if treatment with penicillin is continued. It is thought that the IgG antibody acts as a blocking antibody preventing interaction of penicillin with IgE fixed on the blood basophils and tissue mast cells.

The serum sickness type of reaction

According to Levine (1966) these patients have skin-sensitising antibodies to the minor determinants. They also have IgM or IgG and IgM antibodies of benzylpencilloyl specificity, but owing to the uncertainty of the chemical nature of the minor determinants it is not known whether these patients have IgG or IgM antibodies of these specificities which could act as blocking antibodies.

Classical serum sickness due to protein antigens is almost certainly mediated by immune complexes but it is not known whether this is true for the serum sickness type of reaction due to drug hypersensitivity.

This type of reaction, when due to penicillin, recovers spontaneously in about three-quarters of the affected patients. In the remainder it persists for weeks or months. Apparently some of these patients improve when given a diet restricted in milk and milk products, suggesting that the traces of penicillin in these foods may be sufficient to cause persistence of the reaction (Levine, 1966).

Exanthematic eruptions

These are common, but very little is known about how they are caused. They occur more frequently after treatment with ampicillin than with other penicillins. Like the late urticarial reactions, they may disappear even if treatment is continued. They are remarkable in that they may not recur if a second course of treatment is given after recovery. These two findings could both be due to the development of blocking antibodies. Fellner and colleagues (1973) have claimed that about half the patients who have had exanthematic eruptions due to the penicillins have IgG serum antibodies which react with intercellular epithelial structures. Levine (1966) found that some, but not all, of his patients with this type of rash had very high titres of IgM antibodies of benzylpenicilloyl specificity and in these he thought that the rashes might be mediated by complexes of antigen with IgM antibodies. It is generally agreed that skin tests are often negative and Juhlin and Wide (1972) found tests for penicilloyl-specific IgE antibodies consistently negative. The negative skin tests seem to make the concept that recovery is due to the development of blocking antibodies unlikely. The removal of highly penicilloylated protein contaminants from ampicillin approximately halved the incidence of these rashes, but did not abolish them (Knudsen et al, 1970). Are there therefore two mechanisms involved, one related to the penicilloylated protein impurities and the other to some as yet unidentified factor in the purified ampicillin? The elucidation of the fascinating problem of the exanthematic rashes due to drug therapy awaits further investigation.

Fixed drug eruptions

These have been investigated on a number of occasions using skin autografts. Previously affected skin has been transplanted into an area of normal skin and the normal skin into the previously affected area. After the grafts have healed, the patient has been challenged with the causative drug. Superficial (Thiersch) and full thickness grafts have been used. The results of such experiments have been entirely contradictory and almost every possible result has been observed. In some cases the drug has caused the appearance of the lesion in the transplanted normal skin but not in the transplanted previously affected skin. In others, the drug has caused a reaction in the transplanted previously affected skin but not in the previously normal skin. One group of workers who initially obtained this latter response retested the patient two and a half months later and found that the drug did not produce any lesion in the transplanted previously affected skin but that the transplanted normal skin seemed to react slightly. This might suggest that the previously affected skin took some time to lose its reactivity whilst the previously normal skin took even longer to gain it. However, normal skin has been reported to achieve reactivity quite quickly and has been found to be reactive when first tested less than a month after transplantation. Finally, one group of workers who repeatedly challenged the patient over a period of three years did not observe a recurrence in either grafted site, although the patient continued to react in previously affected areas that had not been transplanted.

Although it is generally thought that fixed eruptions are due to allergic drug hypersensitivity, this is by no means certain and the way in which these eruptions are produced is not known.

Allergic eczematous contact dermatitis

This type of reaction has been extensively investigated, partly because it can easily be reproduced in man by patch testing, and partly because a comparable condition can be produced in the skin of the guinea-pig. The immunological mechanisms are discussed elsewhere (see Chapter 10).

Role of immune complexes in drug hypersensitivity

Diseases caused by immune complexes depend on the interaction of antigen with antibody in antigen excess to form soluble complexes capable of reacting with complement (see Coombs and Gell, 1968). As de Weck (1972) has pointed out, this type of complex is formed only in response to antigens that are multivalent: at least trivalent. In drug hypersensitivity, because there is always a large excess of carrier groups to form complete antigens with drugs (the drugs forming the determinant groups), the probability is that the resulting antigenic complexes will be monovalent. It seems likely, therefore, that immune complexes involving drugs will be found to be rare causes of drug hypersensitivity.

Several workers have claimed to have demonstrated immune precipitate formation by drugs in the sera of patients who have developed various types of drug hypersensitivity, but these claims have not been confirmed. Definite floccular immune precipitates have, however, very rarely been produced by adding the appropriate drug to sera from cases of thrombocytopenic purpura (see Ackroyd, 1964; Karpatkin, 1971) and of combined thrombocytopenia and granulocytopenia (Tullis, 1961) due to drug hypersensitivity. The part played by these precipitins in the genesis of the thrombocytopenia or granulocytopenia is unknown.

Powdered pituitary, inhaled as a snuff, is sometimes used in the treatment of diabetes insipidus. Some patients receiving this treatment develop a syndrome in which the inhalation is followed by wheezing and dyspnoea and the chest x-ray shows a diffuse miliary mottling in the lung fields. This appears to be a true example of a disease caused by immune complexes with a drug. This, however, is a very special case as the drug is a mixture of proteins. The patient's serum contains precipitating antibodies to pituitary extracts and has given positive results in an immunofluorescence complement-fixation test using animal and human pituitary (Pepys et al, 1966).

The most extensively investigated examples of diseases due to immune complexes are serum sickness and immune-complex nephritis. Very little is known about the mechanism by which drugs can cause a condition resembling serum sickness (see above). As already described, in the nephrotic syndrome caused by penicillamine and by gold salts, electron microscopic studies have shown glomerular subepithelial deposits virtually identical with those seen in immune-complex nephritis. Furthermore, complement and immunoglobulin have been demonstrated on the glomerular basement membrane in these conditions. This is highly suggestive evidence that the renal lesions in these cases are due to immune complexes involving the causative drug. Certain difficulties in accepting this explanation are discussed below.

At the beginning of this section it was pointed out that only multivalent antigens can form pathogenic immune complexes. It was also pointed out that drugs probably very rarely form this type of antigen because there is such an excess of carrier macromolecules that drug–macromolecular antigens are probably almost always monovalent. Pencillamine may possibly be an exception partly because it is a highly reactive chemical but mainly, perhaps, because it is given in very large doses (up to 3·0 g or more per day) for long periods. Conceivably, gold may be another exception because it is slowly released from depots thus maintaining high blood levels over long periods.

Delayed hypersensitivity to drugs

This type of reaction has recently been investigated by Redmond and Levine (1968) in cases due to penicillin. They found that the timing and the gross and microscopic appearances of the lesions produced by the intradermal injection of the drug were identical with those of delayed reactions to tuberculin. The significance of this type of hypersensitivity to penicillin is uncertain.

Redmond and Levine (1968) reported that '. . .the great majority of patients with delayed hypersensitivity to penicillin tolerate penicillin therapy without allergic reactions'. In this way, delayed hypersensitivity to penicillin resembles many other immune reactions to drugs; for example, haemagglutinating antibodies to penicillin are often found in patients who are not clinically sensitive to the drug. It can be concluded, therefore, that although delayed hypersensitivity to penicillin may sometimes be demonstrated in patients who are allergic to the drug, it often indicates only that the patient has been exposed to the drug or to an immunochemically related compound and has developed a benign clinically inapparent immunological reaction to it.

Nephropathy

Tubulo-interstitial nephritis. In the extensively investigated case due to methicillin (Baldwin et al, 1968), described above, gamma globulin and the appropriate hapten, but not complement, were demonstrated on the glomerular basement membrane and to a lesser extent on the tubular basement membrane. Hapten and gamma globulin could also be demonstrated in the tubular epithelium and the interstitium. An attempt to show that the gamma globulin and hapten were present as immune complexes was unsuccessful although the possibility was not excluded. Most unfortunately, no electron microscopic studies were made and consequently, although the authors considered that the renal lesion was not caused by immune complexes, minor changes due to such complexes could not be excluded. Their conclusion that the nephropathy was a form of delayed hypersensitivity rested solely on the types of cells in the interstitium and the ultimate cause of this type of renal lesion remains uncertain.

Membranous nephritis. The morbid anatomical changes in the kidneys in membranous nephritis due to drugs have been described above. The subepithelial deposits seen in the glomeruli are identical in appearance with those seen in immune-complex nephritis. Moreover, immunoglobulin and complement have been demonstrated in the glomeruli in a case due to penicillamine (Lachmann, 1968) and in one due to gold (Katz and Little, 1973) which would suggest that these deposits probably consist of immune complexes. However, if they do in fact consist of immune complexes, the nature of the complexes is not clear as it has not so far been possible to show that they are complexes involving the causative drug. Neither mercury nor gold have been seen in the subepithelial deposits in cases due to salts of these metals and Lachmann (1968) was unable to show that the immunoglobulin and complement in the glomeruli in his case due to penicillamine were present as immune complexes involving the drug. It may also be pointed out that Strunk and Ziff (1970) in a study of the effects of gold sodium thiomalate administered intramuscularly, weekly, to rats for periods up to five months, observed that although the kidneys of these animals contained more deposits of gold than did the kidneys of two patients with gold-induced nephropathy, none of the kidneys of the injected rats showed subepithelial deposits resembling those seen in patients with gold nephropathy. The nature of the deposits in membranous nephritis due to drugs remains uncertain. Although they may be composed of immune complexes in which the antigen is the drug or a drug–

macromolecular complex, it seems equally possible that the antigen is a compound present in the body as a result of drug action.

Blood dyscrasias

Thrombocytopenic purpura. An antiplatelet factor can often be demonstrated in the gamma globulin fraction of the patient's serum and plasma. This causes agglutination of the patient's platelets or of normal platelets in vitro, but only in the presence of the drug. The quantity of the drug is not critical and the reaction is not inhibited even by large concentrations of the drug. In the presence of complement the platelets may undergo lysis. This factor is clearly an antibody. The antigen cannot be the platelet alone because platelets are not agglutinated except in the presence of the drug. The most likely explanation for these findings is that the drug acts as a hapten which combines with the platelet envelope to form the complete antigen. This hypothesis is supported by the following observations:

1. If platelets are incubated with the complement-free serum of a sensitised patient in the presence of the drug and are then washed in saline, both antibody and drug are removed from the platelets.
2. If the platelets in the above experiment are washed, not in saline but in a saturated solution of the drug in saline, the antibody remains in contact with the platelets. If the platelets are now dialysed against saline, the drug dialyses away and the platelets separate from the antibody.

The simplest explanation for these findings is that the drug acts as a hapten conferring antigenic properties on the platelets and when the drug (hapten) is removed by dialysis the platelets separate from the antibody because they are no longer antigenic.

An alternative explanation which was suggested by Miescher and Miescher (1952) has been elaborated in considerable detail by Shulman (1958a,b,c, 1963a, b, 1964, 1974). Although in the majority of cases no interaction can be demonstrated between the drug and the serum antibody in the absence of platelets, very occasionally the drug has caused immune precipitate formation (see Karpatkin, 1971). In addition, there have been a few case reports providing evidence of a reaction between the drug and the antibody in the patient's serum although precipitate formation was apparently not observed. It seems that Shulman's patient (1958a, b, c, 1963a) was this type. As a result of a detailed analysis of this case Shulman (1958a, b, c, 1963a, b, 1964, 1974) suggested that the drug formed an immune complex with the antibody and that this complex became adsorbed onto the platelets and in the presence of complement caused their lysis.

One objection to both these hypotheses is that the causative drug is readily removed from platelets and the antibody in the patient's serum by dialysis. This shows that the drug does not combine firmly with platelets or with any constituent of the patient's serum; nor in some cases (for instance, Sedormid) is the causative drug known to have metabolites which could do this. The importance for immunogenicity, of a firm union between the hapten and its carrier macromolecule has already been discussed and it is difficult to see how a hapten which does not form a firm union can have immunogenic properties.

Another objection to these two hypotheses is that hapten inhibition cannot be demonstrated in vitro. No matter how much drug is added, the reaction is not inhibited. Classically, as stated above, if there is an excess of hapten the hapten will combine with the antibody and block the reaction with the complete antigen. Shulman (1963a, b, 1964) attempted to explain the failure of large concentrations of the drug to prevent platelet agglutination in vitro, by postulating that although antibody formation was stimulated by a drug–macromolecular antigen, once the antibody had been formed it could form immune complexes with the drug alone. This explanation is not entirely satisfactory. In fact, neither hypothesis concerning the pathogenesis of drug-induced thrombocytopenic purpura can be accepted without reservation, and it must be admitted that the cause of the platelet destruction in thrombocytopenic purpura due to drug hypersensitivity is still uncertain. For a more detailed discussion of the immunology of this type of drug reaction, see Ackroyd and Rook (1968), Ackroyd (1974), Miescher (1973) and Worlledge (1973b).

The subject of thrombocytopenic purpura due to drug hypersensitivity has recently been reviewed by Karpatkin (1971) and by McVie (1973).

Haemolytic anaemia due to drug hypersensitivity can be caused by several different mechanisms. This subject has recently been reviewed by Worlledge (1973a, b).

Haemolytic anaemia due to drugs which do not form a firm combination with red cells in vitro. This type of haemolytic anaemia has been caused by many different drugs including para-aminosalicylic acid, quinine, quinidine, phenacetin, stibophen and chlorpropamide. Immunologically, it closely resembles thrombocytopenic purpura due to drug hypersensitivity. The patient's serum causes agglutination of his own or of compatible normal red cells only in the presence of the causative drug. Haemolysis has sometimes been observed in the presence of complement. In some cases in which red cell lysis has not occurred, lysis has resulted if trypsinised cells, or cells from cases of paroxysmal nocturnal haemoglobinuria, have been used. The indirect antiglobulin test performed by incubating red cells with the patient's serum and the drug, washing the cells and then exposing them to a broad-spectrum antiglobulin serum has usually been positive as shown by the agglutination of the cells in the antiglobulin serum. This test has usually been negative if a specific anti-gamma globulin serum has been used. The reason for this is that, as with platelets in thrombocytopenic purpura due to drugs, the gamma globulin antibody washes off the cells. The positive result obtained with a broad-spectrum serum can be shown to be due to adsorbed complement. In one reported case, although the union of the drug with the red cells was labile, the red cell–drug–antibody complex was sufficiently stable to withstand washing. In this case, the indirect antiglobulin test using specific anti-gamma globulin serum was, of course, positive.

Haemolytic anaemia due to drugs which form a firm union with red cells in vitro. Penicillin, when given in very large doses (10 megaunits or more a day) is by far the commonest cause of this type of haemolytic anaemia. Recovery follows cessation of therapy, and readministration of large doses of the drug has caused recurrence. The direct antiglobulin test is positive. In this test the patient's washed cells are suspended in antiglobulin serum. A positive result is indicated by agglutination of the red cells showing that the red cells are coated with globulin. In this type of haemolytic anaemia, unlike the type just described in which the red cells do not form a firm union with the drug, the washed red cells are agglutinated by specific anti-gamma globulin serum, thus showing that they are coated with antibody.

The patient's serum in these cases will agglutinate penicillin-coated red cells but not normal red cells. As mentioned above, an antibody capable of agglutinating penicillin-coated red cells can be demonstrated in the majority of normal sera (Levine et al, 1966a). However, whereas this commonly occurring haemagglutinin is inhibited by prior incubation of the serum with penicillin, the haemagglutinating antibody associated with penicillin-induced haemolytic anaemia has not always been completely inhibited by penicillin. This is because the specificity of the antibody in these cases is, in part, to a different penicillin-derived haptenic group. The significance of this difference is not known.

The mechanism by which penicillin causes haemolytic anaemia seems reasonably clear. Large doses of the drug are presumably necessary to ensure adequate coating of the red cells with penicillin, although only a small proportion of patients treated with such doses develop haemolytic anaemia. Penicillin reacts irreversibly with the red cell envelope and provides the antigenic determinant with which the antibody reacts, thus causing the haemolytic anaemia.

Although penicillin is the commonest and most completely investigated cause of this type of haemolytic anaemia, other drugs can form stable antigenic combinations with red cells. These include the chemically closely related antibiotic cephalothin and the analgesic dipyrone (sodium noramidopyrine methanesulphonate).

Haemolytic anaemia due to drugs which cause autoantibody formation. The principal cause of this type of haemolytic anaemia is the antihypertensive drug alpha-methyldopa. Rapid recovery follows withdrawal of the drug. This type of anaemia is rare, but it has been found that about 20 per cent of patients who have been treated with this drug for over a year but who are not clinically anaemic have a positive direct antiglobulin test; they may rarely have a shortened red cell survival time. Antibody is present in the sera and can be eluted from the red cells of patients with a positive direct antiglobulin test, whether or not they have a frank haemolytic anaemia. The antibody has often been shown to have specificity for the Rh locus. Serologically, therefore, these antibodies are indistinguishable from those found in cases of warm-antibody autoimmune haemolytic anaemia. Unlike the other drug-induced haemolytic anaemias described above, the drug is not necessary for the interaction of the antibody with normal red cells.

Alpha-methyldopa is not the only drug which can cause red cell autoantibody formation with Rhesus specificity. The closely chemically related drug L-dopa produces an identical serological picture (Henry et al, 1971) and this drug is now known to have caused the same type of haemolytic anaemia. Very surprisingly, the chemically unrelated drug mefenamic acid has caused an identical type of haemolytic anaemia and any explanation of this type of drug reaction must take into account its production by such dissimilar drugs.

In addition to causing a positive antiglobulin test, alpha-methyldopa and L-dopa have stimulated the formation of antinuclear factors in some patients. So far, antinuclear factors have not been demonstrated in patients being treated with mefenamic acid. Drug-induced autoimmune haemolytic anaemia has recently been reviewed by Worlledge (1969, 1972, 1973a, b).

The nature of haemolytic anaemia due to alpha-methyldopa is even more complicated than the account given above would suggest, for a case has recently been reported in which this drug caused haemolytic anaemia by an entirely different mechanism. In this case the antibody in the patient's serum reacted with red cells only in the presence of the drug and, moreover, the antibody could not be shown to have Rhesus specificity.

It would appear that alpha-methyldopa can cause haemolytic anaemia by at least two mechanisms: by stimulating the formation of an autoantibody active independently of the presence of the drug, or by stimulating the formation of an antibody active only in the presence of the drug.

Positive antiglobulin tests caused by a non-immunological mechanism. The antibiotic cephalothin, which is one of the cephalosporins, produces a positive direct antiglobulin test in a proportion of those patients receiving it. If normal whole blood is incubated with this drug the plasma gamma and beta globulins and albumin become firmly attached to the red cells, and when washed the red cells, because of this non-immunological adsorption of plasma proteins, will give a positive antiglobulin reaction if a sufficiently 'broad spectrum' antiserum is used. Other cephalosporins have a similar activity. The proportion of cephalothin-treated patients who develop this type of direct antiglobulin reaction appears to increase with the dose of the drug and is high in the presence of azotaemia. Most normal sera, however, contain a true anti-cephalothin antibody, comparable with, and often cross-reactive with, the commonly occurring anti-penicillin antibody mentioned above. Spath, Garratty and Petz (1971) have shown that in addition to the non-immunological binding of proteins to red cells caused by cephalothin, cephalothin-treated patients' cells will also specifically bind the anti-cephalothin antibody so that the positive direct antiglobulin test caused by cephalothin therapy may apparently have both a non-immunological and an immunological component. In spite of these remarkable findings, these drugs have not shown a great tendency to cause haemolytic anaemia although, as stated above, cephalothin has on rare occasions caused haemolytic anaemia of the type in which the drug forms a firm union with the red cell.

Agranulocytosis. Much less is known about agranulocytosis than about thrombocytopenic purpura or haemolytic anaemia due to drug hypersensitivity. Hartl (1973) and Pisciotta (1973) have recently reviewed the subject in detail.

In many cases a leucoagglutinin cannot be demonstrated. Occasionally, in the acute stages of the agranulocytosis, the patient's serum may cause agglutination of normal leucocytes. The agglutination can sometimes be increased by the addition of the causative drug to the suspension of white cells in the patient's serum. In the majority of cases the leucoagglutinin is evanescent and disappears during the phase of recovery. Occasionally a case has been reported in which the leucoagglutinin persisted after recovery and then caused leucocyte agglutination only in the presence of added drug. This phenomenon is rare, but has been described in cases of agranulocytosis due to a number of different drugs including sulphapyridine, sulphamethoxypyridazine, amidopyrine, noramidopyrine, naphthylmethylimidazoline and chlorpromazine. In the presence of complement and the drug, loss of amoeboid movement and leucocyte agglutination and lysis have been observed in cases of agranulocytosis due to promazine, chloral hydrate, propranolol and hydroxychloroquine. Lysis of leucocytes by the drug has also been reported in agranulocytosis due to salicylazosulphapyridine, and cell death as measured by the staining of leucocytes by trypan blue has been caused by the drug in the patient's serum in cases of agranulocytosis due to ajmalin, a rauwolfia alkaloid, and to noramidopyrine. The antiglobulin consumption test has been used to detect drug-dependent antibodies to leucocytes in cases due to amidopyrine and phenylindanedione. A positive complement fixation test in the presence of the drug and of the patient's or of normal leucocytes has been reported in a single case due to noramidopyrine in which, in addition, the drug caused leucocyte agglutination and a positive cytotoxicity test using cell staining with trypan blue as an indicator of cell death. A positive lymphocyte transformation test has been reported in two cases due to phenylindanedione in each of which the anti-globulin consumption test was also positive. An extremely interesting technique has recently been applied to the investigation of drug-induced agranulocytosis by McIntyre and her colleagues (1971), in a case due to propylthiouracil and by Pisciotta (1973) in one due to methimazole. These workers observed that the patients' serum taken during the phase of agranulocytosis suppressed the release of carbon dioxide from normal leucocytes during phagocytosis. The suppressive factor in the case due to propylthiouracil was found to be in the IgM fraction of the patient's serum. An attempt to increase this effect by adding the drug propylthiouracil to the incubation mixture was however unsuccessful.

In the first group of cases described above in which leucocyte agglutination occurs during the acute stage of agranulocytosis without added drug, the agglutination is presumably due to the presence of the agglutinin and the drug in the patient's blood. The increase in agglutination sometimes caused by the addition of the drug in vitro supports this view. It is not known why the antibody in drug-induced agranulocytosis should often be so short-lived. This, however, is not peculiar to drug-induced agranulocytosis, for although the antibodies in cases of thrombocytopenic purpura usually persist for much longer, occasional cases have been described in which they were detectable for only a few days. It seems virtually certain that in those cases in which the leucoagglutinin persists after recovery and can then be demonstrated only in the presence of added drug, the mechanism is similar to that which has been discussed in connection with thrombocytopenic purpura due to drug hypersensitivity.

As in drug-induced thrombocytopenia, it is not known whether the drug combines with the white cell to form the antigen or whether the antigen is a drug–macromolecular complex, the cells being destroyed as a result of antigen–antibody interaction in the presence of complement on the cell surface. Apart from a single case of leucopenia and thrombocytopenia due to drug hypersensitivity in which there may have been a drug-dependent precipitin, precipitins do not appear to have been described in agranulocytosis due to drug hypersensitivity; however, one case, due to noramidopyrine, has been reported in which, although a precipitin was not demonstrated, there was evidence that the drug formed a stable union with a serum macromolecule. Leucocyte agglutination occurred in the presence of this complex in the absence of free drug. Apart from a single case due to amidopyrine, leucocyte agglutination has not been inhibited by excess of the causative drug. Finally, a case has been described in which alpha-methyldopa caused agranulocytosis and haemolytic anaemia. The anaemia was autoimmune, like other cases due to this drug, and the antibody had Rhesus specificity. The leucocytes were shown to be coated with gamma globulin, suggesting that the agranulocytosis was due to a similar mechanism to that which caused the haemolytic anaemia.

The drug chlorpromazine, which is a phenothiazine, is one of the compounds mentioned above which can cause agranulocytosis by an immunological mechanism. Much more commonly an antibody cannot be demonstrated, and Pisciotta (1969, 1973, 1974) has accumulated a great deal of evidence to suggest a pharmacogenetic mechanism in these cases. Should this be confirmed, then chlorpromazine, like phenacetin, will have been shown to be able to produce a reduction in circulating blood cells—granulocytes in the case of chlorpromazine and red cells in the case of phenacetin—both by an immunological and a pharmacogenetic mechanism.

Diagnosis

The most important single factor in diagnosis is the recognition by the physician that a patient's unexplained symptom or sign may be due to a drug he has been receiving. Fever is often the first sign of a drug reaction and a careful watch should be kept for this, particularly when treatment is being given with a drug known to cause serious reactions.

The next important factor in diagnosis is the recording of a detailed history of all drugs taken during the previous few months, together with the dates when treatment was started and stopped. It is important to remember that the patient, unless directly questioned, will often not mention drugs regularly consumed, such as aperients or analgesics. These, because he has taken them without trouble in the past, must, in his opinion, be harmless. Furthermore, it is important to enquire about foods, cosmetics etc, which may contain drugs. For instance, more than one case of thrombocytopenic purpura has been caused by quinine in tonic water; the so-called 'cocktail purpura'. Penicillin in milk products has been thought to be a cause of the persistence of urticaria in patients who have had a serum sickness-like reaction due to penicillin. Sensitisation to paraphenylenediamine in hair dyes may sensitise patients to para-amino salicylic acid to mention only a few examples.

The majority of reactions will have appeared in less than four or five days after the last dose of the drug was taken. However, reactions to drugs such as long-acting sulphonamides or drugs administered in a form in which they are slowly released into the gut may take longer to develop, and drugs such as gold salts, which form depots in the tissues, may cause symptoms of hypersensitivity to develop months after they were given. Another cause of delay in the development of symptoms is seen in cases of hypoplastic anaemia due to drug hypersensitivity. If the white cells or platelets are predominantly involved symptoms are likely to appear within a few days, but if the main effect is on the red cells symptoms may not appear for several weeks. The reason for this is that, even when there is complete red cell aplasia, the red cell count is unlikely to fall by more than about one per cent per day and patients rarely complain of symptoms of anaemia until the haemoglobin has fallen to 70 per cent or below.

When a drug reaction is suspected, all drug therapy should, if possible, be stopped. If the symptoms remit this will suggest, but will not prove, that the reaction was due to one of the drugs the patient had been taking. At this point, a knowledge of the potentialities of each drug for causing hypersensitivity reactions is invaluable and the drug least likely to be involved can cautiously be readministered. A scheme for establishing the diagnosis by test dosing in this way is described elsewhere (Ackroyd and Rook, 1968). If the first drug readministered is tolerated in full doses for several days the next least likely cause may be similarly reintroduced. When, however, the reaction is a serious one, it is always better to stop all treatment and to use pharmacologically equivalent drugs which are known not to cross-react with those that have been withdrawn. Penicillin is a case in point. If the patient has developed an immediate-type reaction to penicillin it is better to regard him as allergic to penicillin, even though the evidence is circumstantial, and to substitute another antibiotic which does not cross-react with penicillin, rather than risk precipitating a reaction resembling anaphylactic shock by attempting to reinstitute treatment.

Skin testing

As far as immediate-type reactions are concerned, skin testing is still the most widely practised method of investigation. Test dosing carries too great a risk of precipitating an anaphylactic shock-like reaction. It is too early to assess the value of assaying IgE antibodies. Some workers have been enthusiastic about the value of skin testing in penicillin sensitivity, especially when the use of penicilloyl-polylysine has been combined with the 'minor determinant mixture' which contains, amongst other things, benzylpenicillin (see above). Most clinical immunologists, however, feel that testing with benzylpenicillin is too dangerous, even if scratch testing is performed before proceeding to an intradermal injection. If intradermal testing with benzylpenicillin is undertaken, it should be performed only in a hospital where every resuscitation procedure is available. Skin testing with penicilloyl-polylysine is remarkably safe but, as indicated above, the correlation of a positive reaction with clinical sensitivity to penicillin is not close. In general, skin testing for penicillin hypersensitivity should be regarded as a research procedure and the advice given above should be followed, namely to institute treatment with an antibiotic which does not cross-react with penicillin.

Patch testing is invaluable in the diagnosis of contact dermatitis and eczematous 'contact type' dermatitis. An exhaustive description of the technique is given by Hjorth and Fregert (1972). Patch testing is occasionally positive in cases of thrombocytopenic and non-thrombocytopenic purpura

(Ackroyd, 1952, 1960). The drug causes purpuric haemorrhages in the exposed area.

The action of Trafuril, an ester of nicotinic acid, when applied to the skin, in causing a local increase in skin reactivity to orally ingested allergens has been referred to above. The value of this technique has yet to be established. It seems possible that it might be used to increase the sensitivity of patch testing.

Skin window technique. A drop of a solution of the drug in saline is applied to an abraded area of skin which is then covered with a cover glass. Saline is applied to a control area of skin treated in the same way. When the cover glasses are removed and stained and examined under the microscope, they will be found to be covered with inflammatory cells which have migrated into the area. An eosinophilic response greatly in excess of that seen in the control preparation is apparently seen both in immediate and delayed types of sensitivity while in the latter, a significant increase in basophils may also be seen in the test area. An increase in basophils has also been seen in some cases of immediate-type sensitivity, in addition to the eosinophilic response just mentioned. In the hands of at least two workers, however, this test was found uninformative in cases of suspected drug hypersensitivity and this technique should probably be regarded at present only as a research tool.

In vitro tests

These can conveniently be divided into three groups:

1. Tests dependent on the demonstration of the release of histamine from the patient's whole blood or buffy coat leucocytes or from passively sensitised human lung. These tests are, of course, only applicable to immediate-type sensitivity. They can only be performed in specialised laboratories and their value is at present uncertain. They will not be referred to further.
2. Tests which have been used in the investigation of a wide variety of manifestations of drug hypersensitivity.
3. Tests designed specifically for the investigation of reactions involving the formed elements of the blood.

Tests having a wide applicability

Basophil degranulation tests. Several variants of this test have been described (Shelley and Juhlin, 1961; Shelley, 1963; Perelmutter and Khera, 1970). The theoretical basis of this type of test is that histamine is thought to be released from tissue mast cells and from the basophils in the blood as a result of a reaction involving antibody and the drug to which the patient is sensitive. This type of test attempts to demonstrate degranulation of basophil leucocytes in the blood in vitro during this reaction. Although most workers have considered these tests positive only in immediate-type reactions, Moneret-Vautrin, Grilliat and Pupil (1972) have claimed positive results in some cases of delayed-type reactions, in reactions involving immune complexes and in drug-induced cytopenias.

It is impossible to make any valid statement about this type of test, as some workers have found it diagnostically valuable (Gordon, 1966; Haye, Cooper and Cruickshank, 1968; Moneret-Vautrin et al, 1972) and others consider it useless (Bobitt, Schechter and Pollack, 1964; Feizi, 1967). Striking degranulation of basophils in the presence of the drug is, however, undoubtedly sometimes seen in cases of drug-induced immediate-type sensitivity and this is presumably the basis of the patient's symptoms, but in the hands of most workers, the test has not proved sufficiently reliable to make the results diagnostically valuable.

Lymphocyte transformation test. If lymphocytes from an individual who has been sensitised to an antigen are cultured in the presence of that antigen, some of these cells will undergo blast-cell transformation with an increase in the synthesis of deoxyribonucleic acid (DNA). The proportion of cells undergoing transformation can be estimated morphologically or by measuring the uptake of a labelled nucleoside (usually tritiated thymidine) into the DNA.

This technique has been used extensively in the investigation of drug hypersensitivity, the patient's lymphocytes in his heparinised plasma being cultured in a medium containing the drug to which he is thought to be sensitive.

It might be expected that this test would be positive only in cases of cell-mediated (delayed-type) sensitivity and, indeed, positive results have been reported in cases of contact dermatitis. It is generally accepted, however, that the test is often positive in cases of immediate-type sensitivity, and positive results have been reported in other reactions including cases of agranulocytosis due to drug hypersensitivity.

Unfortunately the results obtained with this test have differed remarkably in the hands of different workers. Thus, Evans (1967) and Ling (1972) have found the test of very little use, whereas Halpern and his colleagues (Halpern, Ky and Amache, 1967; Ky et al, 1970) and Moneret-Vautrin and her collaborators (1972) have found the test invaluable. Halpern, Ky and Amache (1967) originally claimed a 100 per cent agreement with the clinical diagnoses and later Halpern (1970) has claimed a 98·5 per cent agreement with the clinical diagnoses in a thousand cases, these diagnosises being based on the clinical history and sometimes on skin testing. These figures are disturbing because they imply a degree of accuracy in clinical diagnosis that very few clinicians would claim. Most authors have observed lymphocyte transformation in some of their cases, but the results have not been consistent enough for the test to be diagnostically valuable. As an example, Paronetto and Popper (1970) found the test positive in over half the cases of halothane jaundice examined, whereas Sarkany (1972) did not observe a single positive result in 12 cases. This worker has, however, reported some positive results in other conditions (Sarkany, 1968). It cannot even be said that a positive result always indicates clinical hypersensitivity, for Ripps and Fellner (1966) have reported finding several positive responses to penicillin in a control group of patients with no history of penicillin sensitivity, although these patients did have either immediate or delayed-type skin reactions to penicillin or the penicilloyl group. It can only be concluded that, although lymphocyte stimulation undoubtedly occurs in some cases in response to the drug to which the patient is sensitive, the phenomenon is too unpredictable to be of clinical diagnostic value.

Leucocyte migration inhibition test. The patient's peripheral blood leucocytes are placed in capillary tubes and allowed to migrate from the tube onto a glass surface in a suitable medium. After 24 hours the area of migration is measured. The area of migration may be reduced in the presence of antigen to which the patient is sensitive (Bendixen and Søborg, 1969). This test has recently been applied to the diagnosis of drug allergy with encouraging results, but too few investigations have been reported to permit an assessment of the value of the test.

Demonstration of haemagglutinating antibodies to drugs. This test depends on the agglutination by antibody in the patient's serum of red cells which have been coated with a drug. The technique is of wide applicability and has been used in the investigation of antibodies to a number of different drugs, but especially to penicillin and procainamide. The test is of no value in the diagnosis of drug hypersensitivity as it is often positive in patients who are not allergic to the drug they have been taking. A positive result indicates only that the patient has developed antibodies to the drug or to an immunochemically cross-reacting substance. The value of this technique lies in the fact that it enables an assessment to be made of the level in the patient's serum of IgG and IgM antibodies to drugs.

Assay of drug-specific IgE antibodies. Techniques for measuring penicilloyl-specific IgE serum antibodies have been described recently. It is too early to assess their value. Some preliminary results have been discussed by Juhlin and Wide (1972).

Tests for the investigation of reactions involving a reduction in the formed elements in the blood

Unlike many of the tests described above, many of the following tests are highly specific and of considerable diagnostic value.

Thrombocytopenia. The following tests, with the exception of the complement-fixation test with antibody concentration, and the test for drug-dependent precipitins, are most easily performed as soon as the platelet counts have returned to normal as a result of withdrawing the drug. If the platelet count is still low, platelets isolated from compatible normal blood may be added to the patient's blood or plasma. For some reason these tests, when performed in this way, are less sensitive than when autologous platelets are used. The demonstration of a drug-dependent precipitin does not require the presence of platelets. The complement-fixation test with antibody concentration requires the use of platelets from too great a volume of blood for it to be possible, as a rule, to use the patient's platelets.

Inhibition of clot retraction (Ackroyd, 1964). This test is relatively insensitive but technically very simple. The patient's blood is diluted with a solution of the drug in saline and is allowed to clot. The clot retraction is compared with that of blood diluted equally with saline alone. Since clot retraction is a function of platelets, a reduction in retraction in the preparation containing the drug is a measure of the effect of the drug on the platelets.

Sedimentation test (Ackroyd, 1964). This test is also technically very simple. It is much more sensitive than the clot-retraction test. The patient's blood is mixed with a solution of the drug in heparinised saline and is allowed to stand for four or five hours. This test depends on the fact that agglutinated platelets sediment rapidly. A reduction of the platelet count in the supernatant plasma in the drug-containing tube, as compared with a control in which blood is mixed with heparinised saline alone, is a measure of platelet agglutination and possibly also of platelet lysis.

Platelet agglutination and lysis (Ackroyd, 1964). One sample of the patient's platelet-rich heparinised plasma is diluted with a solution of the drug in saline and another, equally, with saline alone. The platelets are observed at intervals for agglutination by phase-contrast microscopy and, if agglutination is not too great to make this possible, they are counted. Platelet lysis is occasionally a very striking feature in such preparations.

Complement-fixation tests (Ackroyd, 1964). (a) Without antibody concentration: The patient's blood is mixed with a solution of the drug in saline and is allowed to clot. The complement in the serum is then titrated. If complement fixation has occurred as a result of a reaction between platelets, antibody and the drug, then the titre will be considerably lower than in a control preparation of the patient's blood diluted with saline.

(b) With antibody concentration: This technique is by far the most sensitive available. It depends on the fact that antibody becomes attached to platelets in the presence of the drug. Washed normal platelets are suspended in as large a volume as possible of the patient's serum which has been freed of complement by heating. A solution of the drug in saline is added to half this preparation and an equal volume of saline is added to the remainder. Each preparation is subsequently centrifuged and equal quantities of the supernatant are removed from each, leaving only the smallest amount required for resuspension of the platelets. After resuspension, equal volumes of guinea-pig serum are added to each preparation and the residual guinea-pig complement is titrated. In this way the antibody in the original large volume of serum is concentrated on the platelets in the remaining much smaller volume, and the degree of complement fixation is thus greatly increased.

Demonstration of a drug-dependent precipitin (Ackroyd, 1964). Drug-dependent precipitins are very rare. If present, they can be demonstrated by adding the drug in saline to the patient's serum. As the relative concentrations of drug and antibody may be critical, as wide a range of concentrations of each as is possible should be investigated.

Antiglobulin consumption test (Dausset and Colombani, 1964). This is a method of detecting immunoglobulin on platelets or leucocytes. In the investigation of drug-induced thrombocytopenia, platelets are suspended in the patient's serum which has been freed of complement by heating. One volume of this suspension is diluted with a solution of the drug in saline, and an equal volume is diluted equally with saline alone. The preparations are centrifuged and the supernatant discarded. The deposited platelets are then washed and resuspended in antiglobulin serum. The antiglobulin titre in each preparation is then measured. If the patient's serum contains a drug-dependent antibody, and if the drug–platelet–antibody complex will withstand washing then the antibody will be fixed onto the platelets in the drug-containing preparation but not in the control preparation. Interaction of this adsorbed drug-dependent immunoglobulin antibody with the antiglobulin antibody in the antiglobulin serum will result in a fall in the antiglobulin titre in the drug-containing preparation as compared with the control.

Liberation of platelet factor 3 (Horowitz, Young and Nachman, 1964; Horowitz et al, 1965). This test measures the release of platelet factor 3 from platelets as a result of damage from interaction of the platelets with drug and antibody. Although this test has been widely used, its value is not established beyond doubt (see Horowitz et al, 1965) and the results should probably not be accepted unless supported by the results of other tests for drug-dependent platelet antibodies.

Timing and choice of in vitro *tests for thrombocytopenic purpura due to drug hypersensitivity.* These tests should be performed as early as possible because, although the antibody may persist practically unchanged for years, it may disappear within a few days. The tests described above are those which have been most widely used. For some reason, not all these tests will be found positive in every case of thrombocytopenic purpura due to drug hypersensitivity. Ideally, therefore, all the tests should be performed in every case. Failing this, the complement-fixation test with antibody concentration is probably the most reliable and the most sensitive.

Haemolytic anaemia. *Red cell agglutination and lysis.* (a) Tests using red cells coated with drugs, in vitro, before being exposed to the patient's serum have already been discussed. As stated above, the demonstration of haemagglutinating antibodies to a drug often means nothing more than that the patient has developed an immunological, but not necessarily a clinical reaction to it. A very sensitive technique for demonstrating haemagglutinating antibodies to penicillin is described by Levine et al (1966a).

(b) Tests using red cells which have not been coated with the drug before being exposed to the patient's serum: The addition of the drug to a suspension of red cells in the patient's serum may cause red cell agglutination. Occasionally lysis will occur in the presence of complement. If lysis does not occur when the patient's cells or normal cells are used, trypsinised red cells or cells from cases of paroxysmal nocturnal haemoglobinuria may be substituted. These undergo lysis more readily and may permit the lytic character of the antibody to be demonstrated. Lysis of these cells also requires complement.

Antiglobulin (Coombs') test. (a) Direct test: The patient's own washed red cells are suspended in a broad-spectrum antiglobulin serum. Agglutination of these cells indicates that they were coated in vivo with immunoglobulin or complement, or both. These can be differentiated by using more specific antisera. As explained above, the antibody and drug may be removed from the red cells during the process of washing but components of complement remain attached to the red cell membrane.

(b) Indirect test: Red cells are suspended in the patient's serum in the presence of the drug. If agglutination or lysis does not occur, the cells are washed and resuspended in antiglobulin serum. If this causes agglutination the significance of this finding can be analysed as described for the direct test.

Exclusion of cases of haemolysis due to enzyme deficiency. Haemolysis due to drugs in patients whose red cells are deficient in the enzyme glucose-6-phosphate dehydrogenase closely mimics haemolysis due to drug hypersensitivity, and this enzyme should be estimated in every case of haemolytic anaemia thought to be due to a drug. Several techniques are available for investigating this enzyme (Beutler, 1967; World Health Organisation Scientific

Group, 1967). A normal level of the enzyme immediately after a haemolytic crisis should not be taken as proof that the patient's red cells are not usually deficient in the enzyme, because in a haemolytic crisis the older cells which are the more enzyme-deficient are destroyed, leaving the younger, less enzyme-deficient cells in the circulation. This has the effect of temporarily raising the level of the enzyme. If, therefore, the first estimation indicates a normal enzyme level, the estimation should be repeated after recovery.

Agranulocytosis. *Leucocyte agglutination.* The patient's serum, taken during the period of agranulocytosis, may contain an agglutinin which agglutinates normal leucocytes in the absence of added drug. This finding is of no diagnostic value as a similar agglutinin may be found in other types of agranulocytosis. The agglutinin disappears as the patient recovers. Evidence that a drug is responsible for the agranulocytosis is occasionally obtained by observing a rise in the leucoagglutinin titre caused by the addition of the drug to the suspension of white cells in the patient's serum. Leucocyte agglutination dependent entirely on the addition of the drug to the patient's serum has only rarely been observed and, when it has, the responsible antibody has often disappeared within a few days. In some cases, however, the antibody has persisted for weeks or months.

Complement fixation test. The complement titre of a suspension of white cells in the patient's serum to which a solution of the drug in saline has been added is compared with that of a corresponding preparation to which saline only has been added. A positive result is indicated by a fall in the titre of the drug-containing preparation as compared with that of the saline control.

Antiglobulin consumption test (Dausset and Colombani, 1964). This test is performed as described above, substituting leucocytes for platelets.

Test for drug-dependent cytotoxic antibodies (Engelfriet and Eijsvoogel, 1965, modified by Magis, Barge and Dausset, 1968). A suspension of leucocytes in the patient's serum is incubated with a solution of the drug in the presence of complement. Trypan blue is then added. Intact cells exclude the dye whereas cells injured by the interaction of the cytotoxic antibody with the drug in the presence of complement are stained. The percentage of stained cells is an indication of the cytotoxicity of the antibody.

Tests involving observations on leucocyte amoeboid movement or phagocytosis. Tests involving the demonstration of a reduction in amoeboid movement, or the inhibition of phagocytosis by polymorphs suspended in the patient's serum, and occurring only in the presence of the causative drug, have occasionally been reported. A test involving a reduction by the drug, of carbon dioxide production during phagocytosis has been referred to above. None of these tests has been used sufficiently to make it possible to assess its value.

Significance of positive skin tests and serological tests in the diagnosis of drug hypersensitivity

In the course of this review it will have become clear that apart from test dosing there are few, if any, infallible tests for drug hypersensitivity. Positive immediate-type skin reactions to penicilloyl-polylysine are common in patients who subsequently tolerate a full course of treatment without trouble (Brown et al, 1964). Delayed-type reactions to intradermally injected penicillin occur in patients without evidence of hypersensitivity to this drug (Redmond and Levine, 1968). Positive results to patch testing sometimes occur in patients who do not develop contact dermatitis when exposed to the allergen with which they were tested (Hjorth and Fregert, 1972). Lymphocyte transformation in the presence of penicillin has been observed in a number of patients not having a history of a drug reaction (Ripps and Fellner, 1966). The drugs alpha-methyldopa, L-dopa and cephalothin frequently cause the recipient's red cells to develop a positive direct antiglobulin test, although overt haemolytic anaemia due to these drugs is quite rare (see above). Probably the most valuable tests at present available are those described above in connection with drug reactions involving the formed elements of the blood. False-positive results are very rare if, as indicated above, tests involving the haemagglutination of red cells coated in vitro with drugs are not considered. False-positive results can, however, occur (see Dausset and Bergerot-Blondel, 1961). False-negative results can occur with any test and are probably due to an insufficient concentration of antibody in the patient's serum.

It will now be clear that the tests described in this chapter should be taken only as providing one part of the evidence on which a diagnosis can be made and, as in other fields in medicine, the most important factor in diagnosis is the clinical history.

Ultimately, if it is essential to establish beyond question the relationship of a drug to the patient's symptoms, recourse may have to be made to test dosing after recovery, with the intention of producing a recurrence of the condition thought to have been caused by the drug. In highly sensitised patients, this can be dangerous, as is evidenced by the occurrence of fatal reactions to intradermal testing (Rose, 1953; Idsøe et al, 1968), or even to scratch testing (Dogliotti, 1968). Test dosing should therefore only be performed when treatment is life saving and no alternative drug can be given. A scheme for undertaking test dosing has been described by the author (Ackroyd, 1964). In highly sensitised patients a reaction may develop within minutes of the administration of a small quantity of the causative drug, but in less sensitive patients there may be no response to a single small dose of the drug and drug administration may have to be continued for several days, or even for two to three weeks, and full doses may have to be given before a reaction develops. If the patient has developed a blocking antibody as is believed to happen in the late urticarial reactions to penicillin (see above), the patient may not develop symptoms even after protracted test dosing.

Treatment

Prophylaxis

The following points should be borne in mind.

Drugs with a high potentiality for causing serious reactions should not be used unless treatment is essential and there is no alternative and safer drug. As Garrod (1958) has pointed out '. . . many unfortunate victims (of aplastic anaemia) have received the treatment (chloramphenicol) for quite trivial conditions'.

If treatment with a drug which is known to cause serious reactions is contemplated, the patient should always be asked if previous administration has caused symptoms and a patient's statement that he is sensitive to a drug should *never* be ignored.

If a patient is receiving treatment with a drug known to cause serious reactions, a careful watch should be kept for even a small spike of fever, as this may herald a reaction, and if treatment is stopped immediately a serious reaction may possibly be avoided.

Specific therapy

In an earlier part of this chapter, the phenomenon of hapten inhibition was mentioned. This phenomenon depends on the hapten being able to react with the antigen-combining sites on the antibody, so preventing reaction of antibody with the complete antigen. De Weck and Girard (1972) have used a synthetic monovalent penicilloyl hapten (benzylpenicilloyl-formyl-lysine) in an endeavour to prevent allergic reactions to penicillin in man. They gave the hapten to a group of patients who were sensitive to penicillin, and reported that 12 of 13 patients were able to continue treatment with penicillin without symptoms, under cover of the hapten. These results clearly need confirmation as de Weck and Girard (1972) point out but, if confirmed, this technique opens up an extremely important advance in therapeutics.

Desensitisation

It has been known for years that the administration of very small, but progressively increasing doses of a drug to which a patient is sensitive sometimes enables him to tolerate the drug. The reason is not known. This procedure is potentially dangerous and should only be attempted when treatment is urgently needed and no effective alternative drug is available. The technique has been described by Smith and Zirk (1961), Crofton (1953) and Alexander (1953).

ACKNOWLEDGEMENT

The general outline of this chapter is similar to that followed by the author in collaboration with Dr Arthur Rook in *Clinical Aspects of Immunology* edited by P. G. H. Gell and R. R. A. Coombs (1968). The author acknowledges with pleasure the contribution made by Dr Rook in that collaborative effort to present in a reasonably orderly fashion the very complex subject of drug hypersensitivity.

References

The following list of references is by no means comprehensive. The sources of many of the statements made in this chapter can be found in Ackroyd, J. F. & Rook, A. J. (1968) Allergic drug reactions. In *Clinical Aspects of Immunology*, 2nd edition, ed. Gell, P. G. H. & Coombs, R. R. A. pp. 693–755. Oxford: Blackwell; and in Ackroyd, J. F. (1974) Immunological mechanisms in drug hypersensitivity, a chapter in the 3rd edition of the same book (in press).

Ackroyd, J. F. (1952) Sedormid purpura: an immunological study of a form of drug hypersensitivity. *Progress in Allergy*, **3**, 531–572.

Ackroyd, J. F. (1953) Allergic purpura, including purpura due to foods, drugs and infections. *American Journal of Medicine*, **14**, 605–632.

Ackroyd, J. F. (1960) The pathogenesis of purpura. In *Lectures on Haematology*, ed. Hayhoe, F. G. J., pp. 217–247. London: Cambridge University Press.

Ackroyd, J. F. (1964) The diagnosis of disorders of the blood due to drug hypersensitivity caused by an immune mechanism. In *Immunological Methods*, ed. Ackroyd, J. F., pp. 453–509. Oxford: Blackwell.

Ackroyd, J. F. (1974) Immunological mechanisms in drug hypersensitivity. In *Clinical Aspects of Immunology*, 3rd edition, ed. Gell, P. G. H., Coombs, R. R. A. & Lachmann, P. J. Oxford: Blackwell.

Ackroyd, J. F. & Rook, A. J. (1968) Allergic drug reactions. In *Clinical Aspects of Immunology*, 2nd edition, ed. Gell, P. G. H. & Coombs, R. R. A., pp. 693–755. Oxford: Blackwell.

Adkinson, N. F. Jr, Thompson, W. L., Maddrey, W. C. & Lichtenstein, L. M. (1971) Routine use of penicillin skin testing on an inpatient service. *New England Journal of Medicine*, **285**, 22–24.

Alarcón-Segovia, D., Worthington, J. W., Ward, L. E. & Wakim, K. G. (1965) Lupus diathesis and the hydralazine syndrome. *New England Journal of Medicine*, **272**, 462–466.

Alexander, L. J. (1953) Desensitisation of the penicillin-sensitive patient. *Archives of Dermatology and Syphilology*, **68**, 323–327.

Baer, R. L. (1954) Cross-sensitisation phenomena. In *Modern Trends in Dermatology* (Second Series), ed. MacKenna, R. M. B., pp. 232–258. London: Butterworth.

Baer, R. L. & Harris, H. (1967) Types of cutaneous reactions to drugs: importance in recognition of adverse reactions. *Journal of the American Medical Association*, **202**, 710–713.

Baker, L. & Miller, M. E. (1967) Depression of immunoglobulin G (IgG) levels associated with diazoxide therapy. *Metabolism*, **16**, 964–966.

Baldwin, D. S., Levine, B. B., McCluskey, R. T. & Gallo, G. R. (1968) Renal failure and interstitial nephritis due to penicillin and methicillin. *New England Journal of Medicine*, **279**, 1245–1252.

Bendixen, G. & Søborg, M. (1969) A leucocyte migration technique for in vitro detection of cellular (delayed type) hypersensitivity in man. *Danish Medical Bulletin*, **16**, 1–6.

Beutler, E. (1967) Glucose-6-phosphate dehydrogenase deficiency: diagnosis, clinical and genetic implications. *American Journal of Clinical Pathology*, **47**, 303–311.

Björnberg, A. & Gisslén, H. (1965) Thiazides: a cause of necrotising vasculitis? *Lancet*, **ii**, 982–983.

Blomgren, S. E., Condemi, J. J. & Vaughan, J. H. (1972) Procainamide-induced lupus erythematosus. *American Journal of Medicine*, **52**, 338–348.

Blomgren, S. E. & Vaughan, J. H. (1968) The immunogenicity of photo-oxidized DNA and of the photoproduct of DNA and procainamide hydrochloride. *Arthritis and Rheumatism*, **11**, 470.

Bobitt, J. R., Schechter, H. & Pollak, V. E. (1964) A critical evaluation of the indirect basophil degranulation test. *Proceedings of the Society for Experimental Biology and Medicine*, **117**, 608–610.

Böttiger, L. E. & Westerholm, B. (1972a) Thrombocytopenia. II: Drug induced thrombocytopenia. *Acta Medica Scandinavica*, **191**, 541–548.

Böttiger, L. E. & Westerholm, B. (1972b) Aplastic anaemia II: Drug induced aplastic anaemia. *Acta Medica Scandinavica*, **192**, 319–321.

Böttiger, L. E. & Westerholm, B. (1973a) Acquired haemolytic anaemia II: Drug induced haemolytic anaemia. *Acta Medica Scandinavica*, **193**, 227–231.

Böttiger, L. E. & Westerholm, B. (1973b) Drug induced blood dyscrasias in Sweden. *British Medical Journal*, **iii**, 339–343.

Brown, B. C., Price, E. V. & Moore, M. B. (1964) Penicilloyl-polylysine as an intradermal test of penicillin sensitivity. *Journal of the American Medical Association*, **189**, 599–604.

Brugmans, J., Schuermans, V., De Cock, W., Thienpont, D., Janssen, P., Verhaegen, H., Van Nimmen, L., Louwagie, A. C. & Stevens, E. (1973) Restoration of host defense mechanisms in man by levamisole. *Life Sciences*, **13**, 1499–1504.

Coombs, R. R. A. & Gell, P. G. H. (1968) Classification of allergic reactions responsible for clinical hypersensitivity and disease. In *Clinical Aspects of Immunology*, ed. Gell, P. G. H. & Coombs, R. R. A., pp. 575–596. Oxford: Blackwell.

Creger, W. P. & Houseworth, J. H. (1954) Erythrophagocytosis and thrombocytopathy occurring during the course of a Henoch-Schönlein syndrome due to quinine. *American Journal of Medicine*, **17,** 423–431.

Criep, L. H. (1971) Allergic vascular purpura. *Journal of Allergy and Clinical Immunology*, **48,** 7–12.

Crofton, J. (1953) Desensitisation to streptomycin and P.A.S. *British Medical Journal*, **ii,** 1014–1017.

Dausset, J. & Bergerot-Blondel, Y. (1961) Étude d'un anticorps allergique actif en présence de para-amino-salicylate de soude (PAS) contre les hématies, les leucocytes et les plaquettes humaines. *Vox Sanguinis*, **6,** 91–109.

Dausset, J. & Colombani, J. (1964) Detection of anti-leucocyte and anti-platelet antibodies by the antiglobulin consumption test. In *Immunological Methods*, ed. Ackroyd, J. F., pp. 575–595. Oxford: Blackwell.

Dern, R. J., Beutler, E. & Alving, A. S. (1955) The haemolytic effect of primaquine. V. Primaquine sensitivity as a manifestation of a multiple drug sensitivity. *Journal of Laboratory and Clinical Medicine*, **45,** 30–39.

de Weck, A. L. (1971a) Drug reactions. In *Immunological Diseases*, 2nd edition, Volume I, ed. Samter, M., pp. 415–440. Boston: Little Brown.

de Weck, A. L. (1971b) Immunological effects of aspirin anhydride, a contaminant of commercial acetylsalicylic acid preparations. *International Archives of Allergy and Applied Immunology*, **41,** 393–418.

de Weck, A. L. (1972) Immunochemical mechanisms in drug allergy. In *Mechanisms in Drug Allergy* (Glaxo Symposium Series) ed. Dash, C. H. & Jones, H. E. H., pp. 2–15. London and Edinburgh: Churchill Livingstone.

de Weck, A. L. & Girard, J. P. (1972) Specific inhibition of allergic reactions to penicillin in man by a monovalent hapten. II. Clinical studies. *International Archives of Allergy and Applied Immunology*, **42,** 798–815.

Dickerman, J. D., Holtzman, N. A. & Zinkham, W. H. (1973) Hemoglobin Zurich: a third family presenting with hemolytic reactions to sulfonamides. *American Journal of Medicine*, **55,** 638–642.

Dogliotti, M. (1968) An instance of fatal reaction to the penicillin scratch test. *Dermatologica*, **136,** 489–496.

Dubois, E. L., Molina, J., Bilitch, M. & Friou, G. J. (1968) Procainamide-induced serologic changes in asymptomatic patients. *Arthritis and Rheumatism*, **11,** 477–478.

Eisen, H. N. (1959) Hypersensitivity to simple chemicals. In *Cellular and Humoral Aspects of the Hypersensitive States*, ed. Lawrence, H. S., pp. 89–119. New York: Hoeber-Harper.

Eisner, E. V. & Kasper, K. (1972) Immune thrombocytopenia due to a metabolite of para-aminosalicyclic acid. *American Journal of Medicine*, **53,** 790–796.

Eisner, E. V. & Shahidi, N. T. (1972) Immune thrombocytopenia due to a drug metabolite. *New England Journal of Medicine*, **287,** 376–381.

Engelfriet, C. P. & Eijsvoogel, V. P. (1965) Cytotoxic iso-antibodies against leucocytes. *Vox Sanguinis*, **10,** 228–233.

Evans, D. A. (1967) The lymphocyte stimulation test in penicillin hypersensitivity. *Journal of Allergy*, **39,** 340–346.

Feizi, T. (1967) The indirect basophil degranulation test for allergy to penicillin. *Transactions of St. John's Hospital Dermatological Society*, **53,** 162–164.

Fellner, M. J., Fukuyama, K., Moshell, A. & Klaus, M. V. (1973) Intercellular antibodies in blood and epidermis. *British Journal of Dermatology*, **89,** 115–126.

Fisher, A. A. (1966) Systemic eczematous 'contact-type' dermatitis medicamentosa. *Annals of Allergy*, **24,** 406–420.

Fregert, S. & Hjorth, N. (1972) The principal irritants and sensitisers. In *Textbook of Dermatology*, ed. Rook, A., Wilkinson, D. S. & Ebling, F. J. G. 2nd edition, Vol. 1. pp. 386–424. Oxford: Blackwell.

Gams, R. A., Neal, J. A. & Conrad, F. G. (1968) Hydantoin-induced pseudo-pseudolymphoma. *Annals of Internal Medicine*, **69,** 557–568.

Garrod, L. P. (1958) The production of bone marrow aplasia by chloramphenicol. In, *Sensitivity Reactions to Drugs*, ed. Rosenheim, M. L. & Moulton, R., pp. 92–99. Oxford: Blackwell.

Gell, P. G. H. & Coombs, R. R. A. (Editors) (1968) *Clinical Aspects of Immunology*, 2nd edition. Oxford: Blackwell.

Gordon, V. H. (1960) The indirect basophil test and drug hypersensitivity. *Annals of Allergy*, **24,** 171–178.

Graham, J. R. (1968) Fibrosis associated with methysergide therapy. In *Drug-Induced Diseases*, ed. Meyler, L. & Peck, H. M., Vol. 3, pp. 249–269. Amsterdam: Excerpta Medica.

Grob, P. J. & Herold, G. E. (1972) Immunological abnormalities and hydantoins. *British Medical Journal*, **ii,** 561–563.

Halpern, B., Ky, N. T. & Amache, N. (1967) Diagnosis of drug allergy in vitro with the lymphocyte transformation test. *Journal of Allergy*, **40,** 168–181.

Halpern, G. (1970) Discussion on Ky et al (1970).

Hartl, P. W. (1973) Drug induced agranulocytosis. In *Blood Disorders Due to Drugs and Other Agents*. ed. Girdwood, R. H., pp. 147–186. Amsterdam: Excerpta Medica.

Haye, K. R., Cooper, J. R. & Cruickshank, C. N. D. (1968) Studies on the degranulation of human basophil leucocytes in vitro. *British Journal of Dermatology*, **80,** 811–821.

Hazlett, B. E. & Yendt, E. R. (1958) Thrombocytopenia following gold therapy with successful treatment. *Canadian Medical Association Journal*, **79,** 31–33.

Henry, R. E., Goldberg, L. S., Sturgeon, P. & Ansel, R. D. (1971) Serologic abnormalities associated with L-dopa therapy. *Vox Sanguinis*, **20,** 306–316.

Hjorth, N. & Fregert, S. (1972) Contact dermatitis. In *Textbook of Dermatology*, ed. Rook, A., Wilkinson, D. S. & Ebling, F. J. G., 2nd edition, Vol. I, pp. 305–385. Oxford: Blackwell.

Hollister, L. E. (1957) Allergy to chlorpromazine manifested by jaundice. *American Journal of Medicine*, **23,** 870–879.

Horowitz, H. I., Young, R. & Nachman, R. L. (1964) Thrombocytopenia due to digitoxin: demonstration of antibody and mechanism of action. *Journal of Clinical Investigation*, **43,** 1236.

Horowitz, H. I., Rappaport, H. I., Young, R. C. & Fujimoto, M. M. (1965) Change in platelet factor 3 as a means of demonstrating immune reactions involving platelets: its use as a test for quinidine-induced thrombocytopenia. *Transfusion*, **5,** 336–343.

Houston, I. B. & Barlow, A. M. (1959) Acute haemolytic anaemia and methaemoglobinuria produced by phenacetin. *Lancet*, **ii,** 1062–1065.

Huguley, C. M., Erslev, A. J. & Bergsagel, D. E. (1961) Drug-related blood dyscrasias. *Journal of the American Medical Association*, **177,** 23–26.

Idsøe, O., Guthe, T., Willcox, R. R. & de Weck, A. L. (1968) Nature and extent of penicillin side-reactions with particular reference to fatalities from anaphylactic shock. *Bulletin of the World Health Organisation*, **38,** 159–188.

Israel, K. S., Brashear, R. E., Sharma, H. M., Yum, M. N. & Glover, J. L. (1973) Pulmonary fibrosis and nitrofurantoin. *American Review of Respiratory Diseases*, **108,** 353–356.

Juhlin, L. & Wide, L. (1972) IgE antibodies and penicillin allergy. In *Mechanisms in Drug Allergy* (Glaxo Symposium Series), ed. Dash, C. H. & Jones, H. E. H., pp. 139–147. Edinburgh: Churchill Livingstone.

Karpatkin, S. (1971) Drug induced thrombocytopenia. *American Journal of Medical Sciences*, **262,** 68–78.

Katz, A. & Little, A. H. (1973) Gold nephropathy: an immunopathologic study. *Archives of Pathology*, **96,** 133–136.

Kirshbaum, M. D. & Beerman, H. (1964) Photosensitisation due to drugs. A review of some of the recent literature. *American Journal of Medical Sciences*, **248,** 445–468.

Knudsen, E. T., Dewdney, J. M. & Trafford, J. A. P. (1970) Reduction in incidence of ampicillin rash by purification of ampicillin. *British Medical Journal*, **i,** 469–471.

Ky, N. T., Chauvin, M. T., Pinon, C. & Halpern, B. N. (1970) Positive immunologic reactions to cephaloridine in patients allergic to penicillin: a study performed with the lymphoblastic transformation test. *Postgraduate Medical Journal*, **46,** Supplement (Cephalosporins), 109–112.

Lachmann, P. J. (1968) Nephrotic syndrome from penicillamine. *Postgraduate Medical Journal*, **44,** Supplement (Penicillamine) 23–27.

Lancet Editorial (1971) Is phenytoin carcinogenic? *Lancet*, **ii,** 1071–1072.

Leemann, W., de Weck, A. L. & Schneider, C. H. (1969) Hypersensitivity to carboxymethyl-cellulose as a cause of anaphylactic reactions to drugs in cattle. *Nature*, **223,** 621–623.

Levin, J. (1974). Effects of oral antidiabetic and diuretic agents on platelets. In *Drugs and Hematologic Reactions* (29th Hahnemann Symposium). ed. Dimitrov, N. V. & Nodine, J. H., pp. 263–270. New York and London: Grune and Stratton.

Levine, B. B. (1966) Immunologic mechanisms of penicillin allergy. *New England Journal of Medicine*, **275,** 1115–1125.

Levine, B. B., Fellner, M. J., Levytska, V., Franklin, E. C. & Alisberg, N. (1966a) Benzylpenicilloyl-specific serum antibodies to penicillin in man. II. Sensitivity of the haemagglutination assay method, molecular classes of the antibodies detected and antibody titers of randomly selected patients. *Journal of Immunology*, **96,** 719–726.

Levine, B. B., Redmond, A. P., Fellner, M. J., Voss, H. E. & Levytska, V. (1966b) Penicillin allergy and the heterogeneous immune responses of man to benzylpenicillin. *Journal of Clinical Investigation*, **45,** 1895–1906.

Ling, N. R. (1972) Lymphocyte transformation in drug allergy. In *Mechanisms in Drug Allergy* (Glaxo Symposium Series), ed, Dash, C. H. & Jones, H. E. H., pp. 171–175. Edinburgh: Churchill Livingstone.

Löbel, H., Machtey, I. & Eldror, M. Y. (1972) Pulmonary infiltrates with eosinophilia in an asthmatic patient treated with disodium chromoglycate. *Lancet*, **ii,** 1032.

McCormick, R. V. (1950) Periarteritis occurring during propylthiouracil therapy. *Journal of the American Medical Association*, **144,** 1453–1454.

MacGibbon, B. H., Loughridge, L. W., Hourihane, D. O'B. & Boyd, D. W. (1960) Auto-immune haemolytic anaemia with acute renal failure due to phenacetin and *p*-amino-salicylic acid. *Lancet*, **i,** 7–10.

McIntyre, P. A., Laleli, Y. R., Hodkinson, B. A. & Wagner, H. N. Jr (1971) Evidence for anti-leucocyte antibodies as a mechanism for drug-induced agranulocytosis. *Transactions of the Association of American Physicians*, **84,** 217–228.

McVie, J. G. (1973) Drug induced thrombocytopenia. In *Blood Disorders Due to Drugs and Other Agents*, ed. Girdwood, R. H., pp. 187–208. Amsterdam: Excerpta Medica.

Magis, C. C., Barge, A. & Dausset, J. (1968) Serological study of an allergic agranulocytosis due to noramidopyrine. *Clinical and Experimental Immunology*, **3,** 989–1003.

Meyler, L. (Editor) (1957) *Side Effects of Drugs: Untoward effects of drugs as reported in the medical literature of the world during the period 1955–56*, Vol. 1. Amsterdam: Excerpta Medica.

Meyler, L. (Editor) (1958) *Side Effects of Drugs: Untoward effects of drugs as reported in the medical literature of the world during the period 1956–57*, Vol. 2. Amsterdam: Excerpta Medica.

Meyler, L. (Editor) (1960) *Side Effects of Drugs: Unwanted effects of drugs as reported in the medical literature of the world during the period 1958–60*, Vol. 3. Amsterdam: Excerpta Medica.

Meyler, L. (Editor) (1963) *Side Effects of Drugs as Reported in the Medical Literature of the World*, Vol. 4. Amsterdam: Excerpta Medica.

Meyler, L. (Editor) (1966) *Side Effects of Drugs: Adverse reactions as reported in the medical literature of the world 1963–1965*, Vol. 5. Amsterdam: Excerpta Medica.

Meyler, L. & Herxheimer, A. (Editors) (1968) *Side Effects of Drugs: A survey of unwanted effects of drugs reported in 1965–1967*, Vol. 6. Amsterdam: Excerpta Medica.

Meyler, L. & Herxheimer, A. (Editors) (1972) *Side Effects of Drugs: A survey of unwanted effects of drugs reported in 1968–71*, Vol. 7. Amsterdam: Excerpta Medica.

Meyler, L. & Peck, H. M. (Editors) (1962) *Drug-Induced Diseases*, Vol. 1. Assen: Royal Vangorcum.

Meyler, L. & Peck, H. M. (Editors) (1964) *Drug-Induced Diseases*, Vol. 2. Amsterdam: Excerpta Medica.

Meyler, L. & Peck, H. M. (Editors) (1968) *Drug-Induced Diseases*, Vol. 3. Amsterdam: Excerpta Medica.

Meyler, L. & Peck, H. M. (Editors) (1972) *Drug Induced Diseases*, Vol. 4. Amsterdam: Excerpta Medica.

Michaëlsson, G., Pettersson, L. & Juhlin, L. (1974) Purpura caused by food and drug additives. *Archives of Dermatology*, **109,** 49–52.

Miescher, P. A. (1973) Drug-induced thrombocytopenia. *Seminars in Haematology*, **10,** 311–325.

Miescher, P. & Miescher, A. (1952) Die Sedormid-Anaphylaxie. *Schweizerische Medizinische Wochenschrift*, **82,** 1279–1282.

Moneret-Vautrin, D. A., Grilliat, J. P. & Pupil, P. (1972) Basophil degranulation in drug allergy. In *Mechanisms in Drug Allergy* (Glaxo Symposium Series), ed. Dash, C. H. & Jones, H. E. H., pp. 159–170. Edinburgh: Churchill Livingstone.

Murray, M. J. (1968) Pulmonary reactions to nitrofurantoin. In *Drug Induced Diseases*, ed. Meyler, L. & Peck, H. M., Vol. 3, pp. 157–160. Amsterdam: Excerpta Medica.

Nagao, T. & Mauer, A. M. (1969) Concordance for drug-induced aplastic anemia in identical twins. *New England Journal of Medicine*, **281,** 7–11.

Nieweg, H. O. (1973) Aplastic anaemia (panmyelopathy): a review with special emphasis on the factors causing bone marrow damage. In *Blood Disorders Due to Drugs and Other Agents*, ed. Girdwood, R. H., pp. 83–106. Amsterdam: Excerpta Medica.

Palva, I. P. & Mustala, O. O. (1970) Drug induced agranulocytosis with special reference to aminophenazone. 1. Adults. *Acta Medica Scandinavica*, **187,** 109–115.

Paronetto, F. & Popper, H. (1970) Lymphocyte stimulation induced by halothane in patients with hepatitis following exposure to halothane. *New England Journal of Medicine*, **283,** 277–280.

Pepys, J., Jenkins, P. A., Lachmann, P. J. & Mahon, W. E. (1966) An iatrogenic autoantibody: immunological responses to pituitary snuff in patients with diabetes insipidus. *Clinical and Experimental Immunology*, **1,** 377–389.

Perelmutter, L. & Khera, K. (1970) A study on the detection of human reagins with rat peritoneal mast cells. *International Archives of Allergy and Applied Immunology*, **39,** 27–44.

Perlman, F. (1965) Value of skin testing for penicillin allergy. *Journal of the American Medical Association*, 192, 64–65.

Pisciotta, A. V. (1969) Agranulocytosis induced by certain phenothiazine derivatives. *Journal of the American Medical Association*, **208,** 1862–1868.

Pisciotta, A. V. (1973) Immune and toxic mechanisms in drug-induced agranulocytosis. *Seminars in Haematology*, **10,** 279–310.

Pisciotta, A. V. (1974) The effect of chlorpromazine on peripheral leucocytes. In *Drugs and Hematologic Reactions* (29th Hahnemann Symposium), ed. Dimitrov, N. V. & Nodine, J. H., pp. 233–247. New York and London: Grune and Stratton.

Redmond, A. P. & Levine, B. B. (1968) Delayed skin reactions to benzylpenicillin in man. *International Archives of Allergy and Applied Immunology*, **33,** 193–206.

Reid, J. M., Stevenson, J. G. & Orr, M. (1969) Non-thrombocytopenic purpura due to chlorothiazide. *Scottish Medical Journal*, **14,** 309–311.

Reynolds, T. B., Lapin, A. C., Peters, R. L. & Yamahiro, H. S. (1970) Puzzling jaundice: probable relationship to laxative ingestion. *Journal of the American Medical Association*, **211,** 86–90.

Reynolds, T. B., Peters, R. L. & Yamada, S. (1971) Chronic active and lupoid hepatitis caused by a laxative, oxyphenisatin. *New England Journal of Medicine*, **285,** 813–820.

Rich, A. R. & Gregory, J. E. (1943) The experimental demonstration that periarteritis nodosa is a manifestation of hypersensitivity. *Johns Hopkins Hospital Bulletin*, **72,** 65–82.

Ripps, C. S. & Fellner, M. J. (1966) Lymphocytes and drug hypersensitivity. *Lancet*, **ii,** 803.

Rodriguez, S. U., Leikin, S. L. & Hiller, M. C. (1964) Neonatal thrombocytopenia associated with antepartum administration of thiazide drugs. *New England Journal of Medicine*, **270,** 881–884.

Rose, B. (1953) Statement on p. 394 in: Boger, W. P., Sherman, W. B., Schiller, I. W., Siegal, S. & Rose, B. Allergic reactions to penicillin. *Journal of Allergy*, **24,** 383–404.

Rosenow, E. C. (1972) The spectrum of drug-induced pulmonary disease. *Annals of Internal Medicine*, 77, 977–991.

Russell, A. S. & Ziff, M. (1968) Natural antibodies to procainamide. *Clinical and Experimental Immunology*, **3,** 901–909.

Samter, M. & Beers, R. F. (1968) Intolerance to aspirin: clinical studies and consideration of its pathogenesis. *Annals of Internal Medicine*, **68,** 975–983.

Sarkany, I. (1968) Clinical and laboratory aspects of drug allergy. *Proceedings of the Royal Society of Medicine*, **61,** 891–894.

Sarkany, I. (1972) Personal communication to Sherlock and Ajdukiewicz (1972).

Shahidi, N. T. (1967) Acetophenetidin sensitivity. *American Journal of Diseases of Children*, **113,** 81–82.

Sheba, C. & Shani, M. (1969) Data on the lack of a particular myelotoxicity of chloramphenicol in Israel. *Haematologica Latina*, **12,** 539–542.

Shelley, W. B. (1963) Indirect basophil degranulation test for allergy to penicillin and other drugs. *Journal of the American Medical Association*, **184,** 171–178.

Shelley, W. B. & Juhlin, L. (1961) A new test for detecting anaphylactic sensitivity: the basophil reaction. *Nature* (London), **191,** 1056–1058.

Sherlock, S. (1968) Drugs and the liver. In *Disease of the Liver and Biliary System*, (ed.) Sherlock, S. 4th edition, pp. 350–386. Oxford: Blackwell.

Sherlock, S. (1971) Progress report: halothane hepatitis. *Gut*, **12,** 324–329.

Sherlock, S. (1972) Liver diseases due to drugs. In *Drug Induced Diseases*, ed. Meyler, L. & Peck, H. M., Vol. 4, pp. 241–260. Amsterdam: Excerpta Medica.

Sherlock, S. & Ajdukiewicz, A. (1972) Hepatic reactions to drugs. In *Mechanisms in Drug Allergy* (Glaxo Symposium Series), ed. Dash, C. H. & Jones, H. E. H., pp. 103–109. Edinburgh: Churchill Livingstone.

Shulman, N. R. (1958a) Immunoreactions involving platelets. I. A steric and kinetic model for formation of a complex from a human antibody, quinidine as a haptene, and platelets; and for fixation of complement by the complex. *Journal of Experimental Medicine*, **107,** 665–690.

Shulman, N. R. (1958b) Immunoreactions involving platelets. III. Quantitative aspects of platelet agglutination, inhibition of clot retraction, and other reactions caused by the antibody of quinidine purpura. *Journal of Experimental Medicine*, **107,** 697–710.

Shulman, N. R. (1958c) Immunoreactions involving platelets. IV. Studies on the pathogenesis of thrombocytopenia in drug purpura using test doses of quinidine in sensitised individuals; their implications in idiopathic thrombocytopenic purpura. *Journal of Experimental Medicine*, **107,** 711–729.

Shulman, N. R. (1963a) Mechanism of blood cell damage by adsorption of antigen–antibody complexes. In *Immunopathology* (Third International Symposium), ed. Grabar, P. & Miescher, P., pp. 338–352. Basel: Schwabe.

Shulman, N. R. (1963b) Mechanism of blood cell destruction in individuals sensitised to foreign antigens. *Transactions of the Association of American Physicians*, **76,** 72–83.

Shulman, N. R. (1964) A mechanism of cell destruction in individuals sensitised to foreign antigens and its implications in auto-immunity. *Annals of Internal Medicine*, **60,** 506–521.

Shulman, N. R. (1974) Drug-induced antibodies to blood cells. In *Drugs and Hematologic Reactions* (*29th Hahnemann Symposium*), (ed.) Dimitrov, N. V. & Nodine, J. H. pp. 187–197. New York and London: Grune and Stratton.

Smith, J. M. & Zirk, M. H. (1961) Toxic and allergic drug reactions during the treatment of tuberculosis. *Tubercle*, **42,** 287–296.

Sorrell, T. C., Forbes, I. J., Burness, F. R. & Rischbieth, R. H. C. (1971) Depression of immunological function in patients treated with phenytoin sodium (sodium diphenylhydantoin). *Lancet*, **ii,** 1233–1235.

Spath, P., Garratty, G. & Petz, L. (1971) Studies on the immune response to penicillin and cephalothin in humans. II Immunohematologic reactions to cephalothin administration. *Journal of Immunology*, **107,** 860–869.

Stewart, G. T. (1973) Allergy to penicillin and related antibiotics: antigenic and immunochemical mechanism. *Annual Review of Pharmacology*, **13**, 309–324.

Strunk, S. W. & Ziff, M. (1970) Ultrastructural studies of the passage of gold thiomalate across the renal glomerular capillary wall. *Arthritis and Rheumatism*, **13**, 39–52.

Symmers, W. St. C. (1958) The occurrence of so-called collagen diseases, and of diseases systemically affecting the connective tissues, as a manifestation of sensitivity to drugs. In *Sensitivity Reactions to Drugs*, ed. Rosenheim, M. L. & Moulton, R., pp. 209–222. Oxford: Blackwell.

Toxicity Bibliography (1968 et seq.) National Library of Medicine Publications, Washington D.C.

Tullis, J. L. (1961) The role of leukocyte and platelet antibody tests in management of diverse clinical disorders. *Annals of Internal Medicine*, **54**, 1165–1180.

Verhaegen, H., De Cree, J., De Cock, W. & Verbruggen, F. (1973) Levamisole and the immune response. *New England Journal of Medicine*, **289**, 1148–1149.

Voss, H. E., Redmond, A. P. & Levine, B. B. (1966) Clinical detection of the potential allergic reactor to penicillin by immunologic tests. *Journal of the American Medical Association*, **196**, 679–683.

Walker, F. B., Smith, P. D. & Maibach, H. I. (1967) Genetic factors in human allergic contact dermatitis. *International Archives of Allergy and Applied Immunology*, **32**, 453–462.

Watkinson, G. & Hillis, B. R. (1947) Photosensitivity to sunlight from use of prophylactic sulphonamides: its relation to vaccination reactions. *British Medical Journal*, **ii**, 609–611.

Williams, D. M., Lynch, R. E. & Cartwright, G. E. (1973) Drug-induced aplastic anaemia. *Seminars in Haematology*, **10**, 195–223.

Williams, W. J., Pioli, E., Horton, J. N. & Waldron, A. (1972) M.I.F. test in halothane jaundice. *British Medical Journal*, **iv**, 47.

World Health Organisation Scientific Group (1967) Standardisation of procedures for the study of glucose-6-phosphate dehydrogenase. *WHO Technical Report Series*, No. 366, p. 53. Geneva.

Worlledge, S. M. (1969) Autoantibody formation associated with methyldopa (aldomet) therapy. *British Journal of Haematology*, **16**, 5–8.

Worlledge, S. M. (1972) Drug allergy and blood pathology. In *Mechanisms in Drug Allergy* (Glaxo Symposium Series), ed. Dash, C. H. & Jones, H. Ξ. H., pp. 112–142. Edinburgh: Churchill Livingstone.

Worlledge, S. M. (1973a) Immune drug-induced haemolytic anaemias. In *Blood Disorders Due to Drugs and Other Agents*, ed. Girdwood, R. H., pp. 11–26. Amsterdam: Excerpta Medica.

Worlledge, S. M. (1973b) Immune drug-induced haemolytic anaemias. *Seminars in Haematology*, **10**, 327–344.

Yunis, A. A. (1973) Chloramphenicol toxicity. In *Blood Disorders Due to Drugs and Other Agents*, ed. Girdwood, R. H., pp. 107–126. Amsterdam: Excerpta Medica.

Yunis, A. A. (1974) Effects of Chloramphenicol on Erythropoiesis. In *Drugs and Hematologic Reactions* (*29th Hahnemann Symposium*) (ed.) Dimitrov, N. V. & Nodine, J. H., pp. 133–140. New York and London: Grune and Stratton.

Yurchak, A. M., Wicher, K. & Arbesman, C. E. (1970) Immunologic studies on aspirin. *Journal of Allergy*, **46**, 245–253.

12. Immunological Aspects of Clinical Organ Transplantation

W. McN. ORR

The importance of kidney transplantation in the management of end-stage renal failure can be recognised by its world-wide acceptance as a therapeutic measure and the current availability of data on some 12 000 recipients in the 11th Report of the ACS/NIH Organ Transplant Registry (Chicago). The increasing number and success of cadaver programmes is related to the improved results obtained over the past ten years using kidneys from this source, although the most predictable and consistent results are still obtained with kidneys from related living donors. Whereas Belzer and Kountz (1973) have reported an 80 per cent success rate in terms of patient survival at one year when one or more cadaver allografts are used, these excellent results have not been universally attained since the cumulative figures from world-wide sources suggest that the average cadaver graft survival at one year is approximately 50 per cent for first grafts. In comparison with the latter, when kidneys are obtained from related living donors such as parents or siblings, graft survival rates of 75 per cent at one year have been observed. Even better results have been reported from some experienced centres using grafts between non-twin siblings of identical tissue-type (HL-A). Moreover, the fact that these improved results between HL-A identical siblings were obtained with less immunosuppression is thought to provide the strongest available evidence of the relevance of histocompatibility matching. However the search for HL-A identical cadaver kidneys by the development of geographically extensive kidney exchange schemes has yielded conflicting results in terms of graft survival and is thought to indicate the existence of additional histocompatibility loci which are not represented by HL-A tissue-typing. The presence of such loci has been given as an explanation of the reactivity observed when the lymphocytes from two such individuals are grown together in culture (mixed leucocyte culture—MLC). Thus the predictability of success in cadaver programmes remains low, particularly so when it is related to histocompatibility matching, and it is clear that the in vitro methods available for assessment of histocompatibility between donor and recipient must be far from complete at the present time. It is also clear that other factors are of importance in successful clinical renal transplantation, namely, the physical condition of the recipient when transplanted and the quality of the transplanted organ with particular reference to the ischaemic damage sustained during procurement. In addition a less readily identifiable influence on graft survival is that of the immunological status of the recipient.

When one turns to grafts other than the kidney, which itself occupies a unique position in terms of the support mechanisms available, one finds that clinical transplantation is still very much in the experimental phase. Whereas grafts of heart, liver, lung, pancreas and bone marrow have now been performed in considerable numbers, relatively few survivors have been reported although encouraging results have been achieved in the case of the heart and liver and latterly in bone marrow transplantation.

The purpose of this chapter is to present a review of current thinking on the mechanism of allograft rejection and the extent to which it may be modified or influenced by immunosuppression and histocompatibility matching. Since three-quarters of the failures in renal transplantation are due to uncontrollable rejection, or death of the patient from infection as a result of immunosuppression, consideration will also be given to methods of assessing immunological reactivity to the graft and in particular to the diagnosis of rejection.

TRANSPLANTATION IMMUNOLOGY AND THE MECHANISM OF THE REJECTION PROCESS

The mechanism of the rejection process has been likened to a nerve reflex arc which consists of afferent, central and efferent limbs. Host sensitisation to the graft occurs by way of the afferent limb and the extent to which it occurs is related to the degree of histoincompatibility that exists between the graft and its host. The central phase consists of the development of an immune response directed against the foreign tissue but which can to some extent be controlled by immuno-suppression. The efferent limb or effector pathway is concerned with the direction of the immune response against the graft resulting in its subsequent destruction, unless modified by immunological means such as tolerance or enhancement.

The dichotomy of the immune response into two main pathways, namely cellular and humoral immunity, has only been clearly separable in experimental situations and the precise and relative role each plays in the various forms of rejection has yet to be defined. In the now extensive experience of human kidney transplantation three main patterns of clinical rejection have been observed. Firstly, there is the least common variety known as *hyperacute* rejection which usually occurs within the first 48 hours after transplantation, and because of its rapid and aggressive onset is thought to be due to the presence of pre-existing humoral antibody, although such antibodies are not always detectable by currently available techniques. It is believed that these pre-existing cytotoxic antibodies are formed in response to a previous blood transfusion, pregnancy or an earlier tissue graft. This type of rejection is largely a vascular phenomenon with consequent thrombosis which almost invariably leads to death of the graft. Secondly, there is the frequently observed *acute* rejection process or 'transplant crisis' which may occur at any time between one week and six months after transplantation. It is usually an acute short-lived episode of varying severity which may result either in complete destruction of the graft, or in recovery but with evidence of permanent damage or return to normal function. The longer the interval between transplantation and this type of rejection, the less likely it is to occur and the more benign and readily reversible it becomes. Acute rejection is characterised histologically by mononuclear cellular infiltration and is believed to be largely due to cell-mediated immunity. The third variety is referred to as *chronic* rejection because it is a much more insidious process and is usually detectable only after several months have elapsed. Selective impairment of function such as proteinuria is often noted to an extent that the condition may clinically resemble the nephrotic syndrome, while little deterioration in the glomerular filtration rate occurs at least initially. The histological appearance consists of glomerular lesions, interstitial fibrosis and progressive narrowing of the blood vessels. The aetiology of chronic rejection is obscure and may be partly mediated by cellular and also by humoral immunity although it should be noted that some humoral factors may be protective, as in enhancement, rather than harmful. The homograft reaction can thus be seen to be a complex process consisting of the combination and interaction of various cellular and humoral immune factors directed towards destruction of the graft and their modification by pre-sensitisation, histocompatibility and immunosuppression.

Antigens involved in sensitisation

Those antigens which are believed to be important in transplantation and to which sensitisation occurs are the ABO red cell antigens, the histocompatibility antigens and there is some evidence to suggest that organ specific antigens may also be relevant. Clinical transplantation is not nowadays performed across the ABO barrier but in earlier experience there was evidence of its importance when on occasion it was believed to be responsible for hyperacute rejection of the homograft. The most important are, however, the histocompatibility antigens that are formed by the histocompatibility genes which are in turn located at histocompatibility or H loci on a single chromosome pair. Since at each locus several alternative genes or alleles may occur which are co-dominant, the degree of polymorphism present will depend on the number of loci and the number of alleles at each locus. Histocompatibility antigens appear also to be associated with the insoluble lipoprotein material in the cell membrane and attempts to extract pure soluble histocompatibility antigens have been made by Davies (1968) and Kahan and Reisfeld (1969). Histocompatibility antigens are probably represented on all nucleated cells including the cell membrane of leucocytes and platelets, thereby providing a convenient source of material for HL-A tissue-typing. It has been suggested that leucocytes may not carry all transplantation antigens (Barker, Lubaroff and Silvers, 1971), since inoculation of adult homologous lymphocytes into neonatal animals did not induce tolerance to all donor tissues, in this case heart and skin grafts respectively. This may mean that skin carries histocompatibility antigens which are not represented on either lymphocytes or heart, or on the other hand it raises the possibility that there may be quantitative differences of these antigens in various tissues. At this point it is perhaps relevant to refer to the concept of the 'passenger leucocyte' and its possible role in the preliminary induction of sensitisation. Guttman, Lindquist and Ockner (1969) and Billingham (1971) suggested that donor leucocytes trapped within the vascular bed of the donor organ might act as the primary and most powerful immunogenic stimulus to the host, and proceeded to demonstrate in rats that kidneys obtained from immunosuppressed donors achieved prolonged survival when transplanted into non-immunosuppressed recipients.

While histocompatibility antigens appear to provide the main stimulus to sensitisation there is also the possibility that organ specific antigens, as distinct from individual specific (histocompatibility) antigens, may on occasion elicit an immune response in the host. This concept of immunological damage to the graft in contrast to that caused by rejection is of more than theoretical interest, since it may provide an explanation for the development of lesions resembling glomerulonephritis in transplanted human kidneys, even when the original disease was not of this variety. If these lesions are caused by humoral antibodies, then the outcome to the graft may depend upon the strength of the recipient's humoral response, being more favourable for low rather than high responders (vide infra). This aspect has been investigated by Milgrom, Klassen and Fuji (1971) in rats where, during rejection of a homograft, they found changes in the animals' *own* kidneys consisting of glomerular basement membrane thickening and some endothelial and mesangial cell proliferation. In addition, globulin deposits were demonstrable along the glomerular capillary walls with the aid of immunofluorescent techniques and when serum from the recipients was layered onto normal kidney sections, staining of the brush border of the cells lining the proximal tubules occurred.

Cell-mediated transplantation immunity

In 1954 Mitchison demonstrated that immunity to first-set homografts is largely cell-mediated by the transfer of immunity to non-sensitised animals with the aid of immunologically competent cells. This process is known as 'adoptive' transfer since it depends upon the presence and continued functioning of previously sensitised donor cells within the recipient. It also follows that only immunologically competent *living* cells such as lymphocytes can be used for this purpose and their ability to transfer immunity provides a method of recognising this property. By means of adoptive transfer both the cell responsible and its route within the recipient could be identified. The similarity between the mechanisms involved in cell-mediated transplantation immunity and the delayed type of hypersensitivity reaction was demonstrated by the work of Brent, Brown and Medawar (1958). These workers showed that guinea pigs sensitised by skin grafts would respond to subsequent intradermal injection of donor specific tissue by a delayed hypersensitivity skin reaction similar to the classic tuberculin reaction. Thus the cellular infiltration which is the most characteristic histological feature of rejection of a first-set homograft can be understood, at least superficially, but it has been shown that most of the cells infiltrating the graft are in fact 'uncommitted' and if this is the case, what is their role? Experimentally it has been shown that dosages of lymph node cells from specifically sensitised animals which would normally transfer the capacity to give 'delayed hypersensitivity reactions' to normal isologous hosts, are ineffective if the *latter* have been previously irradiated. This rather suggests that in non-irradiated hosts immigrant cells (cf. passenger leucocytes) may enter the inoculation sites and furnish the antigenic stimulus.

The first step in the homograft reaction is recognition of the foreign antigen before sensitisation can begin, and where this occurs depends upon the type of graft involved. In the case of orthotopic skin grafts intact lymphatic drainage of the graft site is apparently necessary, for first-set grafts at any rate, to allow recognition to occur. This presumably occurs in the regional lymph node (Barker and Billingham, 1968). However, that peripheral sensitisation does occur in the case of whole organ grafts in which immediate vascular connections are necessary, is evidenced by the work of Strober and Gowans (1965). These workers demonstrated in rats that infusion of an isolated homologous kidney with thoracic duct lymphocytes, which were subsequently returned to the animal from whom they were derived, succeeded in sensitising that animal to tissues of the homologous strain. Alternatively, this ex vivo sensitisation may have been due to the presence of residual passenger cells in the efflux from the kidney perfused with thoracic duct lymphocytes, which in turn were responsible for inducing immunity.

In transplantation immunology, therefore, one can recognise two ways in which lymphocyte participation occurs: firstly, as immunologically competent cells by their ability to identify foreign antigen and to act upon this information; and secondly by their ability to provide the main immunogenic stimulus to the recipient's lymphocytes by virtue of their content of histocompatibility antigens. Both of these aspects were demonstrated by Elkins and Guttman (1968) who showed in rats that Lewis parental strain lymphocytes, deposited beneath the renal capsules of orthotopically transplanted Lewis kidneys to genetically tolerant (BN $\times$ Lewis) F_1 hosts, were capable of causing local invasive and destructive lesions typical of graft rejection. Elkins and Guttman maintained that the donor lymphoid cells were immunologically stimulated by circulating host leucocytes and that the interaction of the two cell populations could result in non-specific damage to the renal parenchyma. Moreover, when Lewis rats received genetically incompatible (BN $\times$ Lewis) F_1 kidneys from animals which had their marrow replaced by cells of Lewis origin (Guttman, Lindquist and Ockner, 1969), rejection was delayed. The capacity of relatively small numbers of passenger leucocytes, as in skin grafts, to present a powerful immunogenic stimulus to the host was demonstrated by Steinmuller (1967) using chimeric mice. He found that transfer of skin grafts from chimeric to normal animals of the same strain resulted in sensitisation of the latter to the strain which donated the cells responsible for inducing chimerism initially. In addition, sensitisation occurred less readily when the chimeric animals were made leucopenic by irradiation beforehand. Thus peripheral sensitisation appears to occur because of close interaction between lymphocytes of donor and recipient origin within the graft itself, and the mechanism is comparable to that seen in local graft-versus-host (GVH) reactions, except that the activity is in the opposite direction. Moreover, the process can be visualised in vitro, as in the MLC reaction, where sensitisation is manifested by morphological alteration of the cells into primitive blast forms.

The central phase of cellular immunity to the homograft depends upon the priming of thymus derived or T lymphocytes which have in turn arisen from stem-cells in the bone marrow initially. Pedersen and Morris (1970) have investigated this aspect in an animal model, by transplantation of kidney homografts to the neck in sheep with cannulation of the hilar lymph vessels to collect the lymphatic effluent from the transplant. Within 24 hours of transplantation, cells appeared in the lymph which transformed into blast forms when cultured in vitro. A few days later, blast cells began to appear in the lymph itself and eventually made up 60 per cent of the total cell population. At four days the substance of the kidney was infiltrated with mononuclear cells and by the time that acute rejection had occurred at one week, up to 60 grams weight of cells had appeared in the lymph draining from the kidney as compared with the few hundred milligrams of cells from control autografts over the same period. When the lymph and its content of cells was diverted from the host, no prolongation of survival of the homografts was obtained although a diminished proliferative response in regional lymph nodes was observed as compared to a control situation. From this experiment one can obtain some idea of the marked cellular activity associated with the destruction of a whole organ homograft in which, as compared with skin, an intact lymphatic efferent pathway is apparently unnecessary.

In the efferent or effector limb of the rejection process small lymphocytes transform into larger blast cells and release various soluble factors, which may in turn augment the immune response by recruitment of macrophages, polymorphs and uncommitted lymphocytes. Several local GVH reaction systems afford fairly convincing evidence of the capacity of lymphocytes to inflict damage directly on target tissue in vivo, as in Winn's (1961) neutralisation assay where he inoculated a mixture of target homologous tumour cells and specifically sensitised lymph node cells into appropriate hosts. Provided that both types of cell were injected into the same site, he obtained inhibition of tumour growth with relatively few sensitised lymphocytes suggesting that close association between effector and target cell was necessary. As the evidence mounted that diffusible agents released from sensitised lymphocytes were in some way associated with the destruction of homografts, efforts were made to identify them more precisely. Meanwhile, attempts to demonstrate adoptive transfer of sensitivity by means of sensitised lymphoid cells imprisoned in millipore chambers were unsuccessful.

The knowledge that sensitised lymphocytes can destroy donor specific target cells in vitro, as described by Goverts (1960) and Rosenau and Moon (1961), has provided a useful in vitro method of assessing cell-mediated immunity. Essentially the technique consists of adding sensitised lymphocytes to target cells in culture, death of the latter being recognised morphologically or by release of a radioactive label from the cells. In addition the lymphocytes cluster around the target cells creating a phenomenon which is known as 'contactual agglutination' (Koprowski and Fernandes, 1962).

The diffusible agents released on stimulation of sensitised lymphocytes, which have already been referred to, have been named according to their various properties. These include macrophage migration inhibition factor (MIF), blastogenic factor, chemotactic factor, factors capable of inciting delayed type inflammatory reactions and lymphotoxins, to all of which Dumonde et al (1969) gave the generic term lymphokines. In addition it should be remembered that non-sensitised lymphocytes may also liberate lymphotoxins both specifically (as in MLC reactions) and non-specifically (in response to phytohaemagglutinin for example). Whether all of these different properties can be ascribed to multiple substances or not is at present unknown, but the activities described appear to be related to large non-dialysable molecules with a molecular weight 20 000 to 80 000. We can now begin to see how, following the arrival and engagement of sensitised lymphocytes in a homograft, diffusible mediators may help by their various activities to augment the locally directed immune response in several ways including the recruitment of additional cell types.

In addition to its use as a method of histocompatibility testing, the mixed leucocyte culture reaction (Bach and Hirschorn, 1964; Bain, Vas and Lowenstein, 1964) has been an important in vitro model of cellular homograft immunity. From it we have learned that although a very small proportion only of the lymphocytes present are initially capable of being sensitised by confrontation with a particular foreign antigen, these sensitised cells can then stimulate a large proportion of the other uncommitted cells to undergo blast formation. Further analogy to the homograft situation was provided by Ginsburg and Sachs (1965), who found that unsensitised lymphocytes underwent blast formation and developed pyronin positive cytoplasm when added to cultures of embryonic homologous cells. Subsequent transferral of these pyroninophilic cells to fresh cultures obtained from the same source brought about the rapid destruction of the latter. These findings appear to provide an in vitro model of cellular homograft immunity since both the afferent and effector limbs of the response take place in vitro.

Humoral mediation of transplantation immunity

Although the capacity of transplantation antigens to evoke a humoral as well as a cellular response has been recognised and serves as a basis for serological tissue-typing procedures, we do not yet know the precise and relative role these antibodies play in homograft rejection. Whereas the humoral immune response to a homograft appeared at first sight to develop later than the cellular one, it has now been shown by more sensitive techniques that these antibodies are present at the time of homograft rejection. However, the evidence incriminating humoral factors as major contributors in the rejection of whole organ homografts remains unsatisfactory. While the destruction of solid tissue grafts is largely mediated by immunologically competent cells, it appears that humoral factors do play a role which is ancillary and probably varies in extent depending upon the type of rejection process taking place.

Whereas antibodies may play a part in the rejection of homografts it also appears that, under carefully controlled experimental situations, antibodies are formed in response to the homograft which are protective rather than destructive. This phenomenon is known as *enhancement* and was described initially in work on tumour immunology. Although enhancing antibodies are protective to the graft, their mode of action is uncertain and there is evidence to suggest an inhibitory action on the immune response at afferent, central and efferent levels.

The best example of the implication of humoral factors in transplantation immunity is in the development of antibodies against histocompatibility or HL-A antigens. Experimentally, antibodies following transplantation can be detected by red cell agglutination or haemolysis, and by cytotoxicity and immunofluorescent techniques. As far as their harmful effects are concerned, it seems that different types of homograft have a variable sensitivity to humoral factors, possibly due to the relative richness of isoantigens in the cell membrane. Data from the study of kidney homografts in man have demonstrated an association between preformed humoral antibodies and hyperacute allograft rejection, and also of circulating antibodies with chronic graft rejection. Jeannet et al (1970) have related the progressive obliterative lesions in allograft blood vessels to the appearance of serum antibodies specific for donor antigens, and Porter et al (1968) had earlier demonstrated the presence of immunoglobulins and complement in these obliterative vascular lesions.

Attempts to recover antibodies from their attachments to graft antigens in transplanted human kidneys were made by Metzgar et al (1972). In approximately one-quarter of the cases studied they succeeded in doing so, and it is of interest to note that they found no correlation between the histology or reaction category and the presence of antibodies. Moreover, they found that the amount of antibody recovered from these kidneys after their removal bore no relation to the level of activity in the recipient's serum beforehand, suggesting that antibodies formed in response to transplantation were removed by the graft from the circulation. Metzgar and his colleagues also drew attention to the importance of using different techniques to detect antibody activity in patients, since only one-third of the positive eluates had antibodies which were demonstrated by all three techniques employed.

There have been several reports of considerable prolongation of kidney allograft survival in animals, especially in rats (Stuart, Saitoh and Fitch, 1968; French and Batchelor, 1969) by the use of active and passive enhancement antibodies. It appears that the rat is a particularly suitable animal in which to induce enhancement, since pre-immunisation in this animal rarely results in hyperacute rejection of a subsequent graft. However, induction of enhancement in other experimental situations has been much more difficult to achieve, although in the sera of human kidney recipients various blocking factors have appeared which are capable of modifying in vitro correlates of cellular allograft immunity. Russell (1971) has maintained that the experimental methods of producing enhancement may prove difficult to apply clinically because of the problem of separating cytotoxic from enhancing antibodies.

The nature of the mechanism whereby some allografts enjoy prolonged survival in the presence of reduced immunosuppression remains uncertain, but can probably be explained in terms of either tolerance or enhancement. Levey (1971) has in fact suggested that these two concepts may be but different facets of the one complex process, whereby the balance between tolerance and enhancement versus immunity depends upon a particular combination of antigen dose, lymphocyte reactivity, and the avidity of antibody formed. The phenomenon of 'adaptation', as described by Woodruff (1961) to explain graft acceptance, appears to be closely related to enhancement.

MODIFICATION OF THE HOMOGRAFT REJECTION PROCESS

In this section we shall attempt to describe the various ways in which the rejection process can be modified and prolonged functional survival of the homograft obtained. Since modification of the rejection process implies manipulation or depression of the immune response of the host concerned we will consider how this can be achieved. Firstly, we will discuss the influence of histocompatibility between donor and recipient and the problems associated with immunological selection of the donor, since highly successful renal transplantation in man has been performed between identical twins without immunosuppression, and between HL-A identical siblings with minimal immunosuppression. Increasing attention is now being given to the less well-defined effect of the immunological status of the recipient upon graft survival, to which reference has been made. The modifying influence of immunosuppression and manipulation of the immune response by tolerance, enhancement and adaptation will also be described.

The study of histocompatibility antigens began in 1916 with the work of Little and Tyzzer on the transplantation of mammary cancer in Japanese waltzing mice. With the aid of such inbred strains or isogeneic animals, Gorer, Lyman and Snell (1948) discovered the H-2 antigen in mice, which by virtue of the fact that it is carried on the red cell membrane and can elicit the production of antibody, is easily investigated by haemagglutination techniques. The fact that histocompatibility antigens could induce the development of circulating antibodies in animals was important because it meant that serological methods could be used for their identification and it also explained the possible role of circulating antibodies in certain rejection phenomena. Using this technique some 30 histocompatibility genes at the H-2 locus were found in mice, and 14 other loci have also been demonstrated. The latter contain variable strength antigens of less importance than those at the H-2 locus, which are the strongest of all histocompatibility antigens in this animal. The number of loci and the alleles at each locus were worked out with the aid of inbred strains and the development of congenic resistant strains of mice, i.e. those which differ at only one histocompatibility locus.

Since the discovery of the first human histocompatibility antigen by Dausset in 1958, intensive research has demonstrated the presence in man of a histocompatibility system (HL-A = human leucocyte locus A) very similar to that in the mouse, although it should be remembered that histocompatibility antigens have not been demonstrated on human red blood cells. In the HL-A system, it has been established that two series of antigens exist, each determined by multiple alleles which occupy two closely linked loci in a particular chromosomal region. The two series are referred to as the LA and the Four series, and to date the WHO have accepted on an international basis the recognition of 8 antigens at the LA sub-locus and 13 antigens at the Four sub-locus.

Various methods have been employed for the identification of these antigens, but mainly by leuco-agglutination and cytotoxicity tests of which the latter is the more sensitive and generally accepted. Other methods which have been used include immunocyto-adherence assay, mixed cell agglutination, complement fixation tests, antiglobulin consumption and inhibition of clot retraction tests in decreasing order of sensitivity. The several ways in which cytotoxicity tests have been evaluated have included study by phase contrast, intracellular penetration of dye and the release of an isotope (^{51}Cr) from labelled cells. Because of the small amount of specific antisera available, a microlymphocytotoxicity test was developed by Terasaki (Terasaki and McClelland, 1964) and is widely used at the present time. Most typing is undertaken on peripheral blood samples, and on lymph node and splenic lymphocytes when these are available. As a result of such tests it has been established that man carries four serologically defined (SD) histocompatibility antigens of which two are located at the first and two at the second sub-locus. Moreover, an individual inherits one chromosome bearing the histocompatibility locus from each parent, and since this chromosome carries two antigens (i.e. one from the first and one from the second sub-locus), it follows that the two antigens on each chromosome are inherited as a block or haplotype (Ceppellini et al, 1967). Because of the block inheritance of the two antigens on a single chromosome, it has been held by some that the haplotype should be considered as a complex product of a single allele rather than two products of two closely linked loci. In support of the latter, very occasional cross-overs between the two series have been reported. Much of this information has been derived from and confirmed by serological testing of whole families, illustrating the remarkable fact that the many different combinations of specificities found are controlled by a single genetic locus. Thus in a family only four types of children are possible from any given mating, so that one quarter of siblings will be HL-A identical, one half will be semi-identical (i.e. share one haplotype), and one quarter will differ by both haplotypes. In spite of the above information, approximately 10 per cent of the genes in both loci remain undetected (Albert, Mickey and Terasaki, 1971) particularly where family studies are not possible, as in cadaveric renal transplantation. Assuming the existence of one further allele at each sub-locus, it has been calculated by Kissmeyer-Nielsen and Thorsby (1970) that 126 different HL-A haplotypes would be possible which in turn could be combined to form 8001 genotypes. The complexity of the situation is increased by the fact that HL-A antigens may have several parts each of which is controlled by separate alleles.

The antisera employed to identify histocompatibility antigens are usually obtained from multiparous women who have been sensitised (probably during labour) to paternal antigens carried by the fetus. It will be obvious that most antisera obtained in this way will be multispecific since the immunisation 'unit' is a haplotype, and that the same problem arises when immunising volunteer donors. The procurement and identification of monospecific antisera for HL-A typing continues to be a difficult and time-consuming but essential process.

Since the object of histocompatibility matching is related to the knowledge that transplants are rejected by an immunological reaction directed against foreign antigens, the two most obvious approaches to the problem are to depress the immuno-competence of the recipient and to provide a graft that is as genetically similar to the recipient as possible. The importance of histocompatibility in relation to subsequent function is demonstrated by the fact that kidney transplants taken from blood relatives fare better than those from unrelated donors (Murray, Barnes and Atkinson, 1970). This distinction has been consistently maintained as the single most important factor governing the outcome of a renal transplant, and clearly overrides the influence of all other variables.

The strongest evidence that HL-A antigens are important histocompatibility antigens comes from the results of renal transplantation between HL-A identical sibling pairs. A graft survival rate of 95 per cent at one year was found within a group of 61 HL-A identical siblings by Mickey et al (1971), and a comparable result was reported from a further collected series of 40 similar cases. It appears therefore that HL-A identical siblings are a privileged group from a transplantation point of view, since they exhibit prolonged skin graft survival and most, but not all, show little or no stimulation on MLC testing. The fact that excellent renal function was obtained in the majority of these cases makes it seem unlikely that additional histocompatibility loci, if present, are comparable in strength to those in the HL-A system.

When one considers further the correlation between HL-A typing and the clinical outcome, difficulties are immediately evident in that it is only in the HL-A identical siblings that there is a clear relationship, whereas in the case of other related and unrelated pairings the situation is still uncertain as to whether or not a positive correlation exists (Dausset and Festenstein, 1973; Belzer et al, 1974; Dausset et al, 1974). This difficulty in predicting the outcome for transplants performed in the latter situation is also seen with MLC testing, where the leucocytes of two individuals are grown together in culture and the immunological response measured. When one-way mixed leucocyte cultures are made in which donor cells are used as the target and the recipient leucocytes are the only responding cells (Bach and Voynow, 1966), it is found that not only do more than 99 per cent of unrelated pairs result in stimulation, but so do a similar proportion of those related pairs who share one haplotype. Since the chances of a successful transplant are considerably greater in the latter group, it is clear that in this situation MLC testing has no value as a predictive test. It is only the identical twins and most of the HL-A identical sibling combinations that do not stimulate each other. Indeed the most useful practical application of MLC testing is in the latter group in identifying, albeit the minority, of HL-A identical sibling pairs that do stimulate and whose transplants are thereby more likely to undergo serious rejection (Etheredge et al, 1974). The difficulty in demonstrating a correlation between HL-A typing and graft outcome for other than HL-A identical siblings may be explained by the presence of a segregant series of antigens of the HL-A system in addition to those at the first or second series. Alternatively the heterogeneity of the HL-A antigen system may be greater than we suspect and we may still be testing for an inadequate number of antigens.

To explain the presence of stimulation of MLC testing in spite of HL-A identity in siblings, a further histocompatibility locus known as the lymphocyte defined (LD) locus has been postulated. Keuning et al (1974) have investigated possible associations between antigens present at this locus and HL-A or SD antigens. They found high linkage disequilibrium (Δ) between certain LD antigens and HL-A 7 or HL-A 8, and suggested that donor recipient pairs matched for either of these two antigens would also be matched for one LD antigen. We have since analysed our own results to see if matching for HL-A 7 or 8 in an unrelated series had any effect on graft survival, and have found a significantly more favourable prognosis for this group of patients (Wentzel et al, 1974).

Thus the predictive value of HL-A typing in terms of graft prognosis for other than HL-A identical siblings still remains controversial, but the excellent results obtained in this special group would not be possible without HL-A typing which enables us to identify these individuals. HL-A typing is also necessary for cross-matching between donor and recipient to reduce the risk of hyperacute rejection, and an additional area in which HL-A typing contributes to clinical transplantation practice is in assessment of the immunological status of the recipient (vide infra).

So far we have discussed the importance of ABO compatibility in clinical transplantation and the relevance and predictive value in terms of graft outcome for HL-A typing and MLC testing. However in any clinical setting the importance of performing a direct cross-match between the donor's lymphocytes and the recipient's serum has been well documented. Hyperacute rejection still occurs in 5 to 10 per cent of cadaver grafts despite a negative cross-match beforehand. Some centres have demonstrated that recipients having antibodies reacting with more than 15 per cent of lymphocytes of the random population have a graft success rate of 30 to 40 per cent, whereas those lacking this reactivity had a frequency of success of 70 to 84 per cent. The influence of blood transfusions in inducing HL-A antibody formation in patients on haemodialysis was investigated by Opelz, Mickey and Terasaki (1972). These workers found that those patients who did not form antibody (in spite of receiving blood transfusions and being on chronic haemodialysis for *more* than a year), had a cadaver graft success rate of 84 per cent at one year whereas for those patients who did not form antibody after being on dialysis for *less* than a year it was 50 per cent. In comparison, the one-year survival rate for cadaver transplants in patients with cytotoxic antibodies was 36 per cent. These results suggested to Opelz and his colleagues that patients who are unresponsive to HL-A incompatible blood transfusions for long periods ('low responders') are also unresponsive to HL-A incompatible kidney transplants. They discussed several possible mechanisms for this unresponsiveness, including the production of enhancing antibodies due to the blood transfusions or alternatively the induction of acquired tolerance. On the other hand, the unresponsiveness of this group of 'low responders' may be due to the fact that the immune competence of this group of patients is less. However, Morris (1973) found in his patients that a reduction in the number of blood transfusions did not result in a decrease in the number of patients developing antibodies. He also investigated the immunological responsiveness of his patients, that is whether they were 'high responders' or 'low responders', by testing the reactivity of their serum against lymphoblastoid cell lines which carry an increased density of HL-A antigens on their cell membrane. Although providing a more sensitive test for the detection of anti-HL-A antibody, these cells also carry antigens peculiar to themselves including the Epstein–Barr virus membrane antigen. Whereas the sera of 95 per cent of normal adult males reacted against these cell lines, only 55 per cent of potential renal recipients did so ('high responders') and graft survival in these patients carried a significantly worse prognosis than in the remaining 45 per cent of recipients who did not react ('low responders'). Sengar, Opelz and Terasaki (1973) have shown that a significant proportion of patients on haemodialysis have serum factors which block the MLC reaction and yet are not cytotoxic to random cell donors. They found that recipients with this type of blocking antibody had an improved early success rate when grafted.

It seems therefore that blood transfusions are capable of producing active immunisation in approximately one-third of potential recipients who in turn will have a low transplant success rate. In contrast, blood transfusions will produce a blocked immune response in the remainder of dialysis patients for whom the chances of a successful graft are greater than in those who have not been transfused.

When we come to consider ways in which the immunological reactivity of the immunosuppressed individual can be measured, we find that very little is available for clinical application at the present time. Apart from detection of blocking factors in the sera of transplant recipients and the responsiveness or otherwise of the individual to foreign HL-A antigens, in vitro methods of measurement of allograft immunity as have been used will be described in the next section. Current methods of immunosuppression by drugs are associated with variable degrees of both specific and non-specific suppression of the immune response, but it is to be hoped that more specific methods of immunosuppression in the future will be capable of being accurately monitored by in vitro techniques. The remainder of this section will be concerned with a description of the concepts which may provide an answer to this problem in the future.

One way in which greater longevity of a homograft might be achieved, at least theoretically, would be by altering its antigenicity but clearly this is not possible in the case of viable homografts. Previous reference has been made to the role of passsenger leucocytes and perhaps other interstitial cell types within the homograft which provide a powerful immunogenic stimulus to the recipient, and experimentally it has been shown in some inbred animals that immunosuppression of the donor has produced prolonged graft survival time in non-immunosuppressed recipients. Guttmann, Lindquist and Ockner (1973) pretreated human cadaver donors with methylprednisolone and cyclophosphamide in an attempt to reduce the immunogenicity of the kidney, but only did so for up to 12 hours before transplantation took place and this interval is probably inadequate. However, these preliminary results suggested that rejection when it did occur was less severe than in a control group of patients and that in the donor pretreated group, improved renal function was also observed.

To return to other experimental methods capable of providing prolonged graft survival, Fabre and Morris (1972a) studied antigen-induced suppression of rejection by intravenous injection of donor blood given before transplantation in rats. They achieved considerable prolongation of survival of renal allografts in some strain combinations by this method, giving support to the possible benefit of blood transfusions before transplantation in man. The mechanism involved was unclear but it might have been due to enhancement, although no donor specific antibody was demonstrable, nor could the effect be transmitted passively. The same workers went on to investigate this specific immunosuppression induced by donor strain blood (Fabre and Morris, 1972b) and found that it was attributable to the injected histocompatibility antigens. Moreover, long surviving kidneys re-transplanted to normal untreated rats of the same strain were rejected much more slowly than controls, suggesting that incomplete graft adaptation had occurred. In addition, fresh kidneys were not rejected by long-term survivors, demonstrating that the immunosuppressive effect had persisted. Fabre and Morris felt that these results favoured enhancement as the mechanism involved, although tolerance could not be excluded.

Antibody-induced suppression of rejection (passive enhancement) has been studied successfully in rats by Stuart, Saitoh and Fitch (1968) and French and Batchelor (1969). In collaboration with Batchelor, Morris tested the hypothesis that suppression of rejection was a competition between protection of the kidney by the passively administered enhancing serum and the cellular immune response of the recipient mediated by T cells, until the animal had produced its own enhancing antibody (Batchelor, Fabre and Morris, 1972). Confirmatory evidence that this was the case was obtained by combined treatment with small doses of antilymphocyte serum (ALS) and enhancing antibody neither of which would have been effective on their own, suggesting that this combination might be profitable in man.

With regard to immunological tolerance, the initial laboratory demonstration was made by Billingham, Brent and Medawar (1953) who injected allogeneic cells into animals in utero and succeeded in producing a tolerant state that was specific and depended upon the persistence of cell chimerism. Subsequently induction of tolerance was shown to be possible in adult animals also and Mitchison (1964) demonstrated that two dosage thresholds for suitable antigens could be used, namely high and low zone tolerance. Chiller, Habicht and Weigle (1971) have shown that T-cell tolerance alone is established in the low zone, whereas in high zone tolerance both T and B cells are made tolerant. Animals can be made tolerant to soluble antigens much more readily than to particulate ones which are taken up rapidly by macrophages, which appear to play a non-specific role (Kölsch and Mitchison, 1968). On the other hand soluble antigens probably interact directly with the receptor sites on the surface of antigen-reactive cells (Weigle, Chiller and Habicht, 1972).

In relation to clinical transplantation, it is obviously the induction of tolerance in adult animals that is of the greatest practical interest. Tolerance may be induced in adult animals by repeated high doses of homologous cells or parabiosis, or alternatively with immunosuppression whether by drugs, whole body irradiation or antilymphocyte serum. In combination with standard immunosuppression, clinical attempts to promote graft tolerance by thymectomy, splenectomy and depletion of thoracic duct lymphocytes via a fistula have not conferred any obvious benefit. However, various experimental studies in which doses of antigen are given together with immunosuppressive drugs have been encouraging, and it may be in time that this will find some clinical application.

It seems that tolerance and enhancement are still some way from clinical practice except in so far that they may already occur in the acceptance of a graft, but it appears that the latter phenomenon is the more likely to be applicable to clinical transplantation.

CLINICAL MANAGEMENT OF THE TRANSPLANT RECIPIENT INCLUDING DIAGNOSIS OF REJECTION

We will now consider the day-to-day management of the patient who has recently received a renal transplant in terms of clinical observations and the possible indications for alteration of immunosuppressive treatment. We shall also discuss the problems associated with the diagnosis of rejection and review the immunological methods for in vitro detection of allograft immunity so far available for monitoring these patients. The problem which presents itself is that most episodes of acute rejection occur within the first few post-operative months and during this period the chances of losing the kidney are at their maximum. Once a three- to six-month interval has elapsed since transplantation and provided that satisfactory renal function is still present, the continuing outlook is much more favourable. Since the assumption is made that prompt and vigorous treatment of these acute rejection episodes is more likely to be successful, much effort has been devoted to finding methods that will provide an earlier diagnosis of rejection.

Initial oliguria and even anuria due to tubular necrosis are commonplace following cadaveric renal transplantation and in such situations there is great difficulty in diagnosing rejection before measurable renal function appears. In the patient who has sufficient renal function to avoid the need for haemodialysis, the diagnosis of rejection can usually be readily made by observing a deterioration in renal function. In these patients, pyrexia where previously there was none, enlargement of the kidney (difficult to quantitate) and increased proteinuria are sufficient evidence to justify anti-rejection therapy. When these features, either singly or combined, are accompanied by an obvious deterioration in renal function (i.e. diminished creatinine clearance), most clinicians would agree on the diagnosis. Although some have advocated percutaneous needle biopsy at this stage, this procedure is not without risk and is probably not indicated since there is poor correlation between the histological appearance of acute rejection and renal function. Other features amongst the many that have been thought to be helpful in reaching a diagnosis have included leucocytosis, thrombocytopenia, enzymuria, increased numbers of mononuclear cells in the urine and hypertension. The appearance of these features in any one case is variable and the parameters that we have found most reliable are pyrexia, enlargement of the kidney and proteinuria together with an element of suspicion in the mind of the clinician.

However, it should be noted with all these parameters that the immunological process is already well advanced when the diagnosis is made and the treatment is commenced.

The diagnosis of rejection in the patient who, in the early post-operative period, is still oliguric from tubular necrosis can be extremely difficult. Even more in this situation is the diagnosis founded upon suspicion of the event particularly when a slight otherwise unexplained fever is observed. Biopsy is not helpful for the reasons just given although it may be indicated in situations of continued non-function of the kidney. Whereas the most common cause of oliguria dating from the time of operation is tubular necrosis, clearly main vessel occlusion is always a possibility and ureteral obstruction also. Urinary fistulae occur early in the post-operative period when they are manifested by wound leakage, but occasionally they are delayed when the leakage will be concealed (extravasation) and the diagnosis less obvious. We frequently undertake isotope renography using ^{131}I Hippuran because it is simple and safe to perform, but have found it of limited usefulness except in so far that it provides an indication of the continued presence or otherwise of a circulation in the transplanted organ. Sharp alterations in renal haemodynamics are reflected in changes in the renogram curve but in common with clinical and biochemical parameters, occur late in the rejection process. In summary, the most important points in the care of the patient at this stage are close and continued observation, particularly if there is pyrexia, when frequently repeated examination by the same individual is best of all. It is important to remember during this early phase that a kidney can probably be lost within 24 hours due to acute rejection if prompt antirejection treatment is not instituted. The size of the problem can be judged by the fact that up to 30 per cent of functioning cadaver kidneys may be lost due to acute rejection that is irreversible by the time that it is treated. It is difficult to tell how many oliguric kidneys with tubular necrosis are lost due to superadded rejection since by the time transplant nephrectomy is performed, advanced ischaemic changes are present. In this latter group of patients it is our practice at about one month post-operatively to perform a full investigative protocol under the one anaesthetic, consisting in chronological order of cystoscopy and retrograde pyelography, renal angiography via a percutaneous transfemoral Seldinger aortogram and finally exploration of the kidney with biopsy or removal of the organ if indicated.

Whatever the organ transplanted, the diagnosis of acute rejection relies upon the observation of functional supported by histological abnormalities in the transplanted organ. Unfortunately the diagnosis is often uncertain because tests reflecting alterations of graft function are usually non-specific and may be due to non-immunological as well as immunological causes. The search for an in vitro indicator of altered immunological reactivity of the host against the graft has until recently been disappointing. MLC reactions are unhelpful in this context for stimulation is observed in the absence of previous sensitisation. For the remainder of this chapter we shall describe the various immunological tests that have or are being evaluated in an attempt to monitor host reactivity towards the graft.

Austen and Russell (1966) observed a slight fall in the second component of complement during clinical episodes of rejection of human kidneys, which returned to normal once the process was reversed. The appearance of antibodies directed against the graft during rejection has been detected by several techniques including antiglobulin consumption (Columbani, Columbani and Dausset, 1964; Ende and Williamson, 1967) and mixed agglutination tests (Milgrom, Kano and Witebsky, 1965). However, neither the appearance of these antibodies nor their timing relative to clinical rejection was consistently observed. Also, a rise in the level of heterophile antibodies in the serum of human renal allograft recipients was noted by Rapaport, Kano and Milgrom (1968) during rejection crises and reduced serum levels of various globulins have been reported during the same period. All these tests suffer from a lack of specificity and none provide an early indication of impending rejection.

The demonstration of increased numbers of blast cells or transformed lymphocytes in the lymph draining from a transplanted kidney during rejection, that are capable of greatly increased incorporation of tritiated thymidine, has led to a search for these cells in the blood. Although an increase in the number of cells can be detected early in rejection crises by the amount of isotope incorporated in a blood sample (Hersh et al, 1970), the effect is not specific and is influenced by the level of corticosteroid therapy.

Other tests that demonstrate specific cell sensitisation, of which several techniques are available, indicate that the host has acquired a specific sensitivity to the donor's antigens. These include mixed leucocyte culture, inhibition of leucocyte migration and cytotoxicity tests. Although MLC reactions between donor and recipient cells will reveal stimulation in most instances irrespective of rejection, Oppenheim, Whang and Frei (1965) reported an increase in the number of transformed cells during rejection crises. However, it is known that the test can be influenced by immunosuppressive drugs and also by the presence of uraemia.

Inhibition of leucocyte migration, that occurs in the presence of antigen to which the cells have previously been sensitised, can be used as an in vitro indicator of specific sensitisation and applied clinically using peripheral blood leucocytes. Various authors have now shown that this test may reflect the specific sensitisation of the recipient occurring during rejection of a graft. Inhibition of migration may be apparent either with donor specific antigens obtained from a variety of tissues, or even with organ specific tissue such as pooled homologous kidney. Current studies in our own Unit (Williams et al, 1974) suggest that this test may be one of the best ways in which to predict the onset of a rejection crisis. Using the test we have found that three to four days before a rejection episode becomes clinically and biochemically manifest, there is marked inhibition of migration which is often preceded by increased migration.

We have used both donor and organ specific tissues as antigens and have found the latter to be of even better predictive value, suggesting that in some instances sensitisation to organ specific antigens may be predominant. The test is read after 24 hours and has to be performed daily for the first few post-operative weeks if its benefit in terms of therapeutic value is to be realised. The result of the test offers useful complementary evidence to that provided by a mild fever in the oliguric patient who is still on dialysis, and may indicate the need for a pulse of high dosage steroid therapy. A further point of interest is that we noted the appearance of blocking factors in the recipient's serum during rejection episodes which were capable of removing the inhibitory effect on cell migration in vitro.

Techniques designed to demonstrate cyotoxicity of the recipient's lymphocytes for donor cells can be performed by the usual methods of studying cytotoxicity using lymphocytes from the peripheral blood. Kahan et al (1974) have recently described an in vitro test for the early diagnosis of rejection from which an answer can be obtained within five hours, thereby making the technique eminently suitable for use in clinical situations. The test is based upon leucocyte aggregation which occurs when donor kidney cells or skin fibroblasts, maintained in tissue culture, are exposed to sensitised recipient leucocytes obtained from the peripheral blood. Kahan and his colleagues studied 23 renal allograft recipients and found that the reactivity observed in the test was specific for donor antigens. Leucocyte aggregation was detected several days before clinical evidence of rejection and disappeared after successful reversal of rejection. On the other hand, if the rejection process could not be reversed and the kidney had to be removed, the patient's leucocytes retained specific reactivity for months. There appeared to be two reaction patterns displayed by patients with renal allografts in situ, one preceding rejection and the other accompanying it. Whereas the former was one of specific reactivity towards donor cells and also target cells possessing HL-A antigens in common or cross-reactive with those of the donor, the marked reactivity during the latter period was quite non-specific. On the basis of this latter observation the authors made the interesting suggestion that broad immune and non-specific activation may occur during rejection once an initial specific triggering event has occurred, and that this may give further support to the need for early treatment of rejection.

A further test that has been employed to monitor the immunological status of renal transplant recipients is the rosette inhibition test as described by Bach and Antoine (1968). The test was initially used to assess the potency of antilymphocyte sera but has since been applied clinically with some success by Munro et al (1971) although the mechanism whereby spontaneous rosette formation occurs is unknown.

CONCLUSIONS

The quality of life following a renal transplant with satisfactory function is virtually normal in terms of physical activity and lack of constraints. However, survival rates for patients on haemodialysis are still better than are those for transplants even though they suffer from the effects of chronic uraemia to a varying degree. One of the problems of renal transplantation is that the prediction of success in the individual case is only high in those that have a related living donor who is willing to donate a kidney, and best of all with HL-A identical siblings. In spite of the lack of correlation between histocompatibility testing and the results in cadaver series, approximately 50 per cent of kidneys do well and clearly there is a need for improved methods of histocompatibility testing.

There is also a need for in vitro tests which provide an early warning system for rejection since closer monitoring of immunosuppression would then be possible.

References

Albert, E. D., Mickey, M. R. & Terasaki, P. I. (1971) Genetics of four new HL-A specificities in the Caucasian and Negro populations. *Transplantation Proceedings*, **111,** 95–100.

Austen, K. F. & Russell, P. S. (1966) Detection of renal allograft rejection in man by demonstration of a reduction in the serum concentration of the second component of human complement. *Annals of the New York Academy of Sciences*, **129,** 657–672.

Bach, F. & Hirschorn, K. (1964) Lymphocyte interaction. A potential histocompatibility test in vitro. *Science*, **143,** 813–814.

Bach, F. H. & Voynow, N. K. (1966) One-way stimulation in mixed leucocyte cultures. *Science*, **153,** 545–547.

Bach, J. F. & Antoine, B. (1968) In vitro detection of immunosuppressive activity of anti-lymphocyte sera. *Nature* (London), **217,** 658–659.

Bain, B., Vas, M. R. & Lowenstein, L. (1964) The development of large immature mononuclear cells in mixed leucocyte cultures. *Blood*, **23,** 108–116.

Barker, C. F. & Billingham, R. E. (1968) The role of afferent lymphatics in the rejection of skin homografts. *Journal of Experimental Medicine*, **128,** 197–221

Barker, C. F., Lubaroff, D. M. & Silvers, W. K. (1971) Lymph node cells: their differential capacity to induce tolerance of heart and skin homografts in rats. *Science*, **172,** 1050–1052.

Batchelor, J. R., Fabre, J. W. & Morris, P. J. (1972) Passive enhancement of kidney allografts. *Transplantation*, **13,** 610–613.

Belzer, F. O. & Kountz, S. L. (1973) The role of clinical transplantation in patients with end-stage renal disease. *Transplantation Proceedings*, **V,** 793–797.

Belzer, F. O., Fortmann, J. L., Salvatierra, O., Perkins, H. A., Kountz, S. L., Cochrum, K. C. & Payne, R. (1974) Is HL-A typing of clinical significance in cadaver renal transplantation. *Lancet*, **i,** 774–777.

Billingham, R. E. (1971) The passenger cell concept in transplantation immunology. *Cellular Immunology*, **2,** 1–12.

Billingham, R. E., Brent, L. & Medawar, P. B. (1953) 'Actively acquired tolerance' of foreign cells. *Nature* (London), **172,** 603–606.

Brent, L., Brown, J. & Medawar, P. B. (1958) Skin transplantation immunity in relation to hypersensitivity. *Lancet*, **ii,** 561–654.

Ceppellini, R., Curtoni, E. S., Mattiuz, P. L., Miggiano, V., Scudeller, G. & Serra, A. (1967) Genetics of leukocyte antigens. A family study of segregation and linkage. In *Histocompatibility Testing*, ed. Curtoni, E. S., Mattiuz, P. L. & Tosi, R. M. pp. 149–185. Copenhagen: Munksgaard.

Chiller, J. M., Habicht, G. S. & Weigle, W. O. (1971) Kinetic differences in unresponsiveness of thymus and bone marrow cells. *Science*, **171,** 813–815.

Columbani, J., Columbani, M. & Dausset, J. (1964) Leukocyte antigens and skin homograft in man. Demonstration of humoral antibodies after homografting by the antiglobulin consumption test. *Annals of the New York Academy of Sciences*, **120,** 307–321.

Dausset, J. (1958) Iso-leuco-anticorps. *Acta Haematologica* (Basel), **20,** 156–166.

Dausset, J. & Festenstein, H. (1973) The long-term fate of cadaver kidney transplants with four defined HL-A antigens (SD1 and SD2 full-house donors). *Transplantation Proceedings*, **V,** (in press).

Dausset, J., Hors, J., Busson, M., Festenstein, H., Oliver, R. T. D., Paris, A. M. I. & Sachs, J. A. (1974) Serologically defined HL-A antigens and long-term survival of cadaver kidney transplants. *New England Journal of Medicine* (in press).

Davies, D. A. L. (1968) Transplantation antigens. In *Human Transplantation*, ed. Rapaport, F. T. & Dausset, J. Ch. 38, p. 618. New York: Grune & Stratton.

Dumonde, D. C., Wolstencroft, R. A., Panayi, G. S., Matthew, M., Morley, J. & Howson, W. T. (1969) 'Lymphokines': Non-antibody mediators of cellular immunity by lymphocyte activation. *Nature* (London), **224,** 38–42.

11th Report of the Human Renal Transplant Registry (1973). *Journal of the American Medical Association*, **226,** 1197–1204.

Elkins, W. L. & Guttmann, R. D. (1968) Pathogenesis of a local graft versus host reaction: Immunogenicity of circulating host leucocytes. *Science*, **159,** 1250–1251.

Ende, N. & Williamson, E. F. (1967) Demonstration by the antiglobulin consumption test of humoral antibodies after homografting. *Transplantation*, **5,** 1525–1528.

Etheredge, E. E., Shons, A. R., Schmidtke, J. R. & Najarian, J. S. (1974) Mixed leukocyte culture reactivity and rejection in renal transplantation in HL-A identical siblings. *Transplantation*, **17,** 537–539.

Fabre, J. W. & Morris, P. J. (1972a) The effect of donor strain blood pretreatment on renal allograft rejection in rats. *Transplantation*, **14,** 608–617.

Fabre, J. W. & Morris, P. J. (1972b) The mechanism of specific immunosuppression of renal allograft rejection by donor strain blood. *Transplantation*, **14,** 634–640.

French, M. E. & Batchelor, J. R. (1969) Immunological enhancement of rat kidney grafts. *Lancet*, **ii,** 1103–1106.

Ginsburg, H. & Sachs, L. (1965) Destruction of mouse and rat embryo cells in tissue culture by lymph node cells from unsensitized rats. *Journal of Cellular and Comparative Physiology*, **66,** 199–207.

Gorer, P. A., Lyman, S. & Snell, G. D. (1948) Studies of the genetic and antigenic basis of tumour transplantation linkage between a histocompatibility gene and 'fused' in mice. *Proceedings of the Royal Society* (London), B, **135,** 499–505.

Goverts, A. (1960) Cellular antibodies in kidney homotransplantation. *Journal of Immunology*, **85,** 516–522.

Guttmann, R. D., Lindquist, R. R. & Ockner, S. A. (1969) Renal transplantation in the inbred rat. IX. Hematopoietic origin of an immunogenic stimulus of rejection. *Transplantation*, **8,** 472–484.

Guttmann, R. D., Beaudoin, J. G. & Morehouse, D. D. (1973) Reduction of immunogenicity of human cadaver renal allografts by donor pretreatment. *Transplantation Proceedings*, **V,** 663–665.

Hersh, E. M., Butler, W. T., Rossen, R. D. & Morgan, R. O. (1970) Lymphocyte activation: A rapid test to predict allograft rejection. *Nature* (London), 226, 757–758·

Jeannet, M., Pinn, V. W., Flax, M. H., Winn, H. J. & Russell, P. S. (1970) Humoral antibodies in renal allotransplantation in man. *New England Journal of Medicine*, **282,** 111–117.

Kahan, B. D. & Reisfeld, R. A. (1969) Transplantation antigens. Solubilised antigens provide chemical markers of biologic individuality. *Science*, **164,** 514–521.

Kahan, B. D., Mittal, K. K., Tom, B. H. & Bergan, J. J. (1974) Immunodiagnostic test for transplant rejection. *Lancet*, **i,** 37–42.

Keuning, J. J., Termijtelan, A., Van den Tweel, J. G. & Van Rood, J. J. (1974) Typing for M.L.C. Paper given at meeting of the British Transplantation Society, London.

Kissmeyer-Nielsen, F. & Thorsby, E. (1970) Human transplantation antigens. In *Transplantation Reviews*, ed. Möller, G. p. 30, Copenhagen: Munksgaard.

Kölsch, E. & Mitchison, N. A. (1968) The subcellular distribution of antigen in macrophages. *Journal of Experimental Medicine*, **128,** 1059–1079.

Koprowski, H. & Fernandes, M. V. (1962) Autosensitization reaction in vitro. Contactual agglutination of sensitized lymph node cells in brain tissue culture accompanied by destruction of glial elements. *Journal of Experimental Medicine*, **116,** 467–476.

Levey, R. H. (1971) Immunological tolerance and enhancement: A common mechanism. *Transplantation Proceedings*, **111,** 41–48.

Little, C. C. & Tyzzer, E. E. (1916) Further experimental studies on the inheritance of susceptibility to a transplantable tumour, carcinoma (J.W.A.) of the Japanese waltzing mouse. *Journal of Medical Research*, **33,** 393–427.

Metzgar, R. S., Seigler, H. F., Ward, F. E. & Rowlands, D. T. (1972) Immunological studies on eluates from human renal allografts. *Transplantation*, **13,** 131–137.

Mickey, M. R., Kreisler, M., Albert, E. D., Tanaka, N. & Terasaki, P. I. (1971) Analysis of HL-A incompatibility in human renal transplants. *Tissue Antigens*, **1,** 57–67.
Milgrom, F., Kano, K. & Witebsky, E. (1965) The mixed agglutination test in studies on human transplantation. *Journal of the American Medical Association*, **192,** 845–848.
Milgrom, F., Klassen, J. & Fuji, H. (1971) Immunologic injury of renal homografts. *Journal of Experimental Medicine*, **134,** 193–207.
Mitchison, N. A. (1954) Passive transfer of transplantation immunity. *Proceedings of the Royal Society* (London), B, **142,** 72–87.
Mitchison, N. A. (1964) Induction of immunological paralysis in two zones of dosage. *Proceedings of the Royal Society of Biological Science*, B, **161,** 275–292.
Morris, P. J. (1973) Histocompatibility in organ transplantation. *Annals of the Royal College of Surgeons of England*, **53,** 324–339.
Munro, A., Bewick, M., Manuel, L., Cameron, J. S., Ellis, F. G., Boulton-Jones, M. & Ogg, C. S. (1971) Clinical evaluation of a rosette inhibition test in renal allotransplantation. *British Medical Journal*, **iii,** 271–275.
Murray, J. E., Barnes, B. A. & Atkinson, J. C. (1970) Eighth Report of the Human Kidney Transplant Registry. *Transplantation*, **11,** 328–337.
Opelz, G., Mickey, M. R. & Terasaki, P. I. (1972) Identification of unresponsive kidney-transplant recipients. *Lancet*, **i,** 868–871.
Oppenheim, J. J., Whang, J. & Frei, E. (1965) The effect of skin homograft rejection on recipient and donor mixed leucocyte cultures. *Journal of Experimental Medicine*, **122,** 651–664.
Pedersen, N. C. & Morris, B. (1970) The role of the lymphatic system in the rejection of homografts: A study of lymph from renal transplants. *Journal of Experimental Medicine*, **131,** 936–969.
Porter, K. A., Andres, G. A., Calder, M. W., Dossetor, J. B., Hsu, K. C., Rendall, J. M., Seegal, B. C. & Starzl, T. E. (1968) Human renal transplants II. Immunofluorescent and immunoferritin studies. *Laboratory Investigation*, **18,** 159–171.
Rapaport, F. T., Kano, K. & Milgrom, F. (1968) Heterophile hemagglutinins in human renal allografts. In *Advance in Transplantation*, ed. Dausset, J., Hamburger, J. & Mathé, G. p. 757. Copenhagen: Munksgaard.
Rosenau, W. & Moon, H. D. (1961) Lysis of homologous cells by sensitized lymphocytes in tissue culture. *Journal of the National Cancer Institute*, **27,** 471–483.
Russell, P. S. (1971) Immunological enhancement. *Transplantation Proceedings*, **III,** 960–966.
Sengar, D. P. S., Opelz, G. & Terasaki, P. I. (1973) Outcome of kidney transplants and suppression of mixed leukocyte culture by plasma. *Transplantation Proceedings*, **V,** 641–647.
Steinmuller, D. (1967) Immunization with skin isografts taken from tolerant mice. *Science*, **158,** 127–129.
Strober, S. & Gowans, J. L. (1965) The role of lymphocytes in the sensitization of rats to renal homografts. *Journal of Experimental Medicine*, **122,** 347–360.
Stuart, F. P., Saitoh, T. & Fitch, F. W. (1968) Rejection of renal allografts: Specific immunologic suppression. *Science*, **160,** 1463–1465.
Terasaki, P. I. & McClelland, J. D. (1964) Microdroplet assay of human serum cytotoxins. *Nature*, (London), **204,** 998–1000.
Weigle, W. O., Chiller, J. M. & Habicht, G. S. (1972) Effect of immunological unresponsiveness on different cell populations. *Transplantation Reviews*, **8,** 3–25.
Wentzel, J., Harris, R., Orr, W. McN. & Mallick, N. P. (1974) HL-A and renal graft survival. *Lancet*, **i,** 1053–1054.
Williams, R. J., Mallick, N. P., Taylor, G. & Orr, W. McN. (1974) The early diagnosis of rejection by the leucocyte migration test in cadaveric renal transplantation. *Clinical Nephrology* **2,** 100–105.
Winn, H. J. (1961) Immune mechanisms in homotransplantation II: Quantitative assays of the immunologic activity of lymphoid cells stimulated by tumor homografts. *Journal of Immunology*, **86,** 228–239.
Woodruff, M. F. A. (1961) The transplantation of tissues and organs. p. 96. Springfield, Illinois: Charles C. Thomas.

Index